Atherosclerosis

METHODS IN MOLECULAR MEDICINE™

John M. Walker, SERIES EDITOR

Atherosclerosis

Experimental Methods and Protocols

Edited by

Angela F. Drew

Children's Hospital Research Foundation
Cincinnati, OH

Humana Press ✳ **Totowa, New Jersey**

Cover art: The cover image shows oil red O stained arteries from typical 20–22-wk-old apoliprotein E-deficient and plasminogen-deficient mice. (*Top left*) Plasminogen-deficient mice have no obvious lipid deposits around the valve cusp. (*Top right*) Apolipoprotein E-deficient mice develop spontaneous lipid-containing fatty streak lesions. Mice with simultaneous plasminogen- and apolipoprotein E-deficiencies develop larger fatty streak lesions (*bottom left*) and more advanced fibroproliferative plaques with organized smooth muscle cell caps and medial disruption (*bottom right*). This illustration was kindly provided by Dr. Qing Xiao.

Cover design by Patricia F. Cleary.

For additional copies, pricing for bulk purchases, and/or information about other Humana titles, contact Humana at the above address or at any of the following numbers: Tel: 973-256-1699; Fax: 973-256-8341; E-mail: humana@humanapr.com, or visit our Website at www.humanapress.com.

Printed in the United States of America. 10 9 8 7 6 5 4 3 2 1

Library of Congress Cataloging-in-Publication Data

Atherosclerosis: experimental methods and protocols / edited by Angela F. Drew.
    p. ; cm. -- (Methods in molecular medicine ; 52)
    Includes bibliographical references and index.
    ISBN 0-89603-751-7 (alk. paper)
    1. Atherosclerosis--Laboratory manuals. I. Drew, Angela F. II. series. [DNLM: 1. Atherosclerosis. 2. Research--methods. WG 550 A86957 2001
    RC692.A7288 2001
    616.19369972--dc21
                                        00-038924

Preface

Atherosclerosis: Experimental Methods and Protocols aims to provide
the reader with a compilation of techniques that will prove useful to active
investigators across the field of experimental atherosclerosis research.
In fact, this volume is unique, the first devoted to a broad spectrum of techniques
and assays, some adopted from other disciplines, not previously brought together
in one book. Our approach is designed to permit researchers to select the
techniques that will answer their particular sets of questions, in any of the
expanding number of both animal models and in vitro systems now available
for studying factors contributing to the development or progression of atherosclerotic lesions. Researchers can only benefit from this collection of relevant
techniques, written and explained by experts in each of these fields.

Both investigators beginning in the field of atherosclerosis studies and
researchers entering the field from related but different areas of study will
benefit from *Atherosclerosis: Experimental Methods and Protocols*. Sufficient
background is provided for a beginner to carry out the techniques described in
the chapters, yet great depth is achieved owing to the special expertise of the
authors. Researchers new to the field of atherosclerosis will appreciate the
benefits of having these techniques gathered in one volume for their investigations. In addition, researchers already in the field of atherosclerosis research
may benefit from the wide array of techniques and ideas provided by enjoying
expanded opportunities to investigate their hypotheses.

Practical information regarding sample collection, choice of model system,
experimental design, and data analysis techniques are each provided in these
chapters. In addition to methods for both well-documented and novel techniques, chapters summarizing general aspects of atherosclerosis research, such
as animal models, are included. A summary of newly emerging animal models, in
particular, genetically manipulated mice, provides sufficient information to
become involved in this exciting new area of research. Assay systems for
serum or plasma determination are becoming increasingly relevant in diagnostic
and epidemiological studies, and have accordingly been described in many of
the chapters. Both traditional and newer methods for identifying and separating classes and subclasses of lipoproteins have been included, along with

assays for more recently identified plasma proteins implicated in atherogenesis, such as cholesteryl ester transfer protein, homocysteine, glycated lipoproteins, and apolipoprotein(a). Chapters describing the isolation and culture of cells and glycosaminoglycans from atherosclerotic plaques follow, and may form the basis of many in vitro assays. In vivo techniques for the collection and analysis of experimental atherosclerotic lesions have been included in the later chapters. Finally, a comprehensive overview describing gene therapies under recent investigation in the field of atherosclerosis/restenosis—along with a practical example of successful implementation of such a therapy in pigs—have been included.

Obtaining a general overview of the material included in *Atherosclerosis: Experimental Methods and Protocols*, prior to a more detailed study of particular chapters, will illuminate many facts broadly related to atherosclerosis that may be useful initially, or later, in the course of a research program. Included in the "Notes" section of each chapter is additional information sufficient for successful application of the technique. Often this kind of detail is lacking from brief methodological descriptions in the literature. From their excellent working knowledge of the techniques described, our authors may save a new researcher much time and effort. The compilation of these techniques into a single volume will hopefully benefit many researchers in pursuit of understanding, diagnosing, and ultimately preventing or treating atherosclerosis.

Angela F. Drew

Contents

Contributors

ROBERTO ACCINNI • *Clinical Physiology Institute of CNR, Section of Milan, Department of Cardiology A. De Gasperis, Ospedale Niguarda Cà Granda, Milan, Italy*

ELENA R. ANDREEVA • *Institute of Experimental Cardiology, Cardiology Research Center, and Institute for Atherosclerosis Research, Russian Academy of Natural Sciences, Moscow, Russia*

GIANNI D. ANGELINI • *Department of Medicine and Therapeutics, University of Glasgow, Glasgow, United Kingdom*

JIM APOSTOLOPOULOS • *Research Department, Australian Red Cross Blood Service, Victoria, Australia*

ANDREW H. BAKER • *Department of Medicine and Therapeutics, University of Glasgow, Glasgow, United Kingdom*

MICHAEL BENDER • *Gustav Embden Centre of Biological Chemistry, Johann Wolfgang Goethe University, Frankfurt-am-Main, Germany*

SHAWN M. CASSIDY • *Division of Pharmaceutics and Biopharmaceutics, Faculty of Pharmaceutical Sciences, University of British Columbia, Vancouver, British Columbia, Canada*

IAN G. DAVIES • *School of Biomolecular Sciences, Liverpool John Moores University, Liverpool, United Kingdom*

RODNEY J. DILLEY • *Morphology Laboratory, Baker Medical Research Institute, Melbourne, Victoria, Australia*

ANGELA F. DREW • *Division of Developmental Biology, Children's Hospital Research Foundation, Cincinnati, OH*

MARISA A. GALLICCHIO • *Department of Medicine, Austin and Repatriation Medical Centre, University of Melbourne, Heidelberg, Victoria, Australia*

SARAH J. GEORGE • *Department of Medicine and Therapeutics, University of Glasgow, Glasgow, United Kingdom*

JOHN M. GRAHAM • *School of Biomolecular Sciences, Liverpool John Moores University, Liverpool, United Kingdom*

BRUCE A. GRIFFIN • *Centre for Nutrition and Food Safety, Department of Biological Sciences, University of Surrey, Guildford, United Kingdom*

WERNER GROSS • *Gustav Embden Centre of Biological Chemistry, Johann Wolfgang Goethe University, Frankfurt-am-Main, Germany*

JOAN A. HIGGINS • *Department of Molecular Biology and Biotechnology, Sheffield University, Sheffield, United Kingdom*

JEFFREY M. ISNER • *Departments of Medicine (Cardiology) and Biomedical Research, St. Elizabeth's Medical Center, Tufts University School of Medicine, Boston, MA*

GEORGE KARAKIULAKIS • *Department of Pharmacology, School of Medicine, Aristotle University of Thessaloniki, Greece*

ALLISON L. KENNEDY • *Division of Pharmaceutics and Biopharmaceutics, Faculty of Pharmaceutical Sciences, University of British Columbia, Vancouver, British Columbia, Canada*

CLINTON T. LLOYD • *Department of Medicine and Therapeutics, University of Glasgow, Glasgow, United Kingdom*

HANNU I. MANNINEN • *Department of Clinical Radiology, Kuopio University Hospital, Kuopio, Finland*

ANDREW C. NEWBY • *Department of Medicine and Therapeutics, University of Glasgow, Glasgow, United Kingdom*

ALEXANDER N. OREKHOV • *Institute of Experimental Cardiology, Cardiology Research Center, and Institute for Atherosclerosis Research, Russian Academy of Natural Sciences, Moscow, Russia*

ELENI PAPAKONSTANTINOU • *Department of Pharmacology, School of Medicine, Aristotle University of Thessaloniki, Greece*

OBERDAN PARODI • *Clinical Physiology Institute of CNR, Section of Milan, Department of Cardiology A. De Gasperis, Ospedale Niguarda Cà Granda, Milan, Italy*

JOSEF R. PATSCH • *Department of Medicine, University of Innsbrück, Innsbrück, Austria*

KATHY D. PETEHERYCH • *Division of Pharmaceutics and Biopharmaceutics, Faculty of Pharmaceutical Sciences, University of British Columbia, Vancouver, British Columbia, Canada*

ANDREAS RITSCH • *Department of Medicine, University of Innsbrück, Innsbrück, Austria*

MICHAEL ROTH • *Institute of Respiratory Medicine, Royal Prince Alfred Hospital, University of Sydney, Camperdown, New South Wales, Australia*

MARCY SILVER • *Departments of Medicine (Cardiology) and Biomedical Research, St. Elizabeth's Medical Center, Tufts University School of Medicine, Boston, MA*

AKIRA TANAKA • *Third Department of Internal Medicine, Tokyo Medical and Dental University, Yushima, Bunkyo-ku, Tokyo, Japan*

KISHOR M. WASAN • *Division of Pharmaceutics and Biopharmaceutics, Faculty of Pharmaceutical Sciences, University of British Columbia, Vancouver, British Columbia, Canada*

QING XIAO • *Center for Cancer Research, Massachusetts Institute of Technology, Cambridge, MA*

1

Animal Models of Diet-Induced Atherosclerosis

Angela F. Drew

1. Introduction

Animals models of atherosclerosis develop lesions either spontaneously or by interventions such as dietary, mechanical, chemical, or immunological induction. Animal models provide a means for studying the underlying mechanisms behind the atherosclerotic disease process, as well as a means for studying the effect of interventions, dietary or otherwise, on the development or regression of disease, while under controlled conditions. The effect of risk factors for atherosclerotic disease development has been evaluated in animal models, with the advantage of excluding other influences. Animal models have provided valuable information regarding diagnostic and therapeutic strategies, with extensive investigation of events occurring in the artery wall throughout these procedures. Animal models have provided information about factors contributing to disease progression and regression that apply to human situations.

It is important to recognize the diversity of animal models that exist for research and the various advantages or disadvantages of each model when choosing the most appropriate model for potential studies. This chapter provides information regarding the benefits and disadvantages of diet-induced models of spontaneous atherosclerosis. Because of the sudden increase in popularity of genetically manipulated mouse models, further information is provided in a later chapter.

2. Models

2.1. Rabbits

Rabbits have become the most popular animal model of atherosclerosis, with New Zealand White (NZW) rabbits being the most widely used. Rabbits have

From: *Methods in Molecular Medicine, vol. 52: Atherosclerosis: Experimental Methods and Protocols*
Edited by: A. F. Drew © Humana Press Inc., Totowa, NJ

been used in studies of lesion characterization, drug interventions, mechanical arterial injury, and arterial metabolism. Rabbits are typically fed 0.5 – 2% cholesterol diets for 4–16 wk, depending on the severity of disease required and the time available for induction. This diet is well tolerated by rabbits, and lesions consistently appear, though with marked variation in lesion size. Lesions occur predominantly in the aortic arch and ascending aorta, but eventually lesions occur throughout the entire aorta *(1)*. Areas of intimal thickenings occur naturally in rabbit arteries, but these areas are free of lipid unless cholesterol or fat is added to the diet.

The advantages of rabbit models include economy, short disease-induction times, availability, and ease in handling. An important disadvantage of utilizing the cholesterol-fed rabbit in atherosclerosis studies is the extreme hyperlipidemia, and subsequent lipid overload, required to produce lesions. This results in a cholesterol storage disease affecting the heart, kidneys, liver, and lungs, which does not typically occur in human atherosclerosis. In addition, rabbits are herbivores and have differences in lipid metabolism compared with man. The resulting lesions are early stage, highly lipid filled, and occur in a different anatomical distribution than in man. However, lesions more closely resembling human atheroma can be induced in rabbits by variations in diet, including fat source *(2)*.

Several genetic variants of the NZW rabbit are currently used in atherosclerosis research because of their hyperresponsiveness to cholesterol feeding or spontaneous hypercholesterolemia. The Watanabe heritable hyperlipidemic (WHHL) rabbit is the best known of these. The WHHL rabbit strain was originally created by Watanabe, by inbreeding rabbits from a single rabbit with high cholesterol *(3)*. It is now known that WHHL rabbits have a defect in the membrane LDL receptor that results in impaired LDL catabolism, creating an animal model for human familial hypercholesterolemia and the first model of endogenous lipoprotein hypercholesterolemia. Lesions are observed at all stages of progression, from fatty streaks to advanced plaques. Lesions are concentrated in the coronary arteries and the aorta, and lipid is contained in both macrophage-derived foam cells and smooth muscle cells.

2.2. Swine Models

Gottleib and Lalich first reported on spontaneous atherosclerosis in swine vessels and intimal thickenings in coronary arteries *(4)*. Animals develop early fatty streaks by 6 mo of age, and advanced lesions occur in pigs older than 1 yr, but no hemorrhage into lesions or thrombosis occurs. Swine are highly suitable models of atherosclerosis, since lesions show a high degree of similarity to human atherosclerosis, including foam cell formation, extracellular fat, and smooth muscle cell proliferation and migration *(5)*. Lesions can be enhanced by feeding high-cholesterol and high-fat diets. Significant genetic variation exists between breeds, and atherosclerotic susceptibility has been characterized as a function of LDL allotype heterogeneity. Swine models provided additional evidence of a link between increased low-density lipoprotein (LDL) levels and atherosclerotic susceptibility. Lesions most closely resemble human lesions after a combination of cholesterol feeding and mechanical arterial injury *(6)*.

Swine models provide significant advantages in atherosclerosis research as their lesions are spontaneous, they consume an omnivorous diet, and they have cardiovascular anatomy similar to man. Their lesions occur with a distribution similar to human lesions, being prominent in the aorta and coronary and cerebral arteries. In addition, swine share similarities with humans in lipoprotein profiles, composition, size, and apolipoprotein content, with the exception that apolipoprotein-AII has not been detected in swine *(7)*. Their large vessels are suitable for most surgical manipulations, and these animals are well utilized in angioplasty and gene therapy research. The disadvantages of using swine models are the expense and difficulty in handling.

Miniature swine provide a more economical model, and some breeds are highly susceptible to diet-induced atherosclerosis. The Yucatan miniature pig is known to be a docile breed, that is susceptible to diet-induced atherosclerosis and develops lesions similar to man. A highly susceptible strain of swine, exhibiting high cholesterol and accelerated atherosclerosis, has been created through inbreeding and extensively studied, the IHLC (inherited hyperlipoproteinemia and hypercholesterolemia) strain *(5)*. These pigs have a reduced rate of catabolism of LDL and spontaneously develop advanced atherosclerosis with intraplaque hemorrhage.

2.3. Nonhuman Primates

Nonhuman primates have the distinct advantage, as an atherosclerosis model, of being phylogenetically similar to humans, and consume an omnivorous diet. The similarities extend into lipoprotein composition and distribution. While primates develop few lesions spontaneously, extensive lesion development occurs after cholesterol feeding. Lesions closely resemble human atheroma and develop into complex lesions with complications such as myocardial infarction. Old World primates develop consistent lesions after cholesterol feeding, with a close anatomical relationship to those of man. Rhesus monkeys have been studied the most extensively and offer the benefits of a convenient size and well-characterized lesions. Rhesus monkeys have been valuable in determining the effects of fats and other dietary manipulations on atherosclerotic development *(8)*. Cynomolgus monkeys are also widely used, as they are also a convenient size and are highly sensitive to dietary cholesterol. New World primates are less widely used, as they tend to develop inconsistent lesions, with an anatomical distribution different from that of man. The disadvantages of primate models include expense, complicated maintenance, decreased availability, and their requirement for special housing *(9)*.

2.4. Avian Models

Birds have been a popular choice with researchers for several reasons. They are inexpensive to maintain and breed well. Some species develop spontaneous atherosclerosis that can be enhanced by high cholesterol diets. In addition, birds have been utilized in genetic studies, since variations between breeds account for differences in susceptibility to atherosclerosis. Pigeons have proven to be the avian model of choice for studying atherosclerotic development, as lesions show a high degree of similarity to human lesions *(10)*. Lesions are most prominent in the thoracic aorta at the celiac bifurcation and in the abdominal aorta. The White Carneau develop spontaneous lesions on a standard grain diet *(11)* and are commonly studied for the complications that develop with their atherosclerosis, such as hemorrhage, medial thinning, and thrombus formation. Pigeons develop myocardial infarctions due to atheromatous embolism *(12)*. Other bird species have been studied, such as the Japanese quail, which is particularly susceptible to atherogenesis. Studies performed on birds have included drug screens, regression studies, and studies of genetic factors involved in the disease process *(13)*.

2.5 Rodents

Mouse and rat models have been investigated as potential models of atheroma development because of their practicality in terms of economy and maintenance. However, their relative resistance to hypercholesterolemia and lesion development, along with the high mortality rates associated with feeding atherogenic diets, has led to their abandonment by most researchers in atherosclerosis research. This situation changed with the recent production of genetically manipulated mouse models of spontaneous atherosclerosis, such as apolipoprotein E-deficient–mice, resulting in a drastic increase in the popularity of mice as models of atherosclerosis (*see* Chapter 3). Atherosclerosis-susceptible strains have allowed investigation of genetic factors in lesion development, by crossbreeding mice with other gene-targeted mice. While genetic manipulation provides numerous opportunities in atherosclerosis research, rodent models have the disadvantage of their different lipoprotein profiles to man and markedly smaller vessel size. Smaller vessel sizes result in different arterial wall morphology, including reduced thickness of the medial layer and lack of vasa vasorum. In addition, certain surgical manipulations, such as balloon catheterization, have not been successfully performed on mouse arteries.

2.6. Cats and Dogs

Cats have not proven to be a broadly suitable model for atheromatous lesion development, as lesions are unlike human atheroma in distribution and characteristics. Neither have dogs been extensively used in atherosclerosis research, although widely used in cardiovascular and surgical studies. Hypothyroidism must be induced to overcome the natural resistance of dogs to hypercholesterolemia or lesion development.

3. Discussion

Ignatowski created the first animal model for atherosclerosis, by feeding rabbits egg yolks, in 1908 *(14)*. After almost a decade of experimental atherosclerosis research, the animals most commonly used have proven to be rabbits, pigeons, swine, and primates. It is notable that animal models that can be genetically manipulated, such as the mouse, are replacing animal models that were previously favored. Mice are becoming increasingly popular since the introduction of atherosclerosis-susceptible strains and the recent availability of gene-targeting technology.

The limitations of using animal models have been outweighed by the benefits of performing studies under controlled conditions—studies that cannot be performed ethically on humans. No animal model is suitable for every study, thus, when choosing an animal model, efforts must be made to optimize study parameters while attempting to maximize similarities with human physiology and atherosclerosis development. Factors such as expense, ease of maintenance and handling, availability, phylogenetic similarity with humans, time to lesion induction, and size of arteries must be prioritized to choose the model that will optimize the study protocol. Some animal models have not been well characterized, which presents difficulties in the interpretation of results. In addition, investigators should note the effect of sex differences on atheroma development, in their model of choice, and the effects of stress, due to unnatural housing conditions.

Animal models are useful for many applications in which results can be extrapolated to human disease, but this is not always the situation. Drug interventions in rats to prevent postangioplasty re-stenosis have not provided reliable data that can be applied to humans. Studies that show great promise in rodent arteries have yielded little benefit in humans. Differences in rodent and human arteries are likely to account for the discrepancy, along with differences in the atherosclerotic process in each species. Such limitations must be kept in mind when interpreting results from animal studies.

References

1. Drew, A. F. and Tipping, P. G. (1995) T helper cell infiltration and foam cell proliferation are early events in the development of atherosclerosis in cholesterol-fed rabbits. *Arterioscler. Thromb. Vasc. Biol.* **15,** 1563–1568.
2. Kritchevsky, D., Tepper, S. A., Kim, H. K., Story, J. A., Vesselinovitch, D., and Wissler, R. W. (1976) Experimental atherosclerosis in rabbits fed cholesterol-free diets. 5. Comparison of peanut, corn, butter, and coconut oils. *Exp. Mol. Pathol.* **24,** 375–391.
3. Watanabe, Y. (1980) Serial inbreeding of rabbits with hereditary hyperlipidemia (WHHL- rabbit). *Atherosclerosis* **36,** 261–268.
4. Gottleib, H. and Lalich, J. J. (1954) The occurrence of arteriosclerosis in the aorta of swine. *Am. J. Pathol.* **30,** 851–855.
5. Rapacz, J. and Hasler-Rapacz, J. (1989) Animal models: The pig, in *Genetic Factors in Atherosclerosis: Approaches and Model Systems* (Lusis, A. J. and Sparkes, S. R.), Karger, Basel, pp. 139–169.
6. Fritz, K. E., Daoud, A. S., Augustyn, J. M., and Jarmolych, J. (1980) Morphological and biochemical differences among grossly-defined types of swine aortic atherosclerotic lesions induced by a combination of injury and atherogenic diet. *Exp. Mol. Pathol.* **32,** 61–72.
7. Mahley, R. W. and Weisgraber, K. H. (1974) An electrophoretic method for the quantitative isolation of human and swine plasma lipoproteins. *Biochemistry* **13,** 1964–1969.
8. Vesselinovitch, D. (1979) Animal models of atherosclerosis, their contributions and pitfalls. *Artery* **5,** 193–206.
9. Armstrong, M. L. and Heistad, D. D. (1990). Animal models of atherosclerosis. *Atherosclerosis* **85,** 15–23.
10. Jokinen, M. P., Clarkson, T. B., and Prichard, R. W. (1985) Animal models in atherosclerosis research. *Exp. Mol. Pathol.* **42,** 1–28.
11. Clarkson, T. B., Middleton, C. C., Prichard, R. W., and Lofland, H. B. (1965) Naturally-occurring atherosclerosis in birds. *Ann. N. Y. Acad. Sci.* **127,** 685–693.
12. Pritchard, R. W., Clarkson, T. B., and Lofland, H. B. (1963) Myocardial infarcts in pigeons. *Am. J. Pathol.* **43,** 651.
13. Vesselinovitch, D. (1988) Animal models and the study of atherosclerosis. *Arch. Pathol. Lab. Med.* **112,** 1011–1017.
14. Ignatowski, A. C. (1908) Influence of animal food on the organism of rabbits. *S. Peterb. Izviest. Imp. Voyenno-Med. Akad.* **16,** 154–173.

2

Mechanical Injury Models

Balloon Catheter Injury to Rat Common Carotid Artery

Rodney J. Dilley

1. Introduction

Removal of arterial endothelium and damage to medial smooth muscle with a balloon embolectomy catheter lead to formation of a thin mural thrombus, platelet adhesion and degranulation, smooth muscle cell migration to the intima, and cell proliferation and matrix synthesis, ultimately producing a thickened neointimal layer. This model was developed initially by Baumgartner and Studer in the 1960s (*1*) and was modified (*2*) and used extensively throughout the 1970s and 1980s to develop our knowledge of vascular smooth muscle and endothelial cell kinetics following injury in adult animals (*3*). In the 1980s and 1990s it was used extensively to explore the effects of pharmacological agents that might influence vascular smooth muscle cell growth (*4–7*).

The model may hold some relationship to the vascular repair responses to angioplasty, but several important differences must be recognized: Injury is to nondiseased vessels with no pre-existing neointimal cell populations, and so responses come predominantly from medial cells, there is little intimal/medial tearing, and low-pressure distention and application of a shearing motion during catheter withdrawal are used. Nonetheless it does represent a widely studied model of endothelial and vascular smooth muscle cell proliferation and migration and as such will likely continue to be used widely.

The injury model has been applied predominantly in the rat, with endothelial removal from either the left common carotid artery or the descending thoracic aorta. Rabbits, guinea pigs, and hamsters have also been used, and

From: *Methods in Molecular Medicine, vol. 52: Atherosclerosis: Experimental Methods and Protocols*
Edited by: A. F. Drew © Humana Press Inc., Totowa, NJ

similar methods have been performed on dogs and pigs. Atherogenesis has been studied in suitable animal models by addition of cholesterol to the diet after balloon injury *(8)*. Numerous other methods have been used to remove or damage endothelium *(9–12)* and to generate a neointima; however, balloon catheter denudation is the most widely used model to date with hundreds of published articles.

In this chapter a procedure is described for endothelial denudation of the rat common carotid artery with a balloon embolectomy catheter. The procedure is simple, requiring little more than introduction of a balloon catheter to the common carotid artery lumen and passage of the inflated balloon to remove the endothelium and damage underlying smooth muscle cells to stimulate a repair response.

2. Materials

1. Animals. Adult male Sprague-Dawley rats, between 350 and 450 g body weight (*see* **Note 1**).
2. Anesthetics. Ketamine (100 mg/mL) and xylazine (20 mg/mL), mixed to the indicated concentration (3:2) and administered by intraperitoneal (ip) injection at a ratio of 0.1 mL/100 g body weight.
3. Catheter. Fogarty arterial embolectomy balloon catheter 2F (Baxter Healthcare, Irvine, CA), with a three-way stopcock and 1 mL syringe attached. All are filled with sterile 0.9% saline, and air is excluded.
4. Antiseptic. Aqueous chlorhexidine solution.
5. Surgical equipment. Surgical lighting, warm pad.
6. Instruments. Scalpel, skin forceps, small (5 cm long) blunt-ended scissors, two pairs of fine, curved forceps for blunt dissection and isolation of carotid artery, one pair of jeweler's forceps for holding the wall of the external carotid artery, fine scissors (e.g., iridectomy scissors), three pairs of artery clamps, needle holders, silk suture material (2/0 and 5/0), skin suture material (e.g., 2/0 Dexon) (*see* **Note 3**).
7. Recovery procedures. Analgesic (Carprofen 5 mg/kg body weight, subcutaneous), warm and quiet recovery space, warm (37°C) saline for rehydration.

3. Methods

1. Weigh rats and anesthetize by ip injection of ketamine and xylazine mixture, with the dose based on body weight (0.1 mL/100 g body weight).
2. When the rat is fully anaesthetised, as demonstrated by absence of a foot withdrawal reflex (about 10 min is usually adequate), shave the ventral surface of the neck between the angle of the jaw and the sternum, swab with antiseptic solution to clean the skin, and remove loose hair.
3. Make a midline skin incision with the scalpel. Using the round-ended small scissors, blunt dissect through the midline between the large mandibular salivary glands, then laterally to the left, via planes of fascia to the bifurcation of the left

common carotid artery. The bifurcation lies approximately at the junction of the stylohyoid, omohyoid, and sternomastoid muscles.

4. Locate the internal carotid artery and blunt dissect under it with small curved forceps so that a loose ligature (2/0 silk) can be placed around the vessel **(Fig. 1A)**. An artery clamp can then be placed on the end of the ligature to lift the carotid artery and hold it aside.
5. Locate the external carotid artery and similarly place two loose ligatures (5/0 silk) around it **(Fig. 1B,C)**.
6. Place a loose ligature on the common carotid artery, proximal to the bifurcation **(Fig. 1D)**.
7. Tie the distal ligature on the external carotid artery **(Fig. 1B)**, leaving at least 2–3 mm from the bifurcation to allow space proximally for a small arteriotomy and another ligature.
8. Apply pressure to lift the ligatures (use artery clamps) on the proximal common carotid and distal external and internal carotid arteries **(Fig. 1A,B,D)**. This will isolate the intervening segment of carotid artery bifurcation from blood flow.
9. With fine scissors make an incision in the external carotid artery, immediately proximal to the distal ligature, ensuring that you leave enough space for the proximal ligature to isolate the arteriotomy (see **Fig. 1E** for placement). This incision must be large enough to admit the balloon catheter, but not so large as to tear the vessel apart (*see* **Note 4**).
10. After checking the catheter assembly **(Fig. 2)** for leaks and correct inflation volume (*see* **Notes 5** and **6**), lift the free edge of the incision with fine forceps and feed the catheter into the external carotid artery, toward the bifurcation.
11. Advance the catheter through to the common carotid artery and continue to the first mark on the catheter (approximately 5 cm) so that the catheter tip lies in the arch of the aorta.
12. Inflate the catheter balloon with 0.02 mL saline.
13. Withdraw the catheter through the common carotid artery to the carotid bifurcation, rotating the catheter between your fingers as you proceed.
14. Deflate the catheter balloon and advance the tip to the aorta again, repeating the injury procedure twice more.
15. Remove the catheter after the third passage and tie the proximal ligature **(Fig. 1C)** on the external carotid artery.
16. Release the remaining loose ligatures **(Fig. 1A,D)** and allow approximately 5 min for full assessment of the blood flow in the common carotid artery. A dilated and pulsating common carotid artery should be evident.
17. Suture-close the skin incision and give parenteral fluids (5 mL warm saline sc) and analgesic (carprofen 5 mg/kg body weight, sc).
18. Animals should be kept warm during recovery for at least 1 h after surgery (*see* **Note 7**).
19. Crushed food pellets and cotton-wool balls soaked with water are placed in the bottom of the cage to allow the animal to feed and drink easily for the first day after neck surgery.

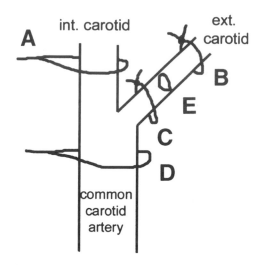

Fig. 1. The carotid artery bifurcation region showing the position of ligatures and arteriotomy during the balloon catheter injury procedure. **(A,D)** Loose temporary ligatures. **(B,C)** Permanent ligatures. **(E)** Arteriotomy.

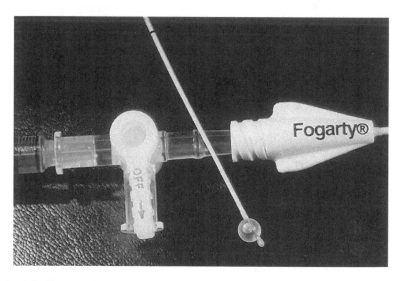

Fig. 2. A balloon catheter assembly showing the syringe filled with 0.02 mL saline **(left)** connected to the catheter **(right)** by a three-way tap **(middle)**. The catheter tip with an inflated balloon is shown **(lower right)**, indicating the length of catheter inserted into the carotid artery by the black mark on the catheter, 5 cm from the tip.

4. Notes

1. Rats of approximately 400 g body weight are convenient to use. The procedure becomes more difficult in small animals (e.g., less than 300–350 g) because of the decreasing size of the external carotid artery.
2. Anesthesia suitable for 30–40 min of surgery is required. Difficult surgerical operations may take longer and require additional anesthetic toward the end of the procedure.
3. Fine and accurate tools are essential.
4. Entry of the catheter through the arteriotomy is the most difficult part of the procedure. There are a number of tips that may be helpful in situations in which it is difficult to place the catheter in the artery.
   a. The arteriotomy should be slightly larger than the tip of the catheter, and the angle of entry must match the angle of the external carotid artery.
   b. When the arteriotomy is too small, gentle outward pressure from the tips of small scissors or forceps will often make the hole large enough.
   c. Use light pressure on the loose ligatures to adjust angles for ease of entry.
   d. It is possible for an assistant to open the arteriotomy with two pairs of fine forceps while the catheter is maneuvered between the forceps into the external carotid artery.
   e. Use a trocar, a 2–3 cm segment of fine tubing, with a diagonal cut on one end. When placed over the catheter tip, the point of the trocar can be used to enter the artery first to guide the catheter into place.
   f. A dissecting microscope may be used, although this is generally not necessary and not always helpful.
5. To enable precise control of inflation volume it is helpful to use a syringe containing only 0.02 mL saline. Different inflation volumes may produce different degrees of injury and thus impact on repair responses, so this method makes it easier to provide a constant level of injury to the artery.
6. It is important to free the syringe and catheter of any air bubbles; these will compress during inflation and thus alter inflation pressure. Air can be removed with a three-way tap between syringe and catheter and a 2-mL syringe used to create a vacuum from the side port. With judicious tapping and alternate application of the vacuum and release of saline into the catheter from the saline filled inflation syringe, the air can be removed from the catheter and inflation syringe.
7. For recovery, fluid and warmth are essential. A humidicrib for recovery over approximately 30–60 min is ideal. Monitor the animals for signs of dehydration, bleeding, or general loss of condition.
8. Thrombosis may occur, especially where flow through vessels is low. If thrombosis rates are found to be unacceptably high, then changing the protocol to minimize handling of the common carotid artery can be helpful in preventing

excessive damage and also in reducing spasm. For example, it is possible to dispense with the ligature on the common carotid artery (**Fig. 1D**) and to use the proximal ligature on the external carotid artery (**Fig. 1B**) to control bleeding, but this can be a more difficult procedure. Thrombosis could be managed with judicious use of anticoagulants, although this should be avoided when possible as some, such as heparin, will have effects on smooth muscle growth responses. Vasodilators (such as topical lignocaine) can also be used to overcome spasm.

9. Aortic balloon injury can be performed with a similar method. An increase in inflation volume to 0.03 mL may be used for this procedure, but it is generally not necessary if the aim is to remove the endothelium. The catheter is advanced to the second mark (10 cm) and inflated before withdrawing, with rotation, to the aortic arch.

10. Retrograde balloon injury from a femoral artery access is also possible, and may be particularly useful for double-injury models in carotid or aorta *(13)*.

11. Larger animals/vessels may require a larger balloon; However, rabbit carotid arteries can be successfully de-endothelialized with the 2F balloon.

12. Successful endothelial removal can be gaged by the intravenous administration of a bolus of Evans blue dye, 60 mg/kg body weight, 20–30 min before sacrifice (Sigma Chemical Company, St. Louis, MO). Denuded areas of artery wall will stain blue, whereas intact endothelium will remain white.

References

1. Baumgartner, H. R. and Studer, A. (1966) Effects of vascular catheterization in normo- and hypercholesteremic rabbits. *Pathol. Microbiol.* **29,** 393–405.
2. Clowes, A. W., Reidy, M. A., and Clowes, M. M. (1983) Mechanisms of stenosis after arterial injury. *Lab. Invest.* **49,** 208–215.
3. Clowes, A.W., Clowes, M. M., and Reidy, M. A. (1986) Kinetics of cellular proliferation after arterial injury: III. Endothelial and smooth muscle growth in chronically denuded vessels. *Lab. Invest.* **54,** 295–303.
4. Jackson, C. L. and Schwartz, S. M. (1992) Pharmacology of smooth muscle cell replication. *Hypertension* **20,** 713–736.
5. Zempo, N., Koyama, N., Kenagy, R. D., Lea, H. J., and Clowes, A. W. (1996) Regulation of vascular smooth muscle cell migration and proliferation in vitro and in injured rat arteries by a synthetic matrix metalloproteinase inhibitor. *Arterioscler. Thromb. Vasc. Biol.* **16,** 28–33.
6. Wong, J., Rauhoft, C., Dilley, R. J., Agratis, A., Jennings, G. L., and Bobik, A. (1997) Angiotensin-converting enzyme inhibition abolishes medial smooth muscle PDGF-AB biosynthesis and attenuates cell proliferation in injured carotid arteries: relationships to neointima formation. *Circulation* **96,** 1631–1640.
7. Ward, M. R., Sasahara, T., Agrotis, A., Dilley, R. J., Jennings, G. L., and Bobik, A. (1998) Inhibitory effects of tranilast on expression of transforming growth factor-beta isoforms and receptors in injured arteries. *Atherosclerosis* **137,** 267–275.
8. Campbell, J. H., Fennessy, P., and Campbell, G. R. (1992) Effect of perindopril on the development of atherosclerosis in the cholesterol-fed rabbit. *Clin. Exp. Pharmacol. Physiol. Suppl.* **19,** 13–17.

9. Webster, W. S., Bishop, S. P., and Geer, J. C. (1974) Experimental aortic intimal thickening: II. Endothelialization and permeability. *Am. J. Pathol.* **76,** 265–284.

10. Clowes, A. W., Collazzo, R. E., and Karnovsky, M. J. (1978) A morphologic and permeability study of luminal smooth muscle cells after arterial injury in the rat. *Lab. Invest.* **39,** 141–150.

11. Lindner, V., Reidy, M. A., and Fingerle, J. (1989) Regrowth of arterial endothelium. Denudation with minimal trauma leads to complete endothelial cell regrowth. *Lab. Invest.* **61,** 556–563.

12. Reidy, M. A. and Schwartz, S. M. (1981) Endothelial regeneration: III. Time course of intimal changes after small defined injury to rat aortic endothelium. *Lab. Invest.* **44,** 301–308.

13. Koyama, H. and Reidy, M. A. (1997) Reinjury of arterial lesions induces intimal smooth muscle cell replication that is not controlled by fibroblast growth factor 2. *Circ. Res.* **80,** 408–417.

3

Genetically Manipulated Models of Atherosclerosis in Mice

Qing Xiao

1. Introduction

Mice are largely resistant to atherosclerosis. However, with dietary intervention or genetic manipulation, mice can be induced to develop atherosclerosis. The focus of this chapter is genetically manipulated models (*see* Chapter 1 for discussion regarding diet-induced atherosclerosis). For a complex genetic disease like atherosclerosis, mouse models provide a suitable means for studying large numbers of animals and a means for manipulating genes thought to be important in lesion development. With the powerful genetic tool that gene-targeted mice provide, we are able to search for the pathogenesis of atherosclerosis, to assess the influence of risk factors, such as elevated plasma glucose or plasma fibrinogen levels, on disease progression. In addition, we can also test the effects of environment, hormones, and drugs on disease progression.

This chapter summarizes currently available mouse models of atherosclerosis, with key features, followed by suggested approaches to choosing an appropriate model, designing a study, and data collection and analysis. Finally, several examples of studies successfully utilizing mouse models are provided to demonstrate experimental designs.

The following paragraph describes the classification of atherosclerotic lesion types throughout the various stages of disease development, in addition to discussing atherosclerotic lesion types occurring in mice and diets commonly used to enhance lesion development in mouse studies.

1.1. Atherosclerotic Lesion Types

Similar to atherosclerotic lesion development in humans, those in mice are found as patchy accumulations of extracellular lipid, matrix deposits, lipid-

From: *Methods in Molecular Medicine, vol. 52: Atherosclerosis: Experimental Methods and Protocols*
Edited by: A. F. Drew © Humana Press Inc., Totowa, NJ

loaded macrophages, inflammatory cells, and smooth muscle cells, within the intima of large or medium-sized elastic or muscular arteries. Lesions are most likely to occur at areas of flow turbulence, such as the bending or branch points of vessels. Lesions can be widespread throughout the whole arterial tree: the aortic root; the coronary, pulmonary, carotid, subclavian, and brachiocephalic arteries; the lesser curvature of the aortic arch; the intercostal, renal, and iliac arteries. Lesions in mice are categorized as fatty streaks, intermediate and advanced lesions, using the classifications described by the American Heart Association for human atherosclerotic lesions *(1–3)*. Briefly, fatty streak lesions are characterized by the presence of lipid-filled macrophages, or foam cells, within the subendothelial space. The intermediate phase is distinguished by the accumulation of smooth muscle cells and extracellular matrix, such as collagen fibers. The advanced lesion has features of extensive fibrosis, thinning of the vessel wall, and the presence of necrotic and calcified tissue, with cholesterol crystals.

1.2. Atherogenic Mouse Diets

Most genetically manipulated mice will not develop atherosclerosis spontaneously on standard low cholesterol, low fat mouse chow, consisting of 5–6.5% (w/w) fat and 0.022–0.028% (w/w) cholesterol (Purina Mills, Inc., St. Louis, MO). There are two types of mouse diet commonly used to induce atherosclerosis: western-type diet and atherogenic diet. Both contain more cholesterol and fat than the regular diet. The western-type diet consists of only 0.15% (w/w) cholesterol and 21% (w/w) fat, while the atherogenic diet contains at least 1% (w/w) cholesterol. Cholic acid, a nondietary component, is added to the atherogenic diet to induce inflammation and, hence, increase atherogenicity. The atherogenic diet is synthesized essentially according to the original composition described by Nishina et al. *(4)*. Several versions of the diet are published with slight variations in the amounts of cholesterol (1–1.25%; w/w), saturated fat (cocoa butter) (15–16%; w/w), and cholic acid (0.1–0.5%; w/w). These diets can be purchased from Harlan Teklad (Madison, WI).

2. Mouse Models

Hypercholesterolemia, diabetes, cigarette smoking, male gender, and hypertension have been identified by epidemiological studies as risk factors for developing atherosclerosis *(5)*. However, only hypercholesterolemia, prolonged accumulation of the cholesterol-rich particles in the circulation, has been proven to be directly atherogenic. Therefore, most successful models of atherosclerosis in mice are established by genetic manipulation of lipid metabolism.

Lipids, including cholesterol, are transported as lipoproteins in the blood. Based on their density, lipoproteins can be divided into very low-density lipoprotein (VLDL), low density lipoprotein (LDL), intermediate-density lipoprotein (IDL), and high-density lipoprotein (HDL) fractions. It is generally accepted that large particles like LDL and IDL are atherogenic whereas HDL is anti-atherogenic.

On a standard chow diet, the cholesterol level in wild-type mice is less than 2.6 mmol/L, most of which is in the HDL fraction, and spontaneous lesions do not develop. Even on a high-cholesterol/high-fat atherogenic diet, the total plasma cholesterol level of wild-type mice rises to only 4.1 mmol/L and lesions still do not result, except in several inbred strains of mice fed the diet for a long time. Altering the lipoprotein profiles by genetic manipulation alone, or a combination of genetic modification and dietary intervention, can lead to the development of atherosclerosis. The following section describes several such models.

2.1. Apolipoprotein E (apoE)-Deficient Mice

ApoE, a ligand for the lipoprotein receptors, is important for lipid clearance, particularly the hepatic uptake of atherogenic chylomicron and VLDL remnants. The deficiency generated by homologous recombination of the gene for apoE leads to the accumulation of atherogenic lipid particles, chylomicrons, VLDL, and IDL remnants. Cholesterol levels in these animals are elevated to 10–23 mmol/L, 5–8 times higher than controls, and they develop spontaneous atherosclerosis (*6,7*). ApoE-deficiency is the only mouse model known to develop severe atherosclerosis on a standard chow diet. The lesions start to appear as early as 8–10 wk in apoE-deficient mice and become widespread as animals get older (*6–9*). Lesions observed are of all stages, varying from fatty streak, intermediate lesion to fibrous plaque, and most importantly, they resemble those of humans (*8,9*). On a standard chow diet, lesions in 3–4 mo old apoE-deficient mice encompass the area of 3×10^3 µm^2. When challenged with a western-type diet for 4–5 wk, apoE-deficient mice develop severe hypercholesterolemia, greater than 46 mmol/L, and lesions are larger (9×10^4 µm^2 cross-sectional area) and more advanced. Cholesterol levels of control mice fed Western-type diets only rise to 4–5 mmol/L, and lesions do not develop (*6*).

2.2. Transgenic Mice Expressing Human APOE*3-Leiden or APOE R142C (Arg142 to Cys)

Expression of defective variants of human APOE: APOE*3-Leiden or APOE R142C (Arg to Cys 142) can transdominantly interfere with normal mouse apoE function. Mice expressing these human genes show abnormal lipid clearance with elevations in chylomicrons and VLDL remnants, on a lesser scale than in apoE-deficient mice. These mice do not develop atherosclerosis on a standard mouse chow diet. However, fatty streaks and fibrous plaques can be observed when mice are fed the atherogenic diet.

2.2.1. Transgenic Mice Carrying Human apoE*3-Leiden

Apolipoprotein E*3-Leiden was identified as a variant of human APOE associated with a dominantly-inherited form of type III hyperlipoproteinemia, which exhibits defective receptor binding *(10,11)*. A genomic DNA segment isolated from the APOE*3-Leiden proband is expressed in mice under the liver-specific regulatory elements *(12)*.

On a standard chow diet, mice with apoE3-Leiden protein develop significantly high levels of total plasma cholesterol and triglycerides, mainly in the HDL fraction, but do not develop lesions *(12)*. However, when mice are fed a high cholesterol, high-fat atherogenic diet (1% cholesterol, 15% cocoa butter, and 0.1 or 0.5% cholic acid) after 8–10 wk, apoE3-Leiden protein becomes distributed in atherogenic VLDL/LDL as well as HDL *(13)*. In addition to the change in protein distribution, lines of mice with high levels of transgene expression develop severe hypercholesterolemia (range from 25–60 mmol/L) along with atherosclerotic lesions in the aortic arch, the descending aorta, and the carotid arteries, after 6 and 14 wk of special dietary treatment, respectively *(13)*. Both fatty streaks and advanced lesions are present in the mice. On average, there are 1–3 fatty streaks and 1–3 advanced plaques observed per mouse *(13)*. Mice on a diet of 0.5% cholic acid have higher occurrence of plaques than mice receiving 0.1% cholic acid *(13)*. Interestingly, quantity of lesions is positively correlated with the serum level of VLDL and LDL *(13)*.

2.2.2. Transgenic Mice Carrying human apoE R142C

Mice expressing human apoE R142C, another defective form of apoE, have elevated levels of total plasma cholesterol, triglycerides, and VLDL on normal diet. Only microscopic fatty streaks are observed at the aortic valves of 4-mo old animals *(14)*. After 3 mo of feeding the atherogenic diet, plasma cholesterol levels are increased mostly in the VLDL fractions, and fatty streak lesions develop.

2.3. Mice with the apoE Gene replaced by Human APOE Alleles

Three main isoforms of human apoE protein differ at the positions 112 and 158 of the protein sequence; apoE2 has a cysteine at both positions, apoE3 has a cysteine at position 112 and an arginine at position 158, and apoE4 has an arginine at both positions. The three isoforms are encoded by APOE allele *2, *3, and *4 at the frequency of 7.3, 78.3, and 14.3%, respectively. APOE*3 is considered the 'normal allele,' while APOE*4 is associated with higher total plasma cholesterol and LDL levels. ApoE2 has only 1% of the receptor-binding affinity of apoE3 and apoE4, and the majority of homozygous individuals display normal plasma cholesterol levels, with the exception of 5–10% that have type III hyperlipoproteinemia.

2.3.1. Transgenic Mice Expressing Human apoE3 Isoform in Place of Mouse apoE

Mice carrying the gene replacement of mouse apoE by the human APOE*3 express human apoE*3 virtually at the same level as that of mouse apoE in control mice *(15)*. When maintained on a standard chow diet, the modification causes only subtle alterations in lipoprotein profiles with notable reduction in the amount of chylomicron and VLDL/LDL remnants *(15)*. Unlike its normal mouse counterpart, human apoE proteins seem to associate with larger lipoprotein particles rather than HDL. No lesions are seen in the majority of the transgenic animals except very small fatty streaks, with an average size of $1 \times 10^3 \mu m^2$, which are found in occasional female mice aged 10–12 mo *(15)*. These animals also metabolize exogenous lipid particles six times slower than controls. Human apoE-expressing mice fed an atherogenic diet (15.8% fat, 1.25% cholesterol, and 0.5% sodium cholate) develop a dramatic fivefold increase in the total cholesterol level, compared with a 1.5-fold increase in control mice *(15)*. Large fatty streak lesions, with a size ranging from 2.4–16.8 $\times 10^4 \mu m^2$, occur in the aortic sinus of the transgenic mice after 12 wk on the diet, while only small fatty streak lesions, of size 2.9–9.2 $\times 10^3 \mu m^2$, virtually the accumulation of a few foam cells, are found in control mice *(15)*.

2.3.2. Transgenic Mice Expressing the Human apoE2 Isoform in Place of Mouse apoE

Expression of human apoE2 causes type III hyperlipoproteinemia in mice fed standard chow, with plasma total cholesterol levels> 5 mmol/L and triglyceride levels 2–3 times higher than in control mice *(16)*. These mice are defective in clearing chylomicron and VLDL remnants, and spontaneous atherosclerotic plaques are seen in female mice in the aortic root at 10 mo of age *(16)*. The cross-sectional lesion areas range from 2×10^4 to $2 \times 10^5 \mu m^2$ *(16)*. Feeding the atherogenic diet for 3 mo accelerates atherosclerotic development, resulting in markedly larger ($5.3 \times 10^5 \mu m^2$) and more advanced lesions, containing small areas of fibrotic and necrotic tissues and cholesterol crystals, in addition to foam cells *(16)*.

2.4. LDL-Receptor Deficient (LDLR) Mice

Disruption of the LDLR gene results in a twofold increase of cholesterol levels to approximately 5 mmol/L, when mice are fed a standard chow diet, compared with control mice *(17)*. On the atherogenic diet, the total plasma cholesterol levels of LDLR-deficient mice are significantly increased to levels greater than 39 mmol/L, as a result of increased levels of VLDL, IDL, and LDL and decreased levels of HDL cholesterol *(17)*. After 7 mo, the LDLR-deficient mice develop massive fatty streaks in the aorta, the opening of the coronary artery, and the aortic valve leaflets *(17)*. Lesions are not found either in wild-type mice fed the same diet or LDLR-deficient mice fed a standard chow diet. On a western-type diet, LDLR-deficient mice develop high cholesterol levels (approx 31 mmol/L), and fatty streaks *(17)*.

2.5. Transgenic Mice Expressing Human apoB, Human apo(a) or Lp(a)

2.5.1. Transgenic Mice Expressing Human apoB

ApoB is the major protein component of the atherogenic lipid particles, including VLDL, IDL, and LDL. Expression of human apoB in mice leads to a modest increase in the amount of LDL. After 4 wk of an atherogenic diet, dramatic changes in the lipoprotein profiles (8–13 mmol/L LDL; 1.5–2.5-fold higher than controls) are seen in the transgenic lines with high levels of human apoB *(18)*. Low-level expression of the transgene (<200 mg/L) in mice seems to have little impact on lesion development *(18)*. Lesions developing in the high expression transgenic mice after 18 wk on the atherogenic diet are significantly larger than in controls. Advanced lesions, containing connective tissue, necrotic core, and cholesterol deposits, develop in the proximal aorta, the aortic arch, the openings of intercostal arteries, and the abdominal aorta *(18,19)*. The most dramatic changes in lesion size are seen in female mice (wild-type mice: 1.4×10^4 μm^2; transgenic mice: 1.6×10^5 μm^2) compared with male mice (wild-type mice: 8×10^3 μm^2; transgenic mice 4.5×10^4 μm^2) *(18,19)*.

2.5.2. Transgenic Mice Expressing Human apo(a)

Lp(a), an LDL-like lipoprotein found in humans but not in mice, contains a unique glycoprotein, apolipoprotein(a), which has many tandemly repeated units resembling the fourth kringle domain of plasminogen, and a single homologue of kringle-5, the protease domain of plasminogen. Apo(a) binds to apoB, a major component of LDL, with a high affinity, forming the lipoprotein, Lp(a). Elevated plasma levels of Lp(a) are associated with increased risk for atherosclerosis. Mice expressing human apo(a) are susceptible to the development of fatty streaks when fed an atherogenic diet, even though only 5% of the plasma apo(a) associates with lipid particles *(20)*. After 3.5 mo of feeding of an atherogenic diet, the mean lesion area for apo(a) transgenic mice is 1000 μm^2, as compared to 100 μm^2 in control mice *(20)*.

2.5.3. Lp(a) Transgenic Mice

Apo(a) binds mouse apoB poorly, hence the majority of apo(a) is expressed in the mice as free plasma apo(a). When both human apoB and apo(a) are introduced into mice, high levels of human-like Lp(a) appear in the circulation. Coexpression of apo(a) and human apoB resulted in an increase in lesion area ($4.7 \times 10^3 \ \mu m^2$) compared with apoB transgenic mice ($3.3 \times 10^3 \ \mu m^2$), apo(a) transgenic mice ($600 \ \mu m^2$) or wild-type mice ($100 \ \mu m^2$), after all mice were fed an atherogenic diet for 14 wk *(21)*. This enhanced atherogenic effect of Lp(a) over apo(a) is further documented in a study of mice fed an atherogenic diet for 18 wk, demonstrating greater lesion area in mice expressing apo(a) together with high levels of human apoB (>200 mg/L; lesion area: 1.9×10^4 μm^2) compared with low levels of apoB (<200 mg/L; lesion area: $8 \times 10^3 \ \mu m^2$) or no expression of apoB (lesion area: $\sim 3 \times 10^3 \ \mu m^2$) *(18)*. Expression of high levels of human apoB alone seem to be sufficiently atherogenic, since coexpression of apo(a) induces only a modest increase in mean lesion size *(18)*.

3. Notes

3.1. Choosing the Right Model for Your Study

To choose a mouse model for atherosclerosis, the following questions should be considered:

a. What is the genetic basis of the model?
b. Do the mice develop spontaneous lesions or is special dietary treatment needed to induce atherosclerosis?
c. When do lesions start to appear?
d. How severe is the disease?
e. Are advanced lesions present? When?

Most of the models develop fatty streaks after feeding of an atherogenic diet for 3–4 mo. ApoE-deficient and LDLR-deficient mice are the most popular models currently used. Depending on the objectives of your study, you may choose different models.

In general, spontaneous models of atherosclerosis are preferred for several reasons: atherogenic diets contain nonphysiologically high levels of fat and cholesterol and the addition of cholic acid, which is not usually present in a diet and can influence the immune system. In addition, a high-fat, high cholesterol diet can complicate the expression and interaction of certain genes. For instance, addition of cholate to the diet can increase both the levels of plasma cholesterol and the expression of apoE3*Leiden. Human apoB expression is also enhanced by 40–90% after 5 wk of an atherogenic diet.

Both apoE-deficient mice and mice with targeted replacement of apoE by human apoE*2 develop spontaneous atherosclerosis. But apoE-deficient mice develop lesions much earlier, and the entire spectrum of lesions is observed. Mice lacking apoE are the most promising models to study the pathogenesis of atherosclerosis, to explore the genetic and environmental modifiers, and to evaluate drugs or therapeutic approaches.

3.2. Maintaining and Breeding of Genetically Manipulated Atherosclerosis-Susceptible Mice

Many varieties of atherosclerosis-susceptible mice can be purchased from Jackson Laboratories (Bar Harbor, ME) or other commercial sources. Mice with specific mutations can be obtained from the investigators who originally made them. For more information about mouse models for human diseases, there are a few databases on the web that I find very valuable, including the mouse knockout and mutation database maintained by BioMedNet (http://www.biomednet.com/db/mkmd) and the mouse models list from the Jackson Laboratories web site (http://jaxmice.jax.org/index.shtml).

Mice are normally housed in the institution facility under specific guidelines. A pathogen-free environment is preferred. Fortunately, the genetic manipulations described above do not affect the survival and reproduction of mice. Viable and fertile atherosclerosis-susceptible mice are relative easy to maintain. To start a colony harboring a specific genetic manipulation, you need to set up a number of breeding cages; each should contain one male and at least one female. In general, females reach sexual maturity at 6 wk whereas males reach maturity at 8 wk. To avoid unplanned mating, progeny should be weaned at age of 3 wk, or at least before sexual maturity, and separated by sex. Males weaned together before maturity can be housed together if there is no exposure to females. One litter should be weaned before the next litter is born, to prevent the younger ones being trampled or starved.

Mice have a gestation period of 18–21 d, and females enter estrus and ovulate every 4–5 d. To maintain a productive colony, mating should be checked after the breeding pair is set up; a whitish vaginal plug in females often indicates successful fertilization. Males can be used to mate with other females after one becomes pregnant. In addition, the litter size from each mating pair should be recorded, and the mating pair should be replaced if they are not productive after 2 mo, produce only small litters, or become older than 9 mo. Moreover, if a male is kept with a pregnant female, she can mate immediately after delivery.

The atherosclerosis-susceptible mutations are screened in mice by PCR or Southern blot analysis using genomic DNA extracted from an ear or tail biopsy. Mutations can be maintained by homozygous breeding, or heterozygous breeding, which results in littermate control mice.

To manage a study efficiently, a mouse log should be constructed using a spreadsheet, which allows data to be entered and sorted easily. Each mouse needs a unique identification number and assignment of a cage card. Mice caged together can be distinguished either by their coat colors or marks on ears or toes. In my experience, the easiest way is to tag mouse ears with a set of metal rings, in which a series of identifying numbers has been engraved. The date of birth, coat color, sex, genotype, and identification numbers of parents (optional) should be recorded on the card. The cards for all of the mice housed in the same cage should be placed together in the same holder. When a mouse is moved from one cage to another, the card should be moved with the mouse, as errors in identification must not occur.

3.3. Experimental Design and Data Collection

Atherosclerosis is such a complex genetic disorder that many variables must be taken into account when an experiment is designed. The first is the genetic background. Many atherosclerosis-susceptible mice are available in an inbred background, such as C57BL6. To minimize the variation in data, mice of inbred strains are recommended. However, all the mice generated by gene targeting, including apoE-deficient and LDLR-deficient mice, were initially created in a mixed genetic background. It is conceivable that strong modifiers of atherosclerosis may be linked to specific background. Therefore, large variability in data is commonly seen in studies with mixed backgrounds, which may lead to wrongful interpretation of experimental results. Until now, most of the atherosclerosis-susceptible mice carrying a targeted inactivation or replacement of a gene have become congenic, which means the original mutation has been backcrossed into an inbred strain for more than nine generations. The genetic background in these congenic mice is almost the same as the inbred ones. In cases in which mixed genetic backgrounds are used, appropriate littermate controls and statistical investigation of data are necessary for proper interpretation of results.

Sex and age should be considered in experimental design. Sex hormones and age do influence the disease. Comparisons can be made only with sex- and age-matched data. For diet-induced atherosclerosis, females are usually chosen, since they respond better than the males.

Lesions can be found at multiple locations and they vary in size and shape at different sites. How can they be compared? Lesions from the proximal aorta are usually measured to quantify atherosclerosis. The anatomical features of this region, aortic valves, and opening of the coronary artery provide an excellent landmark to orient atherosclerotic lesions.

3.4. Applications

3.4.1. Analysis of the Roles of Other Genes in Atherosclerosis

To analyze the roles of chemokines in the initiation and progression of atherosclerosis, apoE-deficient mice have been crossed to CCR2-deficient mice. Decreased lesion formation in CCR2-deficient mice indicates that chemokine-mediated cell trafficking plays an important role in atherogenesis *(22)*. Mice expressing apoAI have been crossed to apoE-deficient mice to test the contribution of HDL to atherosclerosis. As expected, apolipoprotein AI transgene corrects apolipoprotein E deficiency–induced atherosclerosis *(23,24)*.

3.4.2. Test the Effect of Therapeutic Strategy

Bone marrow from wild type mice has been transplanted into apoE-deficient mice and atherosclerosis is prevented *(25)*.

3.4.3. Drug Intervention

The popular cholesterol-lowering drug probucol was fed to apoE-deficient mice to test the efficacy of the drug. Paradoxically, enhancement of atherosclerosis by probucol treatment was seen in apoE-deficient mice *(26)*.

References

1. Stary, H. C., Blankenhorn, D. H., Chandler, A. B., Glagov, S., Insull, W., Jr., Richardson, M., Rosenfeld, M. E., Schaffer, S. A., Schwartz, C. J., and Wagner, W. D. (1992) A definition of the intima of human arteries and of its atherosclerosis- prone regions. A report from the Committee on Vascular Lesions of the Council on Arteriosclerosis, American Heart Association. *Circulation* **85,** 391–405.
2. Stary, H. C., Chandler, A. B., Glagov, S., Guyton, J. R., Insull, W., Jr., Rosenfeld, M. E., Schaffer, S. A., Schwartz, C. J., Wagner, W. D., and Wissler, R. W. (1994) A definition of initial, fatty streak, and intermediate lesions of atherosclerosis. A report from the Committee on Vascular Lesions of the Council on Arteriosclerosis, American Heart Association. *Circulation* **89,** 2462–2478.
3. Stary, H. C., Chandler, A. B., Dinsmore, R. E., Fuster, V., Glagov, S., Insull, W., Jr., Rosenfeld, M. E., Schwartz, C. J., Wagner, W. D., and Wissler, R. W. (1995) A definition of advanced types of atherosclerotic lesions and a histological classification of atherosclerosis. A report from the Committee on Vascular Lesions of the Council on Arteriosclerosis, American Heart Association. *Circulation* **92,** 1355–1374.
4. Nishina P. M., Verstuyft, J., and Paigen, B. (1990) Synthetic low and high fat diets for the study of atherosclerosis in the mouse. *J. Lipid Res.* **31,** 859–869.
5. Ross, R. (1993) The pathogenesis of atherosclerosis: a perspective for the 1990s. *Nature* **362,** 801–809.
6. Plump, A. S., Smith, J. D., Hayek, T., Aalto-Setala, K., Walsh, A., Verstuyft, J. G., Rubin, E. M., and Breslow, J. L. (1992) Severe hypercholesterolemia and atherosclerosis in apolipoprotein E-deficient mice created by homologous recombination in ES cells. *Cell* **71,** 343–353.
7. Zhang, S. H., Reddick, R. L., Piedrahita, J. A., and Maeda, N. (1992) Spontaneous hypercholesterolemia and arterial lesions in mice lacking apolipoprotein E. *Science* **258,** 468–471.

8. Reddick, R. L., Zhang, S. H., and Maeda, N. (1994) Atherosclerosis in mice lacking apo E. Evaluation of lesion development and progression. *Arterioscler. Thromb. Vase. Biol.* **14**, 141–147.

9. Nakashima, Y., Plump, A. S., Raines, E. W., Breslow, J. L., and Ross, R. (1994) ApoE-deficient mice develop lesions of all phases of atherosclerosis throughout the arterial tree. *Arterioscler. Thromb. Vase. Biol.* **14**, 133–140.

10. Havekes, L., de Wit, E., Leuven, J. G., Klasen, E., Utermann, G., Weber, W., and Beisiegel, U. (1986) Apolipoprotein E3-Leiden. A new variant of human apolipoprotein E associated with familial type III hyperlipoproteinemia. *Hum. Genet.* **73**, 157–163.

11. de Knijff, P., van den Maagdenberg, A. M., Stalenhoef, A. F., Gevers Leuven, J. A., Demacker, P. N., Kuyt, L. P., Frants, R. R., Havekes, L. M. (1991) Familial dysbetalipoproteinemia associated with apolipoprotein E3-Leiden in an extent multigeneration pedigree. *J. Clin. Invest.* **88**, 643–655.

12. van den Maagdenberg, A. M., Hofker, M. H., Krimpenfort, P. J., de Bruijn, I., van Vlijmen, B., van der Boom, H., Havekes, L. M., and Frants, R. R. (1993) Transgenic mice carrying the apolipoprotein E3-Leiden gene exhibit hyperlipoproteinemia. *J. Biol. Chem.* **268**, 10540–10545.

13. van Vlijmen, B., van den Maagdenberg, A. M., Gijbels, M. J., van der Boom, H., HogenEsch, H., Frants, R. R., Hofker, M. H., and Havekes, L. M. (1994) Diet-induced hyperlipoproteinemia and atherosclerosis in apolipoprotein E3-Leiden transgenic mice. *J. Clin. Invest.* **93**, 1403–1410.

14. Fazio, S., Sanan, D. A., Lee, Y. L., Ji, Z. S., Mahley, R. W., Rall, S. C. Jr. (1994) Susceptibility to diet-induced atherosclerosis in transgenic mice expressing a dysfunctional human apolipoprotein E(Arg 112,Cys142). *Arterioscler. Thromb. Vase. Biol.* **14**, 1873–1879.

15. Sullivan, P. M., Mezdour, H., Aratani, Y., Knouff, C., Najib, J., Reddick, R. L., Quarfordt, S. H., and Maeda, N. (1997) Targeted replacement of the mouse apolipoprotein E gene with the common human APOE3 allele enhances diet-induced hypercholesterolemia and atherosclerosis. *J. Biol. Chem.* **272**, 17972–17980.

16. Sullivan, P. M., Mezdour, H., Quarfordt, S. H., and Maeda, N. (1998) Type III hyperlipoproteinemia and spontaneous atherosclerosis in mice resulting from gene replacement of mouse Apoe with human APOE*2. *J. Clin. Invest.* **102**, 130–135.

17. Ishibashi, S., Goldstein, J. L., Brown, M. S., Herz, J., and Burns, D. K. (1994) Massive xanthomatosis and atherosclerosis in cholesterol-fed low density lipoprotein receptor-negative mice. *J. Clin. Invest.* **93**, 1885–1893.

18. Callow, M. J., Verstuyft, J., Tangirala, R., Palinski, W., and Rubin, E. M. (1995) Atherogenesis in transgenic mice with human apolipoprotein B and lipoprotein (a). *J. Clin. Invest.* **96**, 1639–1646.

19. Purcell-Huynh, D. A., Farese, R. V. Jr., Johnson, D. F., Flynn, L. M., Pierotti, V., Newland, D. L., Linton, M. F., Sanan, D. A., and Young, S. G. (1995) Transgenic mice expressing high levels of human apolipoprotein B develop severe atherosclerotic lesions in response to a high-fat diet. *J. Clin. Invest* **95**, 2246–2257.

20. Lawn, R. M., Wade, D. P., Hammer, R. E., Chiesa, G., Verstuyft, J. G., and Rubin, E. M. (1992) Atherogenesis in transgenic mice expressing human apolipoprotein. *Nature* **360,** 670–672.
21. Mancini, F. P., Newland, D. L., Mooser, V., Murata, J., Marcovina, S., Young, S. G., Hammer, R. E., Sanan, D. A., and Hobbs, H. H. (1995) Relative contributions of apolipoprotein(a) and apolipoprotein-B to the development of fatty lesions in the proximal aorta of mice. *Arterioscler. Thromb. Vasc. Biol.* **15,** 1911–1916.
22. Boring, L., Gosling, J., Cleary, M., and Charo, I. F. (1998) Decreased lesion formation in CCR2-/- mice reveals a role for chemokines in the initiation of atherosclerosis. *Nature* **394,** 894–897.
23. Plump, A. S., Scott, C. J., and Breslow, J. L. (1994) Human apolipoprotein A-1 gene expression increases high density lipoprotein and suppresses atherosclerosis in the apolipoprotein E-deficient mouse. *Proc. Natl. Acad. Sci. USA* **91,** 9607–9611.
24. Pászty, C., Maeda, N., Verstuyft, J., and Rubin, E. M. (1994) Apolipoprotein AI transgene corrects apolipoprotein E deficiency-induced atherosclerosis in mice. *J. Clin. Invest.* **94,** 899–903.
25. Linton, M. F., Atkinson, J. B., and Fazio, S. (1995) Prevention of atherosclerosis in apolipoprotein E-deficient mice by bone marrow transplantation. *Science* **267,** 1034–1037.
26. Zhang, S. H., Reddick, R. L., Avdievich, E., Surles, L. K., Jones, R. G., Reynolds, J. B., Quarfordt, S. H., and Maeda, N. (1997) Paradoxical enhancement of atherosclerosis by probucol treatment in apolipoprotein E-deficient mice. *J. Clin. Invest.* **99,** 2858–2566.

4

Lipoprotein Isolation and Analysis from Serum by Preparative Ultracentrifugation

Kishor M. Wasan, Shawn M. Cassidy, Allison L. Kennedy, and Kathy D. Peteherych

1. Introduction

Plasma lipoproteins are a heterogeneous population of soluble, macromolecular aggregates of lipids and proteins. They are responsible for the transport of water-insoluble nutrients through the vascular and extravascular fluids from their site of synthesis or absorption to peripheral tissues (1,2). These hydrophobic nutrients (triacylglycerols [TGs] and cholesteryl esters [CEs]) are delivered from the liver and intestine to other tissues in the body for storage or catabolism in the production of energy. Lipoproteins are also known to be involved in other biological processes, including coagulation and tissue repair as well as immune reactions (3,4).

All lipoprotein particles are generally of a spherical shape or form consisting of a nonpolar lipid core (TGs and CEs) surrounded by a surface monolayer of amphipathic lipids (phospholipids and unesterified cholesterol) and specific proteins called apolipoproteins. A number of different phospholipids are incorporated into the coat of the lipoprotein, the most common being phosphatidylcholine, phosphatidylserine, phosphatidylethanolamine, and sphingomyelin. By far, the most abundant of these phospholipids is phosphatidylcholine, which is also utilized as a substrate in the esterification of cholesterol to cholesteryl ester by the enzyme lecithin cholesterol acyltransferase (LCAT). Since lipids generally have lower buoyant densities than proteins, lipoproteins with a larger amount of lipid relative to protein will have a lower density than lipoproteins with a smaller lipid-to-protein ratio (5). Traditionally, plasma lipoproteins are classified and separated according to their density and are divided into five main categories: chylomicrons, very low density lipoproteins (VLDLs), intermediate-density lipoproteins (IDLs), low-density lipoproteins (LDLs), and high-density lipoproteins (HDLs) (**Table 1**).

From: *Methods in Molecular Medicine, vol. 52: Atherosclerosis: Experimental Methods and Protocols*
Edited by: A. F. Drew © Humana Press Inc., Totowa, NJ

Table 1
Density, Size, and Physical Composition of Human Plasma Lipoproteins

Characteristic	Chylomicrons	VLDL	IDL	LDL	HDL
Abbreviation		VLDL	IDL	LDL	HDL
Density (g/mL)	< 0.95	0.95–1.006	1.006–1.019	1.019–1.063	1.063–1.210
Diameter (nm)	75–1200	30–80	25–35	18–25	5–12
Composition (% dry wt)					
Protein	1–2	8	19	22	47
Triglycerides	86	55	23	6	4
Cholesterol	5	19	38	50	19
Phospholipid	7	18	20	22	30
Apoproteins	A1, A2				A1, A2
	B-48	B-100	B-100	B-100	
	C1, C2, C3	C1, C2, C3	C1, C2, C3		C1, C2, C3
	E	E	E		E

Adapted from refs. *1* and *6*.

Chylomicrons, with a diameter of approximately 100 to 1000 nm, are the largest of the lipoproteins and are found in greatest abundance after a meal. They are synthesized by the intestine and are core-rich in TGs derived from dietary fat. VLDLs are the next largest lipoproteins (diameter 3–80 nm) and are also rich in TG. They are synthesized mainly by the liver, but may also be synthesized to a lesser degree by the intestine. IDLs, whose lipid core is comprised mainly of CE with some TGs, are the resultant product of VLDL metabolism. LDLs, in turn, are the product of IDL metabolism in which almost all of the remaining TGs have been hydrolyzed to produce a lipoprotein with a core comprised almost entirely of CE. LDLs are the major cholesterol-carrying lipoprotein and are the second smallest of the lipoproteins, with an average diameter of 18–25 nm. The smallest of the lipoproteins, with a diameter range of 7–12 nm, are the HDLs. These lipoproteins are a diverse population in both structure and function and have a lipid core that contains both CEs and TGs of varying ratios.

The plasma lipoprotein separation techniques currently available were designed to separate, isolate, and purify individual lipoprotein subclasses from plasma. These techniques, including ultracentrifugation, sequential precipitation, size exclusion chromatography, affinity chromatography, fast protein liquid chromatography, and gel electrophoresis, are designed to separate plasma lipoproteins based on their differences in density, molecular size, surface charge or protein content *(6)*.

Ultracentrifugation (UC) appears to be the most acceptable and widely used technique in the separation of different lipoprotein subclasses because of its ease of use, equipment availability, and reproducibility *(7)*. Two main types of UC are used, step-gradient and sequential-density UC. Each UC method has differences in UC time, rotor speed, volume of sample required, and temperature at which the lipoprotein separation occurs, all of which may influence the result *(7)*. Our laboratory *(8)* and others *(7,9)* have done numerous investigations establishing the optimal conditions for lipoprotein separation from plasma with minimal contamination or overlap between lipoprotein fractions.

This chapter describes the separation of human plasma into four major constituents: (1) VLDL — containing the triglyceride-rich components of plasma (chylomicrons and VLDL), (2) LDL — containing the cholesterol-rich LDL and IDL lipoproteins, (3) HDL — comprised of all subfractions of the HDL species, and (4) LPDP — lipoprotein-deficient plasma containing all other components of human plasma with a density greater than 1.21 g/mL. Furthermore, the makeup of these four fractions is elucidated; all lipid constituents and the total protein of each group are quantitated.

2. Materials

2.1. Sample Preparation

To prevent lipoprotein modification during UC we recommend the addition of EDTA (0.04% final concentration), sodium azide (0.05%), and phenylmethylsulfonyl fluoride (PMSF) (0.015%) to freshly prepared plasma.

2.2. Primary Salt Solutions (see Notes 1 and 2)

1. 1.006 g/mL salt solution: Add 11.4 g NaCl + 0.2 g Na_2 EDTA to a 1000-mL volumetric flask. Add ~500 ml H_2O and 1 mL 1M NaOH and mix to dissolve solids. Fill to volume with H_2O + an additional 3 mL H_2O.
2. 1.478 g/mL salt solution: Add 78.32 g NaBr to 100 mL of 1.006 g/mL salt solution.

2.3. Secondary Salt Solutions

1. 1.019 g/mL salt solution: Add 100 mL 1.006 g/mL salt solution to 2.83 mL of 1.478 g/ml salt solution.
2. 1.063 g/mL salt solution: Add 100 mL of 1.006 g/mL salt solution to 13.73 mL of 1.478 g/mL salt solution.
3. 1.21 g/mL salt solution: Add 100 mL of 1.006 g/mL salt solution to 76.1 mL of 1.478 g/mL salt solution.

3. Methods

1. Determine the solvent density of the sample either by calculation or by dialysis against a salt solution of known density. The density of blood bank plasma from whole blood donors can be calculated, since each full plasma unit bag contains 63 mL of acid citrate-dextrose (ACD). It is assumed that all of the ACD added to

the whole blood partitions into the plasma fraction. Information about the ACD content (mL ACD used to process × mL blood) of platelet donor derived-plasma should be obtained for each unit, and density calculated, assuming a hematocrit of 50%. The density of ACD is 1.026 g/mL.

$$\text{ACD plasma density} = ((V_1 * 1.006) + (V_2 * 1.026)) / V_1 + V_2$$

where: V_1 = volume of undiluted plasma
           V_2 = volume of ACD

General equation for solvent density adjustments:

$$V_D = V_s (d_f - d_i) / (d_D - d_f)$$

where: V_D = volume of salt solution to be added to your sample (diluent volume)
           V_s = initial volume of sample
           d_f = desired final density
           d_i = initial density of sample
           d_D = density of solution you are adding to adjust the sample (diluent density)

All other chemicals or reagents not specified otherwise above are from Sigma Chemical Co. (St. Louis, MO), including cholesterol, triglyceride, and protein assay kits. Phospholipid assay kits are from Boehringer Mannheim (Germany).

2. Add 1/ 50 volume of 60 mM EDTA, pH 7.6, to the ACD plasma to give a final EDTA concentration of 1.2 mM (0.04%).

3. Adjust the solvent density (*see* **Table 2**) of the sample as determined by the equation above or by the addition of solid NaBr (*see* **Table 3**) to isolate the lipoproteins of interest. For example, when the solvent density is adjusted to 1.006 g/ mL, VLDL and chylomicron particles are isolated. When the solvent densities are adjusted to 1.019 g/mL, IDL particles are isolated; 1.063 g/mL, LDL particles are isolated; and 1.21 g/mL, HDL particles are isolated.

4. Place adjusted sample into ultracentrifuge tubes and spin as indicated in **Table 4**.

5. Carefully remove tubes from rotor soon after the spin has ended and slice tubes in slicer about 1/4 to 1/3 from the top. If this is the final spin, the tube can be cut closer to the visible, floating lipoprotein fraction. Remove top solution containing floated lipoprotein and rinse tube top and slicer with 2 × 1 mL of the same density salt solution (*see* **Note 3**).

6. If other lipoproteins are required, remove bottom fraction to a graduated cylinder and rinse tube bottom as indicated in **step 5**. The bottom fraction can be discarded if no other lipoproteins are required and skip to **step 9**.

7. Determine volume of bottom fraction, adjust its density as needed using the equation above or solid salt (*see* **Table 3**), and re-spin.

8. Continue at **step 5** and repeat until all desired lipoproteins are isolated (Table 4).

9. Dialyze isolated lipoproteins against 0.9% NaCl, 0.02% Na$_2$ EDTA, pH 8.5, at 4°C. Dialysis should be against 4 changes of buffer of at least 20 volumes for at least 6 h each, with the last dialysis carried out overnight.

Table 2
Density Classification of Lipoproteins

| | Density limits (g/mL) | |
	Lower	Upper
Very Low Density Lipoprotein (VLDL)	———	1.006
Intermediate Density Lipoprotein (IDL)	1.006	1.019
Low Density Lipoprotein (LDL)	1.019	1.063
High Density Lipoprotein (HDL)	1.063	1.21

Table 3
Density Adjustment by Solid NaBr Addition

Initial density	Desired final density	Grams NaBr to be added/mL original solution
1.006	1.019	0.0170
"	1.063	0.0763
"	1.21	0.2945
"	1.25	0.3588
1.019	1.063	0.0589
"	1.21	0.2758
"	1.25	0.3397
1.063	1.21	0.2122
"	1.25	0.2750

Table 4
Ultracentrifugation Times for Lipoprotein Isolation

| | | Centrifugation Time (H) | | | |
| Rotor | Speed | VLDL, IDL, LDL | | HDL | |
		4°C	17°C	4°C	17°C
50.2 Ti	50,000	20	14	30	21
60 Ti	60,000	18	12	26	18
50.3 Ti	50,000	14.5	10	21.5	15

10. Sterile filter and store at 4°C in the dark. Perform chemical analyses for lipids and protein; *see* **Table 5** for typical composition values as a reference point. For every separated lipoprotein and lipoprotein-deficient fraction of each patient plasma sample, a lipid and protein profile is compiled. All lipid and protein concentrations are determined by colorimetric enzyme analysis kits purchased from Sigma and are measured using a UV spectrophotometer. For the determina-

Table 5
Typical Composition of Human Lipoproteins

Lipoprotein	Lipid composition relative to protein content (wt/wt)		
	TC/Prot	PL/Prot	TG/Prot
VLDL	1.0–1.7	1.7–2.1	5.3–6.3
LDL	1.2–1.5	1.0–1.2	0.3–0.5
HDL	0.2–0.4	0.5–0.6	0.08–0.10

TC, total cholesterol; PL, phospholipid; TG, triglyceride; Prot, protein.

tion of total cholesterol, total triglyceride, and total protein in lipoprotein-containing and lipoprotein-deficient plasma, standard curves are created and employed. The total cholesterol and triglyceride standard curves are usually linear over a range of 12.5–200 mg/dL and 15.625–250 mg/dL, respectively. The standard curves for total protein, while not linear, utilized a concentration range of 50–400 μg/mL for total protein determination. The unknown sample concentrations of each of the separated fraction samples are measured directly from their respective standard curves.

The kits for the estimation of triglyceride, cholesterol, protein and phospholipid use the following methods:

3.1. Triglyceride

Briefly, TG is first hydrolyzed by lipoprotein lipase to glycerol and free fatty acids. Glycerol is then phosphorylated by adenosine triphosphate, forming glycerol-1-phosphate (G-1-P) and adenosine-5-diphosphate in the reaction catalyzed by glycerol kinase (GK). G-1-P is then oxidized by glycerol phosphate oxidase to dihydrooxyacetone phosphate and hydrogen peroxide. A quinoneimine dye is produced by the peroxidase catalyzed coupling of 4-aminoantipyrine and sodium N-ethyl-N- (3-sulfopropyl) m-anisidine with hydrogen peroxide. This dye shows a maximum absorbency of 500 nm and is directly proportional to the triglyceride concentration of the sample. Absorbencies of plasma and lipoprotein samples are determined and compared to an external calibration curve for TG (linear range of 10–300 mg/dL; R^2=0.95).

3.2. Cholesterol

In the determination of cholesterol concentrations, cholesterol esters are first hydrolyzed to cholesterol by cholesterol esterase. The cholesterol is then oxidized by cholesterol oxidase to cholest-4-en-3-one and hydrogen peroxide. A quinoneimine dye is produced by the peroxidase catalyzed coupling of 4-aminoantipyrine and *p*-hydroxybenzenesulfonate with hydrogen peroxide. This dye shows maximum absorbency at 500 nm and is directly proportional to the cholesterol concentration of the sample. Absorbencies of plasma and lipoprotein samples will be determined and compared to an external calibration curve for cholesterol (linear range of 10–450 mg/dL; $R^2=0.96$).

3.3. Protein

In the determination of protein concentrations, an alkaline cupric tartrate reagent complexes with the peptide bonds and forms purple dye when the phenol reagent is added. This dye shows maximum absorbency at 750 nm and is directly proportional to the protein concentration of the sample. Absorbencies of plasma and lipoprotein samples will be determined and compared to an external calibration curve for protein (linear range of 5–300 mg/dL; $R^2=0.97$; samples with a greater protein concentration than 300 mg/dL should be diluted prior to assay).

3.4. Phospholipids

Phospholipid concentration measurements (specifically phosphatidylcholine) were performed based on the following test principle. Phospholipids are catalyzed by the enzyme phospholipase D to produce choline and phosphatidic acids. The choline is subsequently oxidized in the presence of choline oxidase to yield betaine and hydrogen peroxide (H_2O_2). The last step of this series of reactions involves a similar reaction previously described for total and free cholesterol determination. H_2O_2 combines with 4-aminophenazone and phenol in the presence of peroxidase to produce 4-(p-benzo-quinone-monoimino)-phenazone (the chromagen) and water *(10)*. The chromagen is a highly colored dye, which has an absorbance maximum at 500 nm. The series of reactions are as follows:

Phospholipid reagent is prepared by dissolving the contents of one enzyme reagent bottle in 40 mL of provided buffer solution. This working reagent solution contains phenol 20 mmol/L, 4-aminophenazone 8 mmol/L, phospholipase D ≥ 1000 U/L, choline oxidase ≥ 1400 U/L, and peroxidase ≥ 800 U/L and is stable for up to 2 wk when stored at 2–8°C. To an appropriately labeled test tube, 10-μL aliquots are added from each separated fraction — VLDL, LDL, HDL, and LPDP. A standard test tube containing 10-μL of a 54.1 mg/dL choline chloride solution (equivalent to 300 mg phospholipids/dL) is also prepared. The reagent blank test tube contains a similar volume of distilled water. To the sample, standard, and reagent blank test tubes, a 1.5-mL aliquot of the previously prepared phospholipid reagent solution is added. The contents of each tube are mixed and incubated at 37°C for 10 min, whereupon the absorbance of the samples (ΔA) and standard (ΔA_{std}) are read against the reagent blank within 2 h. Concentration of phospholipid in each sample is calculated based on the following equation:

$$C = 300 \times \frac{\Delta A}{\Delta A_{std}} \ [mg/dL]$$

4. Notes

1. All glassware and the blade for the tube slicer should be baked overnight at 120°C to eliminate endotoxin contamination. All reagents and dialysates should be prepared with Milli Q water. Use only new plasticware.
2. The density of all stock primary and secondary salt solutions should be verified by weighing 100 mL in a Class A 100-mL volumetric flask.
3. Sometimes you cannot see the colored band for HDL. You can distinguish HDL from the other lipoproteins by its density interface.

Acknowledgments

This work is supported by funds provided by the Medical Research Council of Canada. A. L. Kennedy is supported by a student stipend from the Medical Research Council of Canada. K. D. Peteherych is supported by a University Graduate Fellowship.

References

1. Davis, R. A. and Vance, J. E. (1996) Structure, assembly and secretion of lipoproteins, in *Biochemistry of Lipids, Lipoproteins and Membranes* (Vance, D. E. and Vance, J. E., eds.), Elsevier, New York, pp. 473–483.
2. Harmony, J. A. K., Aleson, A. L., and McCarthy, B. M. (1986) Lipoprotein structure and function, in *Biochemistry and Biology of Plasma Lipoproteins* (Scanu, A. M. and Spector, A. A., eds.), Marcel Dekker Inc., New York, pp. 403–430.
3. Mbewu, A. and Durrington, P. N. (1990) Lipoprotein (a): Structure, properties and possible involvement in thrombogenesis and atherogenesis. *Atherosclerosis* **85,** 1–14.
4. Durrington, P. N. (1989) Lipoprotein function, in *Lipoproteins and Lipids* (Durrington, P. N.,ed.), Wright, London, pp. 255–277.
5. Davis, R. A. (1991) Lipoprotein structure and secretion, in *Biochemistry of Lipids, Lipoproteins, and Membranes* (Vance, D. E. and Vance, J. E., eds.),Elsevier, New York, pp. 403–426.
6. Havel, R. J. and Kane, J. P. (1995) Introduction: Structure and metabolism of plasma lipoproteins, in *The Metabolic and Molecular Basis of Inherited Disease*, vol. 2, (Scriver, C. R., Beaudet, A. L., Sly, W. S., and Valle, D., eds.), McGraw-Hill Inc., New York, pp. 1129–1138.
7. Mackness, M. I. and Durrington, P. N. (1992) Lipoprotein separation and analysis for clinical studies, in *Lipoprotein Analysis: A Practical Approach* (Converse, C. A. and Skinner, E. R., eds.), Oxford University Press, New York, pp. 11–43.
8. Wasan, K. M., Cassidy, S. M., Ramaswamy, M., Kennedy, A., Strobel, F. A., Ng, S. P., and Lee, T. Y. (1999) A comparison of step-gradient and sequential density ultracentrifugation and the use of lipoprotein deficient plasma controls in determining the plasma lipoprotein distribution of lipid-associated nystatin and cyclosporine. *Pharmacol. Res.* **16,** 165–169.

9. Schumaker, V. N. and Puppione, D. L. (1986) Lipoprotein Analysis, in *Methods of Enzymology* (Segrest, J. P. and Albers, J. J., eds.), Academic Press, London, pp. 155–174.

10. Takayama, M., Itoh, S., and Tanimizu, I. (1977) A new enzymatic method for determination of serum choline-containing phospholipids. *Clinica Chim. Acta.* **79,** 93–98.

5

Separation of Plasma Lipoproteins in Self-Generated Gradients of Iodixanol

Joan A. Higgins, John M. Graham, and Ian G. Davies

1. Introduction

The major classes of plasma lipoprotein, very low density lipoproteins (VLDL), low-density lipoproteins (LDL), and high-density lipoproteins (HDL), are characterized on the basis of differences in density and charge (**Table 1**). Centrifugation is the 'gold-standard' for the analysis of plasma lipoprotein classes and beta quantitation, and other analytical procedures *(1–4)*. Lipoprotein classes are separated by flotation of plasma or serum in a series of centrifugation steps in which the density of the plasma is increased sequentially by addition of potassium bromide. Alternatively, plasma is layered beneath a discontinuous gradient and centrifuged to separate the lipoprotein classes in a single step. However, it is impractical to use these methods in a routine analytical or clinical laboratory because of the long centrifugation steps required. It is also necessary to remove the high salt concentrations used before further analysis (e.g., agarose gel electrophoresis or determination of the cholesterol and/or triglyceride levels) can be carried out. The current method used for the assay of LDL and HDL levels in the chemical pathology laboratory involves determination of total plasma cholesterol followed by selective precipitation of HDL and determination of the cholesterol remaining in the supernatant *(1)*. From the data obtained, the LDL and HDL cholesterol levels are indirectly calculated. It is generally accepted that this method is limited and that the results are compromised by modest elevation in levels of plasma triglyceride, such as frequently occurs in clinical samples *(5)*.

From: *Methods in Molecular Medicine, vol. 52: Atherosclerosis: Experimental Methods and Protocols*
Edited by: A. F. Drew © Humana Press Inc., Totowa, NJ

Table 1
Plasma Lipoproteins

Lipoprotein	Protein (%)	PL (%)	Chol (%)	TAG (%)	Mobility	Density	Mean values in serum (mg/dL)
Chylomicrons	2	4	5	89	start	<1.000	<10
VLDL	10	16	17	57	pre-β	<1.006	50–200
LDL	29	24	47	6	β	1.019–1.063	200–300
HDL	49	29	19	5	α	1.063–1.210	200–300

The mean % composition of the major classes of lipoproteins is given: PL, phospholipid; chol, cholesterol and cholesterol ester; TAG, triglyceride. The mobility from the origin is pre-β; β; α see **Fig. 1** for example. The density is the band at which the lipoproteins float from salt gradients.

This chapter describes the use of self-generating continuous gradients of iodixanol for the separation of plasma lipoproteins (6). This method has unique advantages over the current reference method. The centrifugation step is only 2–3 h, the gradients formed are extremely reproducible and stable and, because iodixanol is nontoxic and inert, analysis can be carried out on fractions collected from the gradients without further treatment. The method was developed using a small-volume ultracentrifuge and a near-vertical rotor using approximately 3 mL tubes. It can be readily adapted to larger-volume tubes of similar sedimentation path length <20 mm (6–12 mL tubes) in vertical and near-vertical rotors capable of generating $350,000g_{av}$. However, it must be emphasized that not all rotors are suitable for self-generated gradient formation: for example, tubes in excess of 12-mL volume and >20 mm path length and the use of fixed angle rotors (particularly those that cannot achieve at least $350,000g_{av}$) either may require considerably longer centrifugation times to generate gradients or be completely unsatisfactory. Swing-out rotors are not suitable for self-generated gradients because of their long path length.

2. Materials

2.1. Preparation of Plasma (see Note 1)

1. Conical plastic 15-mL centrifuge tubes.
2. Bench-top centrifuge capable of generating 13,000g with appropriate rotor and tubes.
3. HEPES-buffered saline: 0.8% (w/v) NaCl buffered with 10 mM HEPES NaOH pH 7.4.
4. Automatic pipet (1 or 2 mL) with wide-bore tip prepared by cutting the end from a plastic tip.
5. Metal filling cannulae with Luer fitting (see **Note 2**).
6. 5-mL plastic syringes.
7. Plastic Pasteur pipets.

2.2. Generation of Gradient (see Note 3)

1. Floor-standing ultracentrifuge (at least 65,000 rpm) or microultracentrifuge (e.g., Beckman TLX or Optima Max; Sorvall RC-M120GX or RC-M150GX).
2. Vertical or near-vertical rotor with tube sizes of 2–12 mL volume and <20 mm path length, capable of achieving at least 350,000*g* (e.g., Beckman TLN100, TLV100, or Sorvall RP120VT for microultracentrifuges, or Beckman VTi65.1, NVT65.2, or Sorvall Stepsaver 70V6 for floor-standing machines).
3. Centrifuge tubes for the rotor of choice (*see* **Note 4**).
4. HEPES buffered saline (*see* **Subheading 2.1., item 3**).
5. 5-mL syringe.
6. Metal filling cannulae as in **Subheading 2.1., item 5** (*see* **Note 2**).
7. Liposep iodixanol solution for lipoprotein separation (*see* **Note 5**).

2.3. Gradient Collection

1. Fraction collector capable of collection in 96-well plates or 1.5-mL Eppendorf microtubes.
2. 96-well microtiter plates, with sealable lids if it is intended to store the gradients before analysis, or lidded Eppendorf tubes (*see* **Subheading 2.3., item 1**).
3. Gradient unloader, e.g., Lipotek unloader or Beckman unloader (*see* **Note 6**).
4. Maxidens (*see* **Notes 5** and **7**).
5. Peristalic or isocratic (HPLC) pump (*see* **Note 8**).

2.4. Analysis of Gradient Fractions (see Note 9)

2.4.1. Micromethod for Lipid Analysis (see Note 10)

1. 96-well microtiter plates.
2. Cholesterol assay kit and cholesterol standard (*see* **Note 11**).
3. Triglyceride assay kit and triglyceride standard (*see* **Note 12**).
4. Positive displacement pipets (1–10 µL).
5. 8 or 12 place multipipeter (50–200 µL).
6. Plate reader at about 600 nm (for cholesterol assay) and 500 nm (for triglyceride assay).

2.4.2. Agarose Gel Electrophoresis

1. Agarose gels kits (*see* **Note 12**).
2. Positive displacement micropipets (2–10 µL).
3. Flat-bed electrophoresis and power pack.
4. Hair dryer or drying oven.
5. Destaining solution (45% ethanol in distilled or deionized water).
6. Shallow staining trays approximately 12 × 10 cm.

3. Methods

3.1. Preparation of Plasma (see Note 13).

1. Centrifuge the blood at 2000g for 10 min to pellet the leukocytes and erythrocytes.
2. Remove the plasma from the pellet using a plastic Pasteur pipet and transfer it into a plastic vial, setting aside at least 50 µL for further analysis.
3. Transfer the plasma to a conical centrifuge tube. Carefully layer 0.3 mL of HEPES buffered saline on top.
4. Centrifuge the tubes at 13000g for 20 min (*see* **Note 13**) to float chylomicrons.
5. Carefully remove the chylomicron-containing layer using an automatic pipet with a wide bore tip.
6. Carefully introduce the tip of a metal filling cannula (attached to a 5-mL or 10-mL syringe) to the bottom of the tube (avoiding disturbing any pellet) and remove most (but *not all*) of the plasma from the bottom of the tube. After withdrawing the cannulae from the tube, wipe the outside with a tissue to remove any chylomicrons that might have adhered to its surface (*see* **Note 14**).

3.2. Generation of Gradients (see Note 15)

3.2.1. General Method for Most Centrifuge Rotor Combinations (but see Subheading 2.2.2., Note 3, and Introduction)

1. To 1.0 mL of chylomicron-free plasma add 0.25 mL of Liposep. Keep approximately 200 µL for further analysis.
2. Transfer the plasma/Liposep mixture into an appropriate tube to fill 80% of the usable volume of 2.0-mL tubes and 90% of the volume of all larger tubes. It is permissible to use less than the maximum volume of plasma/Liposep mixture, in which case the volume of HEPES-buffered saline required to fill the tube (see **step 4**) should be increased.
3. In tubes for vertical rotors, underlay the plasma/Liposep mixture with 0.2 mL (tube sizes of less than 3 mL), 0.3 mL (5–6 mL tubes) or 0.5mL (10–12-mL tubes) of 30% iodixanol (50% Liposep, *see* **Note 16**) using a 1-mL syringe and metal filling cannula.
4. Using a 1- or 2-mL syringe and metal filling cannula, layer HEPES-buffered saline on top of the plasma /Liposep mixture to fill all tubes.
5. Seal the tubes according to the instruction manual.
6. Centrifuge the tubes at approximately 350,000g_{av} for 2.5 h at speed (*see* **Note 17**).
7. Allow the centrifuge to slow over a period of about 4 min from 2000 rpm by using the controlled braking program or by turning off the brake. This allows smooth gradient reorientation.

3.2.2. Specific Examples Using Certain Rotor Centrifuge Combinations

3.2.2.1. SEPARATION OF SMALL VOLUMES OF PLASMA(2.5 mL) USING THE TLN100 ROTOR IN THE BECKMAN TLX100 (OR OPTIMA 120 OR OPTIMA MAX ULTRACENTIFUGE)

1. To 2.4 mL chylomicron-free plasma add 0.6 mL Liposep. Keep remaining plasma for further analysis.
2. Transfer 2.6 mL of the plasma-Liposep mixture into an Optiseal tube (2.9 mL) and using a metal cannulae attached to a 2mL syringe layer HEPES-buffered saline on top to fill the tube.
3. Seal the tubes with the plastic stoppers.
4. Centrifuge the tubes at 100,000 rpm (353000*g*) for 2.5 h at speed in the TLN100 rotor at 16°· with slow braking (*see* **Subheading 3.2.1., step 7**).

3.2.2.2. SEPARATION OF LARGER VOLUMES OF PLASMA (~8 mL) IN THE VTI65 ROTOR IN THE BECKMAN L80 OR L7 ULTRACENTRIFUGE

1. To 8 mL chylomicron-free serum add 2.0 mL Liposep. Keep remaining plasma for further analysis.
2. Transfer the mixture to an Optiseal tube (11.2 mL) and underlay with 0.5 mL 1 part Hepes buffer plus 1 one part Liposep using a metal cannula and a 1- or 2-mL syringe.
3. Fill the tube with HEPES-buffered saline using a metal cannula and a 1- or 2-mL syringe.
4. Centrifuge the tubes at 33,000*g* for 3 h at 16° with slow braking (*see* **Subheading 3.2.1., step 7**).

3.3. Gradient Unloading

From the top of the gradient by upward displacement:

1. Carefully remove the stopper from Optiseal tubes (Beckman) or Re-Seal or Easy-Seal tubes (Sorvall) and place the tube in the gradient unloader (*see* **Notes 6 and 20**).
2. Set up the fraction collector with the appropriate time or number of drops and collection vessel (*see* **Notes 18 and 19**).
3. If the Beckman unloader is used, connect the outlet at the top to the fraction collector and the needle assembly at the bottom of the unloader to a pump (*see* **Notes 8 and 19**) (*see* **Fig. 1A**).
4. If the Lipotek unloader is used, connect the inlet to the pump (*see* **Notes 8 and 20**) and the outlet to the fraction collector. The inlet tube should be at the bottom of the gradient in the centrifuge tube and the collar through which the gradient is

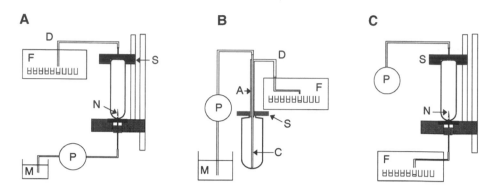

Fig. 1. Gradient unloading formats. The arrangement of the centrifuge tube, pump, fraction collector, and gradient unloader for (**A**) Beckman gradient unloader in upward displacement mode; (**B**) Lipotek gradient unloader in upward displacement mode; (**C**) Beckman gradient unloader in downward displacement mode. A, annulus, through which the gradient is dispaced upward; C, central tube, which is inserted to the bottom of the gradient and delivers Maxidens; D, delivery tube; F, fraction collector; M, Maxidens; N, hollow needle; P, pump; S, seal between the unloader and the centrifuge tube.

    displaced should be at the top of the gradient. This should be set up with an empty tube before collecting a gradient. (**Fig. 1B**).

5. Pump Maxidens (*see* **Note 7**) to fill the pump tubing and the unloader tubing completely to avoid air bubbles disturbing the gradient when the fractions are collected (*see* **Note 20**).
6. Carefully place the tube in the chosen fraction collector. If the Lipotek gradient unloader is used, take care that the disturbance to the gradient is minimal when inserting the inlet metal tube. If the Beckman unloader is used, pierce the bottom of the tube with the needle assembly. While the tube is being pierced keep a slow flow of Maxidens through the needle to avoid air bubbles that would disturb the gradient.
7. Increase the pumping rate. When the tube joining the unloader to the fraction collector is filled with the displaced gradient, begin the collection of fractions.

From the bottom of the gradient by downward displacment using the Beckman gradient unloader:

1. Carefully remove the stopper from the Optiseal tube and place the tube in the gradient unloader (*see* **Note 5**).
2. Set up the fraction collector with the appropriate time or number of drops and collection vessel (*see* **Notes 18,19,21**).
3. If the Beckman unloader is used, connect the inlet at the top to the pump and the needle assembly at the bottom of the unloader to the fraction collector (*see* **Note 8**; **Fig. 1C**).
4. Start the pump. When the tube joining the unloader to the fraction collector is filled with the displaced gradient, begin the collection of fractions.

3.4. Analysis of Gradient Fractions (see Note 9)

3.4.1. Lipid Analysis (see Notes 10 and 11)

1. Transfer 5- and 10-µL aliquots to 96-well microtiter plates, leaving empty wells for standards and blanks.
2. Transfer aliquots of the triglyceride or cholesterol standard to the appropriate wells.
3. Add 200 µL cholesterol or triglyceride assay reagent or follow the manufacturer's instructions.
4. Shake the plates (most plate readers have a plate-shaking facility; alternatively use a flatbed shaker).
5. Allow the color to develop and read the absorbance at 450 nM at 15 and 30 min to ensure the reaction is complete.
6. From the standards, calculate the concentration of cholesterol or triglyceride in the unknown samples and in the plasma samples retained in earlier **steps 3.1.2; 3.2.1.1, 3.2.2.1, 3.2.2.2** (*see* **Note 22**).

3.4.2. Agarose Gel Electrophoresis

1. Make up the electrophoresis buffer and the Sudan stain according to the instructions in the kit.
2. Pour the appropriate volume of buffer into the electrophoresis chamber.
3. Carefully remove the plastic-backed gel from its container.
4. Blot the excess liquid from the gel, using the filter paper strips provided by lining these up with the arrows marked on the edges of the gel.
5. Place the template on the gel, aligning the two outside holes with the arrows marked on the edges of the gel. Two templates are provided, one of which has 8 lanes and the other 10 lanes. For analysis of gradients it is more economical to use the 10-lane template.
6. Apply 2 µL of samples (either plasma or gradient fraction) into the slots in the template.
7. Allow the samples to diffuse into the gel. This takes about 10 min.
8. Remove the template.
9. Place the gel in the electrophoresis tank with the samples on the cathode side, so that the edges of the gel dip about 1 cm into the buffer in each chamber.
10. Plug the chamber into the power supply and run for 90 min at 50 V.
11. Unplug the chamber and remove the gel.
12. Dry the gel, using a hair dryer, for about 20 min. The gel should shrink to a flat layer on the plastic backing. This can be checked by looking at a tilted gel. Undried portions of the gel are raised.
13. Stain the completely dried gel by immersing it for exactly 15 min in the staining solution in the tray.
14. Remove the gel, shake off the excess stain, and destain the gel by immersing it in the destain solution for exactly 5 min.

15. Wash the gel with distilled or deionized water.
16. Blot off the excess water with tissues, and dry the gel with a hair dryer.
17. If necessary, excess stain can be removed from the back of the gel with a tissue soaked in 70% alcohol.
18. Gels can be stored or photographed or the density of the lipoprotein bands measured using a densitometer. The lipoproteins separate in the order from the cathode LDL, VLDL, Lp(a), and HDL (*see* **Note 23**). Chylomicrons remain at the origin. A band of plasma albumin is occasionally visible beyond HDL (**Fig. 2** and **3**).

4. Notes

1. Blood should be taken only by trained personnel using intravenous puncture. Anticoagulants are usually added to the vaccutainer or the syringe used to take blood samples. However, the same results are obtained using either plasma (plus coagulants) or serum (after coagulation).
2. Metal filling cannulae with Luer fittings can be suppled by most surgical instrument suppliers.
3. For rapid formation of self-generating gradients it is necessary to use a vertical or near-vertical rotor. During centrifugation, a gradient forms across the centrifuge tube. Because this is a short-sedimentation path-length the time taken is short compared with gradient formation in most angle rotors. Swing-out rotors are unsuitable unless they are adapted to reduce path length. When the centrifugal force is removed the gradient reorients in the centrifuge tube. A variety of vertical or near-vertical rotors is available, and the method can be adapted for any of these, provided the gradient formed is a similar shape. Several examples are provided in this chapter; however, alternative rotors can be used provided a similar density gradient is established.
4. Vertical and near-vertical rotors use sealed tubes, since the gradient reorients in the tube during acceleration. These tubes are also preferable for reasons of biological safety. The older types of tubes are either heat sealed (Beckman Quick-Seal) or crimp sealed in a metal cap (Sorvall Ultracrimp). More recently, tubes sealed either under pressure by a plastic stopper (Beckman Optiseal) or a plastic crown and central plug (Sorvall Easy-Seal) have become available. Ultracrimp and Optiseal tubes are the easiest to assemble. Both the Quick-Seal and Ultracrimp are best suited for gradient collection from the bottom-dense end first. Otherwise, for upward displacement the tops of these tubes have to be cleanly cut to leave a flat surface to provide a seal against the washer of the gradient unloader. All other tubes, because their sealing device can be removed easily, may be collected by either method, although the sharp flat shoulders of Optiseal tubes compromise collection by upward displacement. However, the conical tops of Sorvall Easy-Seal tubes makes them ideal for collection by this method.
5. Liposep and Maxidens and Lipotek gradient unloader can be purchased from Lipotek Ltd. 34, Meadway, Upton, Wirral, Merseyside CH 49 6TQ, UK, or contact the author JAH.

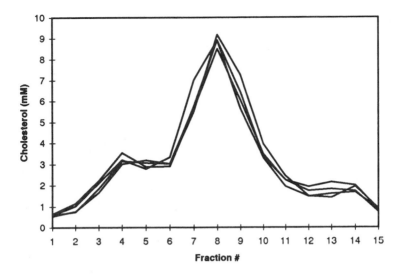

Fig. 2. Reproducibility of separation. Four aliquots of the same plasma were separated in four separate gradients; 15 fractions were collected from each gradient, and the concentration of cholesterol was determined. Each line indicates the cholesterol concentration for a single gradient.

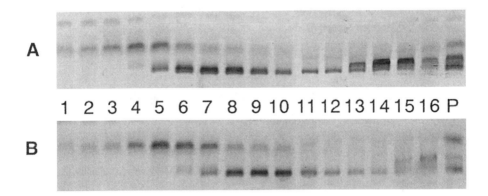

Fig. 3. Examples of separation of plasma lipoproteins from clinical specimens. Plasma was separated as in **Fig. 5**, except that 16 fractions were collected. The lipoproteins in each fraction were analysed by electrophoresis. P is the total plasma, and fraction 16 is the bottom of the gradient. The lipoproteins separate as HDL, VLDL, and LDL from the top of the gel. Compared with the sample in **Fig. 5**, which is from a normal volunteer, in (**A**) there is increased VLDL and LDL, both of above-average density. In (**B**) the LDL has lower density. This illustrates the sensitivity of the separation.

6. The Lipotek gradient unloader does not involve tube-piercing and can be used only to collect gradients from the top by upward displacement. The Beckman gradient unloader incorporates a tube piercer and can be used to collect from the bottom of the gradient (by downward displacement). The Lipotek gradient unloader is considerably cheaper. The choice of equipment will depend on the needs of the investigator and his or her budget.

7. Maxidens is a low-viscosity, high-density, inert liquid.

8. The choice of pump depends on the budget and requirements of the investigator. To collect equal-sized samples it is best to use the fraction collector set at time. However, this requires a constant flow rate, which is achieved only by using a nonpulsing isocratic pump (or HPLC pump). Alternatively, samples also can be collected by drop-number, and either pump is appropriate. There is some small difference in the size of the drops from different regions of the gradients because of the difference in iodixanol concentration. Therefore, to calculate recoveries of lipoproteins from the gradient in this case, it may be necessary to measure the volume of each sample. This is time consuming. The isocratic pump is considerably more expensive than the peristalic pump.

9. It is usual to quantify lipoprotein fractions by measuring the cholesterol and/or triglycerol content. Lipoproteins can be identified by separation by agarose gel electrophoresis. Methods for these procedures are described. However, as iodixanol is inert, fractions from the gradients can also be used directly for a variety of protocols, including enzyme assays and quantification or identification of apolipoproteins by ELISA or SDS-polyacrylamide gel electrophoresis, respectively.

10. Plasma cholesterol and triglyceride are analyzed using enzyme-based reagent kits available with full instructions from a variety of suppliers. To minimize use of these relatively expensive reagents we use a micromethod in which the color is developed in microtiter wells and read with a plate reader. If the investigator has access to automated equipment, e.g., the Cobra Miras autoanalyzer, this can be used. The gradients should be collected in the appropriate tubes for the analyzer used. Cholesterol is assayed using enzyme-based kits obtainable from a number of suppliers (Boerhinger-Mannheim, Sigma).

11. Triglyceride is assayed using enzyme kits obtainable from a number of suppliers (Boehringer Mannheim, Sigma, Wako Chemicals).

12. Although it is possible to prepare agarose gels on microscope slides, far better results are obtained using preprepared agarose gels from Sebia. These are supplied in a kit with the electrophoresis buffer, application templates, and Sudan black for staining the gels

13. The purpose of the centrifugation step prior to running the gradient is to remove chylomicrons. If the samples are particularly rich in chylomicrons the plasma may be centrifuged at a higher g force in a suitable rotor and centrifuge (e.g., 50,000 rpm in the TLA100.4 rotor of the TLX100 ultracentrifuge). This step may be omitted if fasted samples are used.

14. No matter how carefully the plasma is aspirated into the syringe the residual chylomicrons at the meniscus tend to fall slowly into the infranatant as the meniscus descends. Leaving about 0.3 mL plasma in the tube guards against contamination of the infranatant by chylomicrons.

15. In inital experiments, tubes containing iodixanol diluted with HEPES-buffered saline in place of plasma should be centrifuged and the gradients collected. By determination of the refractive index of the gradient fractions, the density of iodixanol throughout the gradient can be determined from density =3.459 ρ-3.266 (where ρ is the refractive index). This can be used to determine the density of the lipoprotein fractions and also as an internal control. If alternative rotors are used, the gradient shape should be the same. Examples of gradients generated are shown in **Fig. 4**.

16. Because the density of plasma proteins in iodixanol is approximately 1.26 g/mL, these macromolecules will band at the bottom of a gradient. If they sediment to the wall of the tube, they will tend to contaminate the entire gradient when it is harvested. To avoid this in a vertical rotor, a small cushion is included. This cushion forms a sharp dense gradient adjacent to the wall of the tube. This is not required in a near-vertical rotor in which any sediment material is located close to the bottom of the tube.

17. In some of the rotors that are capable of generating g forces higher than $350,000g_{av}$, it should be possible to reduce the centrifugation time more or less proportionally.

18. The volume and number of fractions taken from a gradient will depend on the investigation in hand. If the aim is to measure the major lipoprotein bands or to prepare lipoproteins in bulk, relatively large fractions will suffice. However, greater resolution and more information is obtained by taking smaller fractions. Examples of separations are shown in **Figs. 3** and **5**.

19 If a suitable fraction collector is not available, the fractions can be collected manually in equivolume aliquots from a burette filled with Maxidens either by gravity or by connecting the buret to a pump connected to the centrifuge tube. Alternatively, the fractions can simply be collected manually, drop-wise, into Eppendorf tubes from a bottom-pierced tube, by gravity. All of these methods are labor-intensive and not applicable if large numbers of gradients are collected.

20. The conical neck of Sorvall Re-seal tubes ends in a small tube-like projection, which can simply be connected to the collecting tubing of the fraction collector and thus eliminate any requirement for a sealing device, which would indeed be difficult to apply. In this case, the Maxidens must be introduced by a needle into the bottom of the tube.

21. An efficient peristaltic pump can be used to pump air as the downward displacing force. Alternatively, if the internal diameter of the tubing in the pump is no more than 0.6 mm, then the pump can be placed in line from the bottom of the tube.

22. Standards for triglyceride and cholesterol are in mg/dL (or mmoles/L in the UK). The values for the analysis of the lipids are therefore obtained in these units of concentration. If recoveries of lipids in fractions are required, these can be calculated by measuring the volume of the fraction and determining the absolute amount of lipid, using the calculation:

volume of fraction (mL) × concentration (mg/dL) / 100 = mg lipid in aliquot measured

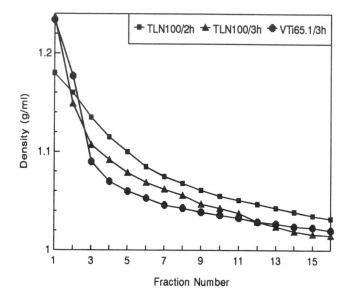

Fig. 4. Examples of gradients generated from 12% iodixanol in different rotors centrifuged at different times.

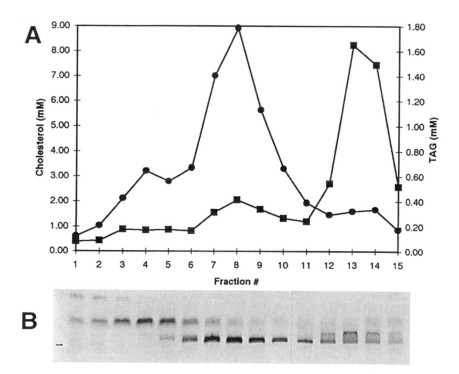

Followed by mg lipid in aliquot (µL) × volume of fraction (µL) / volume of the aliquot to give the amount of lipid in each fraction. Using these calculations the recovery of lipid in each fraction can be calculated. Using agarose gels to identify the lipoproteins in the gradients, the recovery of each lipid in each lipoprotein class can be calculated, and from the volume of plasma originally used, the cholesterol or triglyceide content of lipoprotein classes or subclasses can be determined. Once a standard protocol is established these calculations can be carried out automatically. Examples of lipid distribution on gradients is shown in **Fig. 5. Fig. 2** shows the results of cholesterol distribution of the same plasma sample separated on four separate gradients to demonstrate the reproducibility of the separation

23. The banding density of the lipoprotein classes in iodixanol differs slightly from that in salt gradients, because the proteins retain their native hydration in iodixanol, while in salt gradients water is lost, resulting in an increase in the density of the lipoprotein particles. The banding densities in iodixanol gradients are <1.006 g/mL for VLDL, 1.01–1.03 g/mL for LDL; and 1.03–1.14 g/mL for HDL.(*see* **Table 1** for densities in salt gradients)

References

1. Macness, M. and Durrington, P. N. (1992) Lipoprotein separation and analysis for clinical studies, in Lipoprotein Analysis: A Practical Approach. (Converse, C. A. and Skinner, E. R. eds.), IRL Press at Oxford University.
2. Lindren, F. T., Jensen, L. C., Hatch, and F. T. (1979) Isolation and quantitation of serum lipoproteins, in Blood Lipids and Lipoproteins; Quantitation, Composition and Metabolism. (Nelson, G. J., ed.), R.E. Kreiger Publishing, Huntington, NY.
3. Chapman, M., Goldstein, J., LaGrange, D. and Laplaud, P. M. (1981) A density gradient ultracentrifugation procedure for the isolatation of the major lipoprotein classes from human plasma. *J. Lipid Res.* **22,** 339.
4. Kelley, J. L. and Kruski, A. W. (1986) Density gradient ultracentrifugation of serum lipoproteins in a swinging bucket rotor. *Methods Enzymol.* **128,** 170.
5. McNamara, J. R., Cohn, J. S., Wilson, P. W. F., and Schaeffer, E. J. (1990) Calculated values for low densitylipoprotein cholesterol in the assessment of lipid abnormalities. *Clin. Chem.* **36,** 36–42.
6. Graham, J. M., Higgins, J. A., Gillott, T., Taylor, T., Wilkinson, J., Ford, T., and Billington, D. (1995) A novel method for the rapid separation of plasma lipoproteins using self-generating gradients of iodixanol. *Atherosclerosis* **1345,** 125–135.

Fig. 5. Separation of plasma lipoproteins in the TLN100 rotor. Plasma was mixed with iodixanol (final volume 12%) and centrifuged as described in Subheading 3.2.2.1., step 1; 15 fractions were collected, with fraction 15 the bottom of the gradient. In (**A**) the cholesterol (●) and triacylglycerol (■) were determined and plotted as m*M* concentration in each fraction. In (**B**) the lipoproteins in each fraction were analyzed by electrophoresis. The lipoproteins separate as HDL, VLDL, and LDL from the top of the gel. Thus, fractions 1–5 contain HDL, fractions 6–12 contain LDL, and fractions 13–15 contain all of the VLDL and a trace of LDL.

6

Fractionation of Lipoprotein Subclasses in Self-Generated Gradients of Iodixanol

John M. Graham, Bruce A. Griffin, Ian G. Davies, and Joan A. Higgins

1. Introduction

Chapter 5 described the use of self-generated gradients of iodixanol for the fractionation of human plasma lipoproteins into the major classes: high-density, low-density, and very low density (HDL, LDL, and VLDL). During the metabolism of plasma HDL and LDL, the lipid and apoprotein composition of the lipoprotein particles changes in such a manner that a series of subclasses exists, each with a distinctive range of densities (1). Thus, in KBr gradients, the two major subclasses, HDL_2 and HDL_3, have densities of 1.063–1.125 g/mL and 1.125–1.21 g/mL, respectively (1). In some individuals a third subclass (HDL_1) is recognized (1.055–1.063 g/mL). Electrophoretic (2) and immunological (3,4) techniques have identified additional subfractions. Likewise, subclasses of LDL have been identified and isolated using shallow KBr gradients (5,6). The major LDL subfractions are LDL_1, LDL_2, and LDL_3, which have densities of 1.025–1.034 g/mL, 1.034–1.044 g/mL, and 1.044–1.060 g/mL, respectively (6), and electrophoretic analysis has identified more subfractions (7). The subfractions of LDL are of particular interest, as the presence of small, dense LDL particles in the plasma appears to be associated with a predisposition to cardiovascular disease, and they are recognized as a major causative factor in atherosclerosis (8). Methods for monitoring the LDL subclass pattern in population studies and in dietary and drug intervention trials are thus of considerable interest. This chapter is concerned primarily with the subfractionation of LDL. Although HDL subfractionation systems using iodixanol self-generated gradients have not yet been validated by direct comparison with other methods (e.g., gradient gel electrophoresis or KBr gradient centrifugation), a protocol is included.

From: *Methods in Molecular Medicine, vol. 52: Atherosclerosis: Experimental Methods and Protocols*
Edited by: A. F. Drew © Humana Press Inc., Totowa, NJ

The shallow KBr gradients required to resolve LDL subclasses *(6)* are not suited to a routine laboratory technique. Self-generated iodixanol gradients, on the other hand, are extremely easy to customize to specific separation requirements as their density profile can be easily modulated, either by changing the centrifugation parameters and/or changing the starting concentration of iodixanol. Some profiles are best created, not by using a single starting density but by using two layers of iodixanol of different concentrations. **Fig. 1** shows some of the variations in density gradient profile that can be obtained using either two uniform densities of 12.5% or 15% (w/v) iodixanol or equal volumes of 6% and 12.5% or 12.5% and 20% iodixanol.

Efficient gradient formation and rapid banding of the lipoprotein particles require the short sedimentation path lengths that are achievable only with vertical and near-vertical rotors. However, the creation of high-resolution systems depends not only on the choice of the proper gradient formation conditions, but also on the modes of collection and fractionation of the gradient. During deceleration of the rotor to rest, the gradient reorients in the tube; hence, if the long axis of the tube is greater than its diameter, the gradient becomes more shallow after reorientation. Consequently, the lipoprotein bands become more spread out, and coupling this with the collection of the gradient in small volume fractions enhances the resolution achieved *(9)*. Thus, tall tubes for rotors such as the Beckman VTi65.1 or the Sorvall Stepsaver 65TV13 are ideal; they have sedimentation path lengths of less than 18 mm and volumes of 5–13 mL. Nevertheless, it is also possible to obtain LDL subfractionation in the smaller-volume tubes of vertical and near-vertical rotors for microultracentrifuges if sufficiently small volume fractions are collected and analyzed. The larger-volume tubes can be used to provide LDL subclasses on a preparative basis for further analysis, the smaller tubes can be used diagnostically to check the predominant density of the LDL particles in individual plasma samples.

Two-layer iodixanol systems (12% + 6% or 12% + 9%) are particularly suited to LDL subfractionation, while at the same time giving improved separation of the LDL from HDL and VLDL if whole plasma is fractionated. Although in some rotors such as the Beckman NVT65.2 (5-mL tubes), single-phase systems using a starting concentration of 9% (w/v) iodixanol are also satisfactory for subfractionation of LDL; the lightest LDL does band very closely to the VLDL. If this is not a problem, then a single-phase system has the merit of simplicity. A two-phase system overcomes this problem and results in an even greater spread of the LDL. In small-volume rotors such as the Beckman TLN100, a two-layer system is a more strict requirement.

2. Materials

See **Subheadings 2.1.** and **3.1.** of Chapter 5 for materials and method of preparing chylomicron-free plasma. *See* **Subheadings 2.3., 2.4., 3.3.,** and **3.4.** of Chapter 5 for details of gradient collection and analysis.

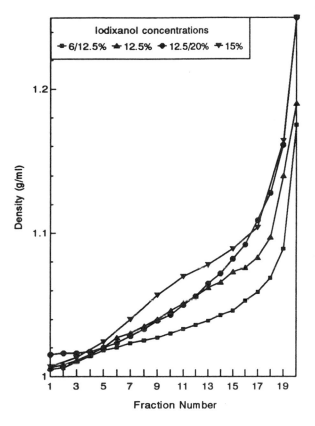

Fig. 1. Effect of iodixanol concentration and the use of two layers of iodixanol on the density profile of self-generated gradients in the Beckman VTi65.1 vertical rotor. Optiseal tubes were either filled with a uniform concentration of iodixanol (12.5 or 15%) or equal volumes of 6 and 12.5% or 12.5 and 20% (w/v) iodixanol and centrifuged for 3 h at 350,000g. All gradients were unloaded low-density-end first by upward displacement with Maxidens (*see* **Note 2**).

1. HEPES-buffered saline (HBS): 0.85% NaCl, 10 mM HEPES-NaOH, pH 7.4.
2. Metal filling cannulae with Luer fitting (approx 0.8 mm id).
3. Plastic syringes (2 and 5 mL).
4. Chylomicron-free plasma (*see* **Subheadings 2.1.** and **3.1.** of Chapter 5) (*see* **Note 1**).
5. Liposep (*see* **Note 2**).
6. Floor-standing ultracentrifuge (capable of at least 65,000 rpm) or microultracentrifuge.
7. Vertical or near-vertical rotor, with tube sizes of 3–12 mL, capable of achieving at least 350,000g. The separations described use a Beckman TLN100 (3.3-mL tubes), NVT 65.2 (5-mL tubes), or VTi65 (11.2-mL tubes). For the use of other rotors *see* **Note 3**.
8. Beckman Optiseal tubes or similar (*see* **Note 4**).

3. Methods

3.1. LDL Subfractionation Using a One-Layer System in the Beckman NVT65.2.

1. Add 1.5 vol of Liposep to 8.5 vol of chylomicron-free plasma.
2. Transfer 4.5 mL plasma/Liposep mixture to a 4.9-mL Optiseal tube and overlayer (to fill the tube) with HBS.
3. Centrifuge at $350,000g_{av}$ for 3 h.
4. Allow approx 4 min for rotor to decelerate from 2000 rpm to 0 rpm (use a controlled braking program or turn off the brake).

3.2. LDL Subfractionation Using Two-Layer Systems in the Beckman NVT65.2 or TLN100.

1. Prepare Solution A by diluting 1.5 vol of Liposep + 8.5 vol of HBS.
2. Add 1 vol of Liposep to 4 vol of chylomicron-free plasma.
3. Transfer 2.2 mL (NVT65.2) or 1.4 mL (TLN100) of Solution A to appropriate Optiseal tubes and underlayer, using a syringe and filling cannula, with an equal volume of the plasma/Liposep mixture (*see* **Note 5**).
4. Overlayer (to fill the tube) with HBS.
5. Centrifuge at $350,000g_{av}$ for 3 h; if possible use a controlled acceleration program to allow a slow, smooth acceleration to 2000 rpm.
6. Allow approx 4 min for rotor to decelerate from 2000 rpm to 0 rpm (use a controlled braking program or turn off the brake).

3.3. LDL Subfractionation Using Two-Layer System in the Beckman VTi65.1

1. Prepare Solution B by diluting 1 vol of Liposep with 9 vol of HBS.
2. Add 1 vol of Liposep to 4 vol of chylomicron-free plasma.
3. Transfer 5 mL of Solution B to an Optiseal tube (11.2 mL) and underlayer, using a syringe and filling cannula, with an equal volume of the plasma/Liposep mixture (*see* **Notes 5** and **6**).
4. Overlayer (to fill the tube) with HBS.
5. Centrifuge at $350,000g_{av}$ for 3 h. If possible, use a controlled acceleration program to allow a slow, smooth acceleration to 2000 rpm.
6. Allow approx 4 min for rotor to decelerate from 2000 rpm to 0 rpm (use a controlled-braking program or turn off the brake).

3.4. HDL Subfractionation Using a One-Layer System in the Beckman NVT65.2.

1. Add 1 vol of Liposep to 4 vol of chylomicron-free plasma.
2. Transfer 4.5 mL plasma/Liposep mixture to a 4.9-mL Optiseal tube and overlayer (to fill the tube) with HBS (*see* **Note 7**).
3. Centrifuge at 350,000g_{av} for 3 h.
4. Allow approx 4 min for rotor to decelerate from 2000 rpm to 0 rpm (use a controlled-braking program or turn off the brake).

3.5. Gradient Collection

1. Collect the gradients in Optiseal tubes, dense-end first or by upward displacement with Maxidens (*see* **Note 2**) according to one of the methods described in **Subheading 3.3.** of Chapter 5, but see **Note 4** for information about the limitations on gradient collection imposed by tube types.
2. Collect fractions of the following maximum volume aliquots: 0.14 ml (TLN100), 0.2 mL (NVT65.2), or 0.5 mL (VT65.1) (*see* **Note 8**).

3.6. Gradient Analysis

1. Carry out chemical analysis for cholesterol and triacylglycerol and/or agarose gel electrophoresis (*see* **Note 9**) as required (*see* **Subheading 3.4.** of Chapter 5). Some of the separations that can be obtained with the Beckman VTi65.1, TLN100, and NVT65.2 rotors are discussed in **Notes 10, 11,** and **12,** respectively.

4. Notes

1. Although removal of chylomicrons is not strictly necessary if the sole object of the fractionation is to investigate the LDL profile of the plasma, the tendency of the chylomicrons to adhere to the surface of the tube after they have floated up through the gradient means that they can contaminate gradient fractions during collection.
2. Liposep and Maxidens can be purchased from Lipotek Ltd, 34 Meadway, Upton, Wirral, Merseyside, CH49 6JQ, UK.
3. The subfractionation of LDL and the simultaneous resolution of the densest LDL from the lightest HDL (and the lightest LDL from VLDL) is more dependent on the generation of the correct gradient profile than is the separation of the major lipoprotein classes (*see* Chapter 5). Although other rotors may be prove to be successful, it may be necessary to perform a number of preliminary experiments

to adapt the technique to a new rotor type. Whether the smallest-volume rotors are suitable depends very much on the ability to use a fractionation system that will permit the collection of very small volume fractions without disturbing the gradient. Thus, for floor-standing ultracentrifuges the Beckman NVT65, NVT 90, NVT100 and Sorvall Stepsaver 65V13, Stepsaver 70V6, TV865, or TV1665 should all provide very satisfactory resolution. For microultracentrifuges the Beckman TLV100 and Sorvall RP120VT, RP100-VT, and S120-VT (approx 2-mL tubes) should also be satisfactory, but the 1.2-mL tubes of the Beckman TLN120 may be more difficult to unload satisfactorily. Many of the microultracentrifuge fixed-angle rotors may also be suitable for this procedure, but although these have been used successfully for the separation of the major lipoprotein classes, they have not yet been used for LDL subfractionation. and again there may be problems in devising a suitable unloading system.

4. Any suitable tubes can be used. The contents of heat-sealed or crimp-sealed tubes are not easily collected by upward displacement, although other tubes with a flat top can be unloaded in this manner, which is probably the method of choice for LDL subfractions, as there is less contamination by HDL (note, however, that the very flat shoulders of Beckman Optiseal tubes often cause some contamination of light LDL by VLDL). Re-Seal tubes for the Sorvall RP120VT have been successfully unloaded from the top by upward displacement with Maxidens introduced to the bottom of the tube by tube puncture. *See* **Subheading 3.3.** and **Fig. 1** of Chapter 5 for more details on gradient collection. The thick-walled tubes of fixed-angle rotors cannot be unloaded in any mode that involves tube puncturing. Small-volume (<3 mL) tubes are not suited to upward displacement in which a tube is inserted through the gradient to deliver a dense liquid to the bottom of the tube.

5. Although confinement of the plasma sample to the lower layer of a two-layer system is recommended, both layers can actually be formed by diluting plasma with Liposep. The subfractionation of LDL is normally unaffected if both layers are formed from plasma, but resolution from HDL may be slightly impaired. Confinement of the plasma to the lower layer allows the LDL to float into a plasma-protein- and HDL-free gradient.

6. The relative volumes of the two layers in the VTi65.1 system can be altered within certain limits: The volume of the lower layer can be reduced from 5 mL to 2 mL but increases beyond 7.0 mL are not recommended.

7. For HDL, better resolution from the LDL is obtained when the plasma is confined to the layer of the two-phase system (*see* also **Note 5**).

8. There is no reason why smaller-volume fractions cannot be collected; the volumes chosen provide approx 20–24 fractions from any centrifuge tube. The data discussed in the following Notes attest to the adequacy of this regimen.

9. Unlike KBr gradients, it is not possible to visualize the LDL banding profile simply by measuring the A_{280} profile of the gradient, as iodixanol absorbs strongly in the UV, and direct spectrophotometric measurements can be made only above 340 nm.

10. That these shallow iodixanol gradients are able to discriminate different density subclasses of LDL in the same manner as shallow KBr gradients has been tested

in the following experiment. The LDL of the plasma from six individuals was fractionated in shallow KBr gradients, and the peak LDL fractions from these KBr gradients was then diluted with an equal volume of HEPES-buffered saline and then treated as described in **Subheading 3.3.** After centrifugation in a VTi65.1 rotor, the cholesterol distribution in the gradient was measured **(Fig. 2)**. Three of the plasmas showed a peak density of 1.025 g/mL (**A, C,** and **F** in **Fig. 2**); one had a lower density of 1.021 g/mL (**E** in **Fig. 2**), and two displayed a higher dens:.y of 1.035 g/mL (**B** and **D** in **Fig. 2**). The relative densities of the six plasma samples in KBr showed exactly the same pattern.

11. The system described in **Subheading 3.2.** in the TLN100 is an effective means of spreading out the LDL **(Fig. 3)**, and although the separation from HDL and VLDL may not be as great as with the larger volume rotors, it can discriminate different LDL banding patterns in plasma samples from different individuals (data available from the authors).

12. The three gradients systems run in the NVT65.2 rotor **(Fig. 4)** demonstrate how changing the density profile of the gradient can be tailored to specific requirements. The **Subheading 3.1.** method **(Fig. 4A)** gives a good spread of the LDL and would be an excellent diagnostic gradient, although the densest LDL and the lightest IIDL overlap slightly (in particular, in fraction 9). The **Subheading 3.2.** method spreads the LDL even more and at the same time reduces the overlap with the IIDL **(Fig. 4B)**. A 12% system in the NVT65.2 is potentially a good candidate for HDL subclass detection, not only is HDL spread over a large number of fractions, there is evidence from the agarose gel of two distinct HDL regions, a minor one in fractions 4 and 5 and a major one in fractions 7–11 **(Fig. 4C)**. This separation, however, has not yet been validated by comparison with separations in KBr gradients or by gradient gel electrophoresis, nor have specific clinical samples been studied.

References

1. Skinner, E. R. (1992) The separation and analysis of high-density lipoprotein (HDL) and low-density lipoprotein (LDL) subfractions, in *Lipoprotein Analysis — A practical approach.* (Converse, C.A. and Skinner, E.R., eds.), IRL Press at Oxford University Press, Oxford, UK, pp. 85–118.
2. Blanche, P. J., Gong, E. L., Forte, T. M., and Nichols, A.V. (1981) Characterization of human high density lipoprotein by gradient gel electrophoresis *Biochim. Biophys. Acta* **665,** 408–419.
3. Cheung, M. C. (1986) Characterization of apolipoprotein A-containing lipoproteins. *Methods Enzymol.* **129,** 130–145.
4. Gibson, J. C., Rubinstein, A., Ginsberg, H. N. and Brown, V. G. (1986) Isolation of apolipoprotein E-containing lipoproteins by immunoaffinity chromatography. *Methods Enzymol.* **129,** 186–198.
5. Chapman, M. J., Laplaud, P. H., Luc, G., Forgez, P., Brickest, E., Goulinet, S., and Lagrange, D. (1988) Further resolution of the low density lipoprotein spectrum in normal human plasma: physicochemical characteristics of discrete subspecies isolated by density gradient ultracentrifugation. *J. Lipid Res.* **29,** 442–458.

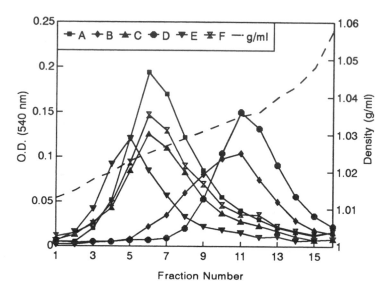

Fig. 2. The cholesterol profiles in iodixanol gradients of peak LDL fractions isolated from KBr gradients (6) from six individuals *(A–F)*. LDL fractions from the KBr gradients were treated according to the method described in **Subheading 3.3.** All gradients were unloaded low-density end first by upward displacement with Maxidens (*see* **Note 2**). The cholesterol profile is given as the optical density (O.D.) measured in a standard spectrophotometric assay. See text for further details.

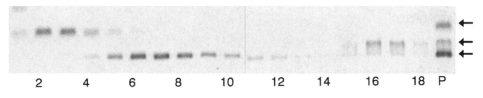

Fig. 3. LDL subfractionation in the Beckman TLN100 near vertical rotor. Agarose gel electrophoresis of fractions collected from the gradient system described in **Subheading 3.2.** (plasma was present only in the lower layer) after centrifugation at 350,000*g* for 3 h. Fractions (1–18) were unloaded dense-end first by tube puncture; **P** is the original plasma, and the three arrows (**top** to **bottom**) indicate the location of HDL, VLDL, and LDL on the gel. See text for further details.

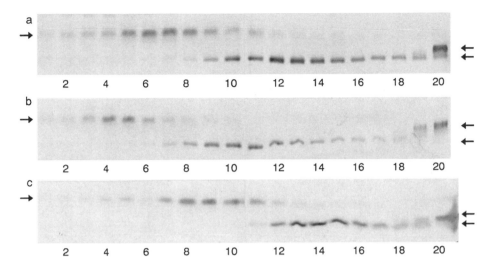

Fig. 4. LDL subfractionation in the Beckman NVT65.2 near-vertical rotor. Agarose gel electrophoresis of fractions from **(a)** method described in **Subheading 3.1.**, **(b)** method described in **Subheading 3.2.** iodixanol (plasma only in the dense layer), and **(c)** method described in **Subheading 3.4.** after centrifugation at 350,000*g* for 3 h. All gradients were collected in 20 fractions, dense-end first, by tube puncture. The **arrow** on the **left** of each gel indicates the location of HDL, and the **two arrows** on the **right** indicate **(top to bottom)** VLDL and LDL on the gels. See text for further details.

6. Griffin, B. A., Caslake, M. J., Yib, B., Tait, G. W., Packard, C. J., and Shepherd, J. (1990) Rapid isolation of low density lipoprotein (LDL) subfractions from plasma by density gradient ultracentrifugation. *Atherosclerosis* **83,** 59–67.
7. Campos. H., Blijlevens, E., McNamara, J. R., Ordovas, J. M., Posner, B. M., Wilson, P. W., Castelli, W. P., and Schaefer, E.J. LDL particle size distribution. Results from the Framingham offspring study. *Atherosclerosis Thrombosis* **12,** 1410–1419.
8. Krauss, R.M. (1994) Heterogeneity of plasma low density lipoproteins and atherosclerosis risk. *Curr. Opin. Lipidol.* **5,** 339–349.
9. Graham, J. M., Higgins, J. A., Gillott, T., Taylor, T. , Wilkinson, J., and Billington, D. (1996) A novel method for the rapid separation of plasma lipoproteins using self-generating gradients of iodixanol. *Atherosclerosis* **124,** 123–133.

7

Detecting Cholesteryl Ester Transfer Protein in Plasma

Andreas Ritsch and Josef R. Patsch

1. Introduction

Transport of triglycerides (TGs) and cholesteryl esters (CEs) in plasma can be viewed as taking place via two major groups of lipoproteins, the TG-rich lipoproteins (chylomicrons and VLDL), on one hand, and the cholesterol-rich lipoproteins (LDL and HDL), on the other. The metabolism of these groups is linked by exchange processes, catalyzed mainly by a plasma glycoprotein referred to as lipid transfer protein I (LTP-I) *(1)* or cholesteryl ester transfer protein (CETP) *(2–5)*.

With the crucial role that CETP holds for the distribution of CEs and TGs among plasma lipoproteins and, thus, for cholesterol metabolic routing to body tissues, extensive studies will be necessary if we are to understand how CETP is regulated in certain clinical settings. For such studies, a basic requirement is the ability to accurately quantify the concentration of CETP in plasma. Measurement of CETP-activity has been made available *(6)* and has proved helpful and informative *(7)*. However, this approach has limitations inherent in activity measurements in general, in which exogenous substrates have to be prepared and partial loss of activities is difficult to control for. Measuring enzyme mass directly avoids such problems and is more feasible for everyday use. Various assays for measurement of CETP mass have indeed been developed *(8–12)*. These procedures employed monoclonal and polyclonal antibodies raised individually against CETP to establish solid-phase radioimmunoassay (RIA) and enzyme-linked immunosorbent assay (ELISA) procedures; valuable information was gained on CETP, including plasma levels in normolipidemic and hyperlipidemic individuals and various other clinical settings, and correlations were established between CETP levels and other plasma lipid transport parameters.

From: *Methods in Molecular Medicine, vol. 52: Atherosclerosis: Experimental Methods and Protocols*
Edited by: A. F. Drew © Humana Press Inc., Totowa, NJ

We have used novel approaches for developing specific antibodies, employing gene technology *(13)*: cDNAs encoding recombinant antibody fragments were cloned employing mRNA preparations from lymphocytes of immunized animals. CETP-specific recombinant antibody fragments for CETP ELISA were successfully employed and are described in this chapter.

The focus of this report, however, will be description of CETP-activity and CETP-mass measurements using assays that were demonstrated to be applicable and useful in clinical studies. Included also are the preparation of exogenous substrate for CETP-activity assay, isolation of CETP from human plasma, and preparation of CETP–specific polyclonal antibody employed in the ELISA.

2. Materials

2.1. Measurement of CETP Activity

2.1.1. Radiolabeling of LDL

2.1.1.1. PREPARATION OF LIPOPROTEIN-DEFICIENT PLASMA (LPDP)

1. Blood samples were collected from donors after an overnight fast into tubes containing EDTA to give a final concentration of 1.6 mg/mL. Human plasma was collected after centrifugation at 1500*g* for 10 min at 4°C and stored at 4°C.
2. $MnCl_2 \cdot 4 \cdot H_2O$ p.a. (Nr. 5927.1000, MERCK).
3. $MQ-H_2O$: water prepared by Milli-RO 12 Plus and Milli-Q Plus PF (Millipore).
4. DS: 10 % (w/v) dextran sulfate sodium salt (Code No. 17-0340-01, Pharmacia Biotech) in $MQ-H_2O$, freshly prepared.
5. $BaCl_2 \cdot 2 H_2O$ ACS reagent (B-6394, Sigma; toxic).
6. 0.45 μm filter Millex-HA (Millipore).
7. J2-HS centrifuge, JLA-10.5 rotor (Beckman).

2.1.1.2. PREPARATION OF SYNTHETIC VESICLES CONTAINING ^{14}C-CHOLESTERYL-OLEATE

1. PC: 100 mg/mL L-α-phosphatitylcholine Type III-E from egg yolk in hexane (P-5388, Sigma), store at –20°C.
2. BHT: 2 m*M* butylated hydroxytoluene (B-1378, Sigma) in chloroform, store at –20°C.
3. ^{14}CE: cholesteryl[1-^{14}C]oleate, 56.0 mCi/mmol (CFA256 B58, Amersham Life Science).
4. VB: 50 m*M* Tris-HCl, 0.01% EDTA, pH 7.4.
5. Megason Ultrasonic Disintegrator (Ultrasonic Instruments International, Inc., New York).

2.1.1.3. LABELING OF LDL

1. LP-B: 100 m*M* NaCl, 10 m*M* Tris-HCl, 1 m*M* EDTA, 1 m*M* NaN_3 (toxic), pH 7.4.
2. SDS-B: 10% sodium dodecyl sulfate in LP-B.

3. PB: 0.1 *M* NaH$_2$PO$_4$, pH 7.4.
4. DTNB-B: 11 mg/mL DTNB (D-8130, Sigma) in PB, store at 4°C (LCAT inhibitor).
5. LDL: low-density lipoprotein is isolated by zonal ultracentrifugation (as described by Patsch et al.) *(14)* and stored in LP-B at 4°C.
6. Shaking water bath, SW-20C (Julabo Labortechnik GMBH, Seelbach, Germany).

2.1.1.4. ISOLATION OF LABELED LDL

1. Ultra clear™ tubes, 14 × 89 mm (Beckman).
2. NaBr (S-9756, Sigma), NaBr solutions are prepared in MQ-H$_2$O.
3. Cholesterol CHOD-PAP Kit (1489232, Roche): measurements are performed according to the manufacturer's instructions, optical density at 505 nm is measured in a spectrophotometer.
4. Dialysis membrane Spectra/Por6, MWCO 50.000 (132542, Spectrum Medical Industries, Inc., Los Angeles, CA).
5. Liquid scintillation (LSC) cocktail: Ultima Gold XR (Packard, Groningen, The Netherlands).
6. LS 6500 Multi purpose Scintillation Counter (Beckman).
7. DU 640 Spectrophotometer (Beckman).
8. L8-60 M Ultracentrifuge (Beckman), SW41 swinging bucket rotor (Beckman).

2.1.2. Measurement of CETP Activity of Plasma Samples

1. Precipitation mix 1: 4 mL 4% Na-phosphotungstic acid (Nr. 583, Merck) in 160 m*M* NaOH + 1 mL 2 *M* MgCl$_2$·6H$_2$O (Nr. 1.05833, Merck).
2. HDL$_3$: high-density lipoprotein 3 is isolated by zonal ultracentrifugation (as described by Patsch et al.) *(14)* and stored in LP-B at 4°C.
3. Microfuge: Mikro 24–48 R (Hettich Zentrifugen, Tuttlingen, Germany).

2.1.3. Fast CETP Activity Assay

1. PBS: 0.2 g/L KCl, 0.2 g/L KH$_2$PO$_4$, 8.0 g/L NaCl, 2.16 g/L Na$_2$HPO$_4$·7H$_2$O, pH 7.4.
2. BSA: Bovine Albumin Fraction V (A-4503, Sigma).
3. Precipitation mix 2: 1 mL 2 *M* MnCl$_2$ + 1 mL heparin 5000 I.E./mL (Novo Industri A/S, Copenhagen, Denmark).

2.2. Measurement of CETP Mass

2.2.1. Isolation of CETP from Human Plasma

2.2.1.1. HYDROPHOBIC INTERACTION CHROMATOGRAPHY

1. Phenyl Sepharose Column: 100 mL Phenyl Sepharose High Performance (17-1082-01, Pharmacia Biotech, Uppsala, Sweden).

2. NTE: 2 *M* NaCl, 10 m*M* Tris-HCl, 1 m*M* EDTA, pH 7.6.
3. Gradifrac System including Control Unit UV-1, Recorder Rec 102, Pump P-50, Conductivity monitor, and Mixer 1.6 mL (Pharmacia Biotech, Uppsala, Sweden).

2.2.1.2. Ion Exchange Chromatography (Fig. 1A)

1. CM sepharose column: 50 mL Fractogel TSK CM-650 (M) (Merck).
2. CB: 10 m*M* citric acid trisodium dihydrate, pH 5.5 (C-8532, Sigma).
3. CA: 2 *M* citric acid (Nr. 818707, Merck).

2.2.1.3. Concentration of CM Pool

1. Bradford reagent: 100 mg Coomassie Brilliant Blue G 250 (BIO-RAD, Richmond, CA) in 50 mL methanol + 100 mL 85% (v/v) phosphoric acid (Merck), dilute 1:4 in MQ-H$_2$O prior to use (= diluted Bradford reagent).

2.2.1.4. Exclusion Size Chromatography (Fig. 1B)

1. HW 55 column: 270 mL Fractogel TSK HW55 (S) (Merck).
2. Dialysis membrane Spectra/Por6, MWCO 15.000 (132560, Spectrum Medical Industries, Inc., Los Angeles, CA).

2.2.2. Raising of CETP–Specific Polyclonal Antibodies

1. Freund's Adjuvant Incomplete (F-5506, Sigma).
2. 20 gage needle: 20G × 11/2" (Braun, Melsungen, Germany).
3. 1 mL syringe: Inject F 1 mL (Braun, Melsungen, Germany).
4. EDTA-tube: 2.7 mL S-Monovette KE (Sarstedt, Nümbrecht, Germany).

2.2.3. Detection of Anti-CETP Antibodies
2.2.3.1. Dot Blot Analysis

1. TBS: 0.02 *M* Tris-HCl, 0.15 *M* NaCl, pH 7.5.
2. TBS/SM: 2% skim milk powder (902887, ICN Industries, Inc., Aurora, Ohio) in TBS.
3. TBS/T: 0.1% Tween-20 (Sigma) in TBS.
4. TBS/SM/T: 2% skim milk powder + 0.1% Tween-20 in TBS.
5. AP-B: 100 m*M* Tris-HCl, 100 m*M* NaCl, 50 m*M* MgCl$_2$, pH 9.5.
6. Substrate solution: 45 µL NBT (1383213, Boehringer Mannheim; toxic) + 35 µL X-phosphate (1383221, Boehringer Mannheim; toxic) in 10 mL AP-B.
7. Nitrocellulose membrane Protran BA 83 (Schleicher & Schuell, Dassel, Germany).

2.2.3.2. Measurement of Antibody Titer (ELISA)

1. Coating buffer: 0.01 *M* NaHCO$_3$ (Merck) buffer, pH 9.6.

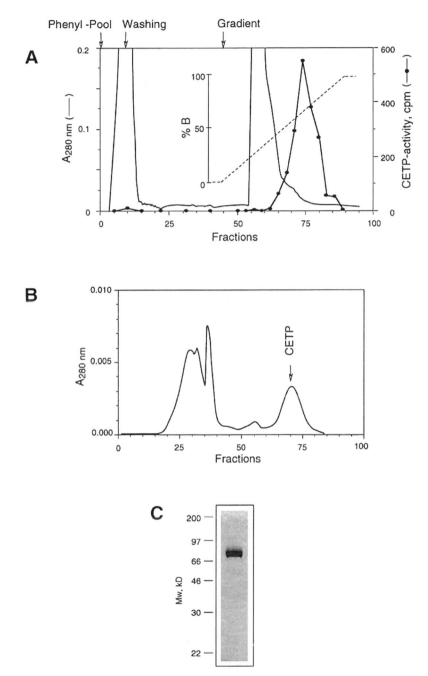

Fig. 1. Isolation of CETP from human plasma. (**A**) Ion exchange chromatography: Phenyl pool was applied to a CM sepharose column. After washing with 10 m*M* citrate, pH5.5, a 100-mL gradient ranging from 0 (buffer A) to 1 *M* NaCl (buffer B) was

2. TBS/BSA: 2% BSA in TBS.
3. Anti-rabbit IgG-AP: Goat anti-rabbit IgG/alkaline phosphatase ImmunoPure®
   (Nr. 31342, Pierce, Rockford, IL).
4. PNPP-B: 0.1% 4-nitrophenylphosphate (107905, Boehringer Mannheim) in 1 M
   diethanolamine (Merck), 0.5 mM MgCl$_2$, 0.02% NaN$_3$, pH 7.4.
5. Microtiter plate: F96 Maxisorp Immuno-Plate (Nunc, Roskilde, Denmark).
6. Plate washer 812 SW1 (SLT Lab Instruments, France).
7. Plate reader Spectra III (SLT Lab Instruments, Austria).

2.2.4. Affinity Purification of CETP Specific Antibodies

2.2.4.1. PREPARATION OF CETP SEPHAROSE

1. CNBr-activated sepharose 4B (17-0430-01, Pharmacia Biotech).
2. Coupling buffer: 0.1 M NaHCO$_3$ (Nr. 6329, Merck), 0.5 M NaCl, pH 8.3.
3. Acetate buffer: 0.1 M Na-acetate, 0.5 M NaCl, pH 4.0.
4. Tris-buffer: 0.1 M Tris-HCl, 0.5 M NaCl, pH 8.0.
5. PBS/TH: 0.02 % thimerosal (Sigma) in PBS.
6. Column C 10/20 (Pharmacia Biotech).
7. Red Rocker (Hoefer Scientific Instruments, San Francisco).

2.2.4.2. AFFINITY CHROMATOGRAPHY

1. Elution buffer: 0.1 M glycine, pH 2.7 (808822, ICN Industries, Inc., Aurora, OH).
2. Dialysis membrane Spectra/Por6, MWCO 15.000 (132560, Spectrum Medical
   Industries, Inc., Los Angeles, CA).

2.2.6. CETP-ELISA

1. TBS/BSA/T: 2% BSA + 0.2% Tween-20 in TBS.
2. DeltaSoftIITM software (BioMetallics, Inc.)

---

applied to the column. Protein concentration was monitored by measuring absorbance
at 280 nm. Eluted fractions were analyzed for CETP activity. The gradient is indicated
by a dotted line. (B) Exclusion size chromatography: Mini phenyl pool was applied
via injection loop to HW55 sepharose column. Protein concentration was monitored
by measuring absorbance at 280 nm. CETP elutes as a single peak at 0.6 column
volume. (C) SDS-PAGE analysis of purified CETP. 500 ng of CETP was applied to a
10% SDS-PAGE and visualized by Coomasie-blue staining. The positions of marker
proteins are indicated.

3. Methods

3.1. Measurement of CETP Activity

To assay for CETP activity, the transfer of ^{14}C-cholesteryl oleate from LDL to HDL is quantified. In addition to measurement of CETP activity of plasma samples *(6)*, a fast assay for measuring CETP-activity of various fractions, in the course of the CETP purification procedure, is included (**Subheading 3.1.3**).

3.1.1. Radiolabeling of LDL

LDL particles are radiolabeled by incubation with synthetic vesicles containing ^{14}C-cholesteryl oleate. Lipoprotein-deficient plasma is used as CETP source for radiolabeling of LDL.

3.1.1.1. PREPARATION OF LIPOPROTEIN-DEFICIENT PLASMA (LPDP)

1. Supplement 10 mL of fresh human plasma with 0.375 g $MnCl_2$ and 1.35 mL DS and centrifuge at 4400*g* in a Beckman JLA10.5 rotor for 20 min.
2. Collect supernatant, supplement with 0.118 g $BaCl_2$ and centrifuge as before.
3. Collect supernatant and pass through a 0.45-μm filter (= LPDP).

3.1.1.2. PREPARATION OF SYNTHETIC VESICLES CONTAINING ^{14}C-CHOLESTERYL-OLEATE

1. Combine 10 μL PC, 5 μL BHT, and 10 μCi ^{14}CE and gently vortex.
2. Evaporate total liquid under gaseous nitrogen on ice.
3. Resuspend pellet gently in 1 mL vesicle buffer (VB).
4. Generate synthetic vesicles by sonication for 5 min, three times, on ice (Megason Ultrasonic Disintegrator, intensity 4), with two intervening incubations for 5 min on ice between rounds of sonication (= synthetic vesicle mix).

3.1.1.3. LABELING OF LDL

1. Combine 40 μL SDS-B, 350 μL DTNB-B, 3 mL LPDP, and 25 μm LDL. Make up to a final volume of 6 mL by addition of LP-B (= reaction mix).
2. After addition of 1 mL synthetic vesicle mix, incubate the whole mixture for 18 h in a 37°C water bath with gentle shaking (= labeling mixture).

3.1.1.4. ISOLATION OF LABELED LDL

1. After addition of 2.28 g NaBr, dispense half of the labeling mixture into two Ultra-Clear™ centrifuge tubes.
2. Overlay each tube with 3.5 mL 0.063 g/mL NaBr, 3.5 mL 0.019 g/mL NaBr, and 3 mL 0.006 g/mL NaBr.
3. Centrifuge at 151,000*g* for 24 h at 12°C in a SW41 rotor, then isolate the thin

orange layer in the upper half of the centrifuge tube and dialyze against LP-B ($= ^{14}$C-LDL) (*see* **Note 1**).

4. Determine specific radioactivity by measuring total cholesterol (Total Cholesterol Kit) and radioactivity (10 µL ^{14}C-LDL in 1 mL LSC-cocktail). Samples should be within range of 1000–2000 cpm /µg LDL-cholesterol.

3.1.2. Measurement of CETP Activity of Plasma Samples

1. Add 6.25 µL precipitation mix 1 to 50 µL of human EDTA-plasma, followed by immediate vortexing and centrifugation at 11,000*g* for 10 min in a microfuge at 4°C.
2. Use supernatant directly as probe for the CETP-activity assay.
3. Make up reaction mixture by combining 20 µL probe, 350 µL PB, 50 µL DTNB-B, 200 nM HDL$_3$-cholesterol, 10.000 cpm ^{14}C-LDL, and unlabeled LDL to give a final amount of 500 nM LDL cholesterol. Add LP-B and a final volume of 700 µL.
4. Mix by turning 10 times end over end, and incubate 16 h in a 37°C water bath with gentle shaking.
5. Add 300 µL PB and 167 µL 0.1 *M* MnCl$_2$, vortex and incubate for 10 min at RT.
6. Centrifugation at 11,000*g* for 30 min at 4°C, then add 800 µL of supernatant to 10 mL of LSC-cocktail and measure cpm for at least 5 min.
7. Take measurements in duplicate. C$_0$ and C$_{37}$ controls consist of lipoprotein buffer as probe and incubation at 0°C and 37°C, respectively (*see* **Note 2**).
8. Calculate CETP activity of plasma samples using **Equation 1**:

$$\text{CETP-activity:} = (\text{cpm}_{\text{probe}} - \text{cpm}_{\text{c37}}) \times 500 \text{ nmol} / 10.000 \text{ cpm} / 0.02 \text{ mL} / 16 \text{ h}$$

$$= (\text{cpm}_{\text{probe}} - \text{cpm}_{\text{c37}}) \times 0.156 \text{ nmo} / \text{h} / \text{mL}$$

3.1.3. Fast CETP-Activity Assay

1. Make up reaction mixture by combining 100 µL of sample, 80 µg HDL$_3$-cholesterol, 10,000 cpm ^{14}C-LDL, and unlabeled LDL to give a final amount of 95 µg LDL cholesterol. Add 6% BSA/PBS to give a final volume of 475 µL (*see* **Note 3**).
2. Mix by turning end over end 10 times and incubate for 2 h in a 37°C water bath with gentle shaking.
3. Add 25 µL precipitation mix 2, vortex, and incubate for 30 mins on ice.
4. Centrifuge at 11,000*g* for 20 min at 4°C, and add 400 µL of supernatant to 5 mL LSC-cocktail, then measure cpm for at least 5 min.

3.2. Measurement of CETP Mass

3.2.1. Isolation of CETP from Human Plasma

Repeated purification procedures, as described below, are necessary to obtain CETP in quantities sufficient for immunization of rabbits (**Subheading 3.2.2.**), preparation of CETP sepharose (**Subheading 3.2.4.1.**) and for CETP standards used in the CETP ELISA **(Subheading 3.2.6.)**. All chromatography procedures are performed on a Gradifrac system including UV and conductivity monitoring and automatic fraction collection.

3.2.1.1. HYDROPHOBIC INTERACTION CHROMATOGRAPHY

1. Equilibrate the phenyl sepharose column with 2 column volumes MQ-H_2O and 2 column volumes NTE.
2. Supplement LPDP, prepared from 1 L human plasma as described above **(Subheading 3.1.1.1.)**, with NaCl (final concentration of 2 M) and apply to the column.
3. Wash with 500 mL NTE and 500 mL 100 mM Tris-HCl, pH 7.5, and elute bound proteins with 3 mM Tris-HCl, pH 7.5.
4. Collect fractions within the elution peak (= phenyl pool).
5. Column parameters:

Volume	100 mL
Diameter	5 cm
Flow rate	5 mL/min
Absorbance	2.0
Fraction size	5 mL

3.2.1.2. ION EXCHANGE CHROMATOGRAPHY (**FIG. 1A**)

1. Equilibrate CM sepharose column with 2 column volumes CB.
2. Supplement phenyl pool with 1/100 volume of 100 × CB, adjust to pH 5.5 using CA, and apply to column.
3. Wash column with 5 column volumes CB.
4. Apply 100-mL gradient ranging from 0 (buffer A) to 1 M NaCl (buffer B) in CB to the column.
5. Analyze eluted fractions for CETP activity (*see* **Subheading 3.1.3.**) and pool fractions within the CETP peak (= CM pool).
6. Column parameters:

Volume	50 mL
Diameter	2.6 cm
Flow rate	2 mL/min
Absorbance	0.2
Fraction size	5 mL

3.2.1.3. CONCENTRATION OF CM POOL

Concentration of CM pool is performed manually using a Mini phenyl sepharose column (volume: 1 mL, diameter: 1 cm) applying static pressure, without UV and conductivity monitoring, without automatic fraction collection, and at an approximate flow rate of 1 mL/min.

1. Rinse column with 10 mL MQ-H_2O and 10 mL NTE.

2. Supplement CM pool with 1 *M* NaCl and apply to the column, then rinse with 5 mL 100 m*M* Tris-HCl, pH 7.5.
3. Elute bound proteins with 3 m*M* Tris-HCl, pH 7.5 and collect 10 0.5-mL fractions (*see* **Note 4**).
4. Analyze fractions for their protein concentration by pipeting 2 μL of each fraction into a 40-μL droplet of diluted Bradford reagent on a parafilm.
5. Pool 3–4 fractions showing highest protein concentrations and supplement with 1/10 volume of 10 × PBS (= Mini phenyl pool).

3.2.1.4. EXCLUSION SIZE CHROMATOGRAPHY (FIG. 1B)

1. Rinse HW55 column with PBS overnight. Apply Mini phenyl pool via injection loop.
2. CETP elutes as a single peak at 0.6 column volume.
3. Pool fractions within the peak and concentrate as described for concentration of CM pool (*see* **Subheading 3.2.1.3.**) using a Mini phenyl column.
4. Dilute 6 μL of each fraction eluted from the Mini phenyl column 1:10 in MQ-H$_2$O and measure OD$_{205}$ of diluted samples using a 60-μL microcuvet. Calculate protein concentrations using Equation 2:

$$C^{mg/mL} = OD_{205}/30.5 \text{ (see Note 5) (15)}.$$

5. Pool 3–4 fractions containing highest CETP concentrations, dialyze against PBS, and store in aliquots at –80°C.
6. By analyzing purified CETP on a 10% SDS-PAGE, only a single band at ~66 KD should be detectable (*see* **Note 6**; **Fig. 1C**).
7. Column parameters:

Volume	270 mL
Diameter	1.9 cm
Flow rate	0.5 mL/min
Absorbance	0.01
Fraction size	2.5 mL

3.2.2. Raising CETP–Specific Polyclonal Antibodies

1. Mix 0.15 mL CETP solution (0.2 mg/mL in PBS) with an equal volume of Freund's incomplete adjuvant by repeated passages through a 20-gage needle connected to a 1-mL plastic syringe until a viscous water-in-oil emulsion forms (*see* **Note 7**).
2. Inject the emulsion intracutaneously in the back area of an adult female rabbit at 8–10 sites.
3. Repeat the injection procedure after 2 mo and 4 mo.
4. Bleed the rabbit before and 7 d after each immunization procedure. Blood is obtained from the marginal vein of the ear.
5. Two weeks after the last immunization, bleed the rabbit and store serum in 5-mL aliquots at –80°C (= anti-CETP serum) (*see* **Note 8**).

3.2.3. Detection of Anti-CETP Antibodies

Dot blot analysis using CETP fixed to cellulose nitrate membrane represents an easy way for detecting CETP-specific antibodies in plasma, whereas concentration of CETP-specific antibodies is measured by CETP ELISA.

3.2.3.1. DOT BLOT ANALYSIS

1. Dot 1 µL CETP solutions, of concentrations between 100 and 0.1 ng/mL, in TBS, and 1 µL 0.1% BSA/TBS (negative control), onto a cellulose nitrate membrane and allow to dry.
2. Block membrane in TBS/SM for 1 h.
3. Wash with TBS/T three times then incubate with secondary antibody (anti-rabbit IgG conjugated to alkaline phosphatase) diluted 1:2000 in TBS/T for 2 h.
4. Wash with TBS/SM/T, three times for 10 min, then equilibrate the membrane in AP-B and incubate in substrate solution.
5. After sufficient color development, rinse membrane three times with MQ-H$_2$O and subsequently dry on filter paper.
6. All incubations are carried out with continuous shaking (except for color development) at RT.

3.2.3.2. MEASUREMENT OF ANTIBODY TITER (ELISA)

1. Coat wells of a microtiter plate with 0.1 mL CETP solution (10 µg/ mL in coating buffer). Incubate overnight at 4°C and wash 3 times with TBS/T.
2. Block free sites on the plate with TBS/BSA for 0.5 h.
3. Apply 0.1 mL serum, serially diluted in PBS from 1:10 to 1:100 000, to each well and incubate for 2 h, then wash three times with TBS/T.
4. Apply 0.1 mL of antirabbit IgG-AP, diluted 1:2000 in TBS/T, for 2 h, then wash three times with TBS/T.
5. Add 0.1 mL of PNPP-B. Measure optical density at 405 nm after sufficient color development has occurred.
6. All incubation steps are kept out at room temperature (except coating of plate at 4°C), and all washes are performed using an automatic microtiter plate washer.

3.2.4. Affinity Purification of CETP-Specific Antibodies

CETP-specific antibodies are isolated from rabbit plasma by affinity chromatography using a CETP sepharose column.

3.2.4.1. PREPARATION OF CETP SEPHAROSE

1. Swell 3 g CNBr-activated sepharose in 20 mL 1 mM HCl for 15 min at RT (*see* **Note 9**).
2. Wash the gel on a sintered glass filter with 400 mL 1 mM HCl, then suspend in 20 mL 1 mM HCl and transfer to a 50-mL reaction tube.

3. After centrifugation at 2200g in a JLA-10.5 Beckman rotor, replace supernatant with coupling solution, consisting of 0.5 mg purified CETP in 10 mL coupling buffer (save 0.1 mL coupling solution for measurement of coupling efficiency).
4. Rotate the mixture containing ligand and swollen gel end over end overnight at 4°C.
5. After centrifugation at 2200g in a JLA-10.5 Beckman rotor, supernatant is replaced by 10 mL 0.1 M Tris-HCl, pH 8.0, followed by incubation for 2 h at 4°C to block excess active groups (save 0.1 mL supernatant for measurement of coupling efficiency).
6. Transfer CETP-sepharose to a chromatography column and wash 3 times with 30 mL acetate buffer followed by 30 mL Tris-buffer.
7. Wash CETP sepharose with 10 volumes PBS and store in PBS/TH at 4°C.
8. Measure protein concentration of coupling solution before addition to activated sepharose and after coupling reaction, by the method of Lowry *(16)*. Less than 5% of CETP should remain in the supernatant after the coupling reaction.

3.2.4.2. AFFINITY CHROMATOGRAPHY

Affinity chromatography is performed on a Gradifrac system (Pharmacia) with a flow rate of 1 mL/min. Protein concentration is monitored by measuring absorbance at 280 nm; 2-mL fractions are collected automatically.

1. Wash the CETP sepharose column with 10 volumes PBS.
2. Dilute 2 mL anti-CETP serum, 1:5 in PBS, pass through a 0.45-μm filter, and apply to the column.
3. Wash with 10 mL PBS, and elute bound IgG with elution buffer.
4. Pool samples of the elution peak, dialyze against PBS, and store in aliquots at –80°C.

3.2.5. Preparation of CETP-Deficient Plasma

CETP-deficient plasma is used as dilution reagent for preparation of CETP standards in the CETP ELISA and is obtained by passing plasma through an anti-CETP sepharose column.

1. Prepare anti-CETP sepharose according to the preparation of CETP sepharose (*see* **Subheading 3.2.4.1.**), except use 1.5 mg of freeze-dried CNBr-activated sepharose 4B and 4.6 mg of affinity-purified anti-CETP IgG (*see* **Note 9**).
2. Pass 50 mL EDTA-plasma and the respective eluates through the anti-CETP IgG sepharose column three times. Between passages, wash the column with 3 column volumes of elution buffer.
3. Demonstrate absence of CETP by CETP-activity measurement (*see* **Subheading 3.1.**), and store CETP-deficient plasma in aliquots at –80°C.

3.2.6. CETP ELISA

1. Coat wells of a microtiter plate with 0.1 mL anti-CETP IgG solution (10 μg/mL in coating buffer). Incubate overnight at 4°C then wash three times with TBS/T.

2. Block free sites on the plate with TBS/BSA for 0.5 h.
3. Wash 3 times with TBS/T and add 50 µL of TBS/BSA/T to each well of the plate.
4. Create a set of at least 6 standards by repeated threefold dilutions of a CETP master sample, prepared by addition of purified CETP to CETP-deficient plasma (*see* **Notes 10** and **11**). Prepare plasma samples by diluting EDTA plasma of patients in CETP-deficient plasma.
5. Add 50 µL of each sample to the wells.
6. Incubate for 2 h, and wash 3 times with PBS/T.
7. Apply 0.1 mL anti-rabbit IgG-AP diluted 1:2000 in TBS/T for 2 h, then wash 3 times with TBS/T.
8. Add 0.1 mL of PNPP-B. After sufficient color development, measure optical density at 405 nm using a microtiter plate reader.
9. Perform parameter curve fit (with software such as DeltaSoft™) and use to calculate CETP concentration of plasma samples.
10. Measure all samples in duplicate. Intraassay and interassay coefficients of variation on 10 samples and 10 subsequent measurements of the normal plasma pool at ~1.2 µg CETP/mL are represented by SD values expressed as a percentage of the mean value and should not exceed 5% and 10%, respectively (*see* **Notes 12** and **13**).
11. Dilute plasma samples such that measurements are taken within the steepest part of the standard curve, representing the range of maximal precision, which can be estimated graphically as shown in **Fig. 2**.
12. All incubation steps are carried out at RT (except coating of plate at 4°C) and all washes are performed using an automatic microtiter plate washer.

4. Notes

4.1. Measurement of CETP Activity

1. If no swinging bucket rotor is available, isolation of radiolabeled LDL also may be performed using angle head rotors. The labeling mixture is supplemented with NaBr to give a density of 1.019 g/mL and centrifuged at 270,000g for 12 h at 12°C in a Type 50.4 Beckman rotor. The orange layer at the bottom of the tube is collected, supplemented with NaBr to give a density of 1.063 g/mL, and centrifuged as before. Labeled LDL may be isolated from the orange layer in the upper half of the tube *(17)*.
2. C_0 and C_{37} controls are included in CETP-activity measurements, not only for background subtraction, but also to check the quality of the substrate. C_0 represents CETP-independent transfer of cholesteryl oleate from LDL to HDL, including stability of radiolabeled LDL, and should not exceed 100 cpm/800 µL. C_{37} - C_0 serves as an indicator of CETP traces contained in HDL$_3$ used as acceptor lipoprotein and should be no more than 100 cpm/800 µL.
3. High concentrations of BSA are necessary to stabilize CETP in samples of low protein concentrations in the course of the CETP-purification procedure. Without addition of BSA, no CETP activity is detectable in such preparations.

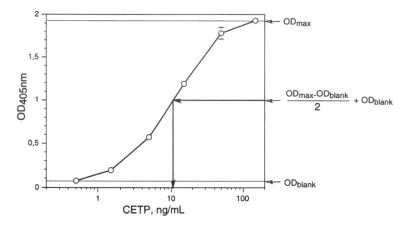

Fig. 2. CETP ELISA: Point of best precision can be estimated graphically as the point of intersection between the standard curve and the OD value middling those of highest standard and blank, respectively. A typical standard curve using CETP standards containing 0.5, 1.5, 5, 15, 50, and 150 ng/mL is shown. Standard deviations of duplicate measurements exceeding 3% of mean are indicated by error bars. In this ELISA, samples (averaging 1.1 µg CETP/mL plasma) should be diluted 1:100 to perform measurements of best precision.

4.2. Measurement of CETP Mass

4. Elution of CETP from Mini phenyl sepharose column should be performed at very low flow-rate to ensure elution within 2 or 3 fractions. Mini phenyl sepharose may be prepared by replacing Sephadex G-50 of prepacked NICK columns (Pharmacia Biotech, Code No. 17-0855-01) by 1 mL phenyl sepharose high performance.

5. For estimation of protein concentration in the course of the purification procedure we employed the method of Lowry, using bovine albumin as a standard. However, when assaying purified CETP by the Lowry method, 3.7-fold higher values were obtained when compared to those from amino acid analysis. Therefore, we used the method described by Scopes, which is based on the peptide bond absorbance; with this procedure, values only 6% higher than those from the amino acid analysis were obtained. In several measurements, extinction coefficient for CETP averaged 30.5 and is therefore used in **Equation 2 (Subheading 3.2.1.4.).**

6. On SDS-PAGE gels of high resolution, CETP appears to be a duplex band. As both bands are detected by anti-CETP antibodies, these bands most likely represent different glycosylated forms of CETP.

7. Antigen emulsion used for immunization of rabbits is prepared by passing the antigen/Freund's incomplete adjuvant mixture through a 20-gage needle. Because of high viscosity a great deal of pressure is to be exerted for the last passages of the emulsion through the needle. The formation of a water-in-oil emulsion can be tested by pipeting a small droplet onto water, which should stay discrete for several hours.

8. Blood samples of immunized rabbits should be collected into tubes containing EDTA to give a final concentration of 1.6 mg/mL, since yield of plasma is higher when compared to that of serum.

9. Rather high amounts of CNBr-activated sepharose, in relation to amount of ligand, were used for preparation of CETP sepharose and anti-CETP IgG sepharose, as this ensures avoidance of steric hindrances during affinity chromatography.

10. Using our CETP-specific polyclonal antibody as coating and detection antibody, standards containing 0.5, 1.5, 5, 15, 50, and 150 ng/mL CETP worked very well to create a sigmoidal standard curve.

11. CETP standards for the ELISA, prepared by addition of purified CETP to CETP-deficient plasma, may be replaced by corresponding diluted samples of normolipidemic plasma pool, whose CETP concentration had been determined accurately in repeated CETP ELISA measurements. To obtain a normolipidemic plasma pool, plasma samples from each of 50–100 normolipidemic donors are combined and stored in aliquots at –80°C.

12. Precision of the CETP ELISA may be enhanced by the following measures: (1) After washing microtiter plates using an automatic microtiter plate washer, remaining liquid should be removed by tapping the plate on filter paper, thereby avoiding unwanted and unequal dilution of the following reagent. (2) Color development should be continued until the optical density of the most concentrated standards is within a range of 1 and 2 OD_{405nm}. (3) Usage of a multichannel pipet ensures dispensing constant volumes of blocking, antibody and substrate solutions. (4) Do not use Triton X-100 as detergent instead of Tween-20, as it may distort precision of the ELISA because of its instability during storage.

13. CETP–specific mouse monoclonal antibody (2E7) and recombinant antibody fragments with high affinity for CETP have been successfully employed as both coating and detection antibody in the CETP ELISA. Because of their high binding affinity to CETP, their ability to recognize epitopes different from those of our polyclonal CETP antibody, and their ready access and unlimited supply, recombinant antibody fragments appear to be very useful tools for the performance of CETP quantification procedures. In routine CETP measurements, we used recombinant antibody fragment 1CL8 in the coating step and our polyclonal antibody in combination with an enzyme-linked anti-rabbit antibody as detection reagent. Using this combination, CETP concentrations in the range between 0.1 and 10 µg/mL can be detected with an intra-assay coefficient of variation of 3.8%. Because of high affinity ($KD = 4.36 \times 10^{-9}$ M) and purity (isolated by affinity chromatography) of 1CL8, coating concentrations as low as 0.3 µg/mL were sufficient to reach maximal signal in the ELISA.

Acknowledgments

We wish to thank Ronald W. Clark, Department of Cardiovascular and Metabolic Diseases, Pfizer Inc., for kindly providing the monoclonal anti–CETP antibody 2E7. This work was supported by grants S-4606 (J.R.P.) and S07106-MED (J.R.P) of the Austrian Fonds zur Förderung der Wissenschaftlichen Forschung.

References

1. Albers, J. J., Tollefson, J. H., Chen, C. H., and Steinmetz, A. (1984) Isolation and characterization of human plasma lipid transfer proteins. *Arteriosclerosis* **4,** 49–58.
2. Jarnagin, A. S., Kohr, W., and Fielding, C. J. (1987) Isolation and specificity of a Mr 74.000 cholesteryl ester transfer protein from human plasma. *Proc. Natl. Acad. Sci. USA* **84,** 1854–1857.
3. Barter, P. J., Hopkins, G., and Calvert, G. D. (1982) Transfers and exchanges of esterified chlosterol between plasma lipoproteins. *Biochem. J.* **208,** 1–7.
4. Hesler, C. B., Swenson, T. L., and Tall, A. R. (1987) Purification and characterization of human cholesteryl ester transfer protein. *J. Biol. Chem.* **262,** 2275–2282.
5. Morton, R. E. and Zilversmit, D. B. (1982) Purification and characterization of lipid transfer protein(s) from human lipoprotein-deficient plasma. *J. Lipid Res.* **23,** 1058–1067.
6. Groener, J. E. M., Pelton, R. W., and Kostner, G. M. (1986) Improved estimation of cholesterylester transfer/exchange activity in serum or plasma. *Clin. Chem.* **32,** 283–286.
7. Dullaart, R. P. F., Groener, J. E. M., Wijk, H., Sluiter, W. J., and Erkelens, D. W. (1989) Alimentary lipemia-induced redistribution of cholesteryl ester between lipoproteins. *Arteriosclerosis* **9,** 614–622.
8. Marcel, Y. L., McPherson, R., Houge, M., Czarnecka, H., Zawadzki, Z., Weech, P. K., Whitlock, M. E., Tall, A. R., and Milne, R. W. (1990) Distribution and concentration of cholesteryl ester transfer protein in plasma of normolipidemic subjects. *J. Clin. Invest.* **85,** 10–17.
9. Fukasawa, M., Arai, H., and Inoue, K. (1992) Establishment of anti-human cholesteryl easter transfer protein monoclonal antibodies and radioimmunoassaying of the level of cholesteryl ester transfer protein in human plasma. *J. Biochemistry* **111,** 696–698.
10. Ritsch, A., Auer, B., Foger, B., Schwarz, S., and Patsch, J. R. (1993) Polyclonal antibody-based immunoradiometric assay for qualification of cholesteryl ester transfer protein. *J. Lipid Res.* **34,** 673–679.
11. Clark, R. W., Moberly, J. B., and Bamberger, M. J. (1995) Low level quantification of cholesteryl ester transfer protein in plasma subfractions and cell culture media by monoclonal antibody-based immunoassay. *J. Lipid. Res.* **36,** 876–889.
12. Ritsch, A., Doppler, W., Pfeifhofer, C., Sandhofer, T., Bodner, J., and Patsch, J. R. (1999) Cholesteryl ester transfer protein gene expression is not specifically regulated by CCAAT/Enhancer-binding protein in HepG2-cells. *Atherosclerosis*, **146,** 11–18.
13. Winter, G., Griffiths, A. D., Hawkins, R. E., and Hoogenboom, H. R. (1994) Making antibodies by phage display technology. *Annu. Rev. Immunol.* **12,** 433–455.
14. Patsch, J. R. and Patsch, W. (1986) Zonal Ultracentrifugation. *Methods Enzymol.* **129,** 3–26.
15. Scopes, R. K. (1974) Measurement of protein by Spectrophotometry at 205 NM. *Anal. Biochem.* **59,** 277–282.
16. Lowry, O. H., Rosebrough, N. J., Farr, A. L., and Randall, R. J. (1951) Protein measurement with the Folin phenol reagent. *J. Biol. Chem.* **193**, 265–275.
17. Kaser, S. (1998) Untersuchungen des Cholesterinester-Transfers in Humanen Plasmen, Thesis. University of Innsbruck.

8

Determination of Plasma Homocysteine

Roberto Accinni and Oberdan Parodi

1. Introduction

A number of epidemiological and clinical studies have linked elevated plasma homocysteine (Hcy) to atherosclerotic vascular disease affecting coronary, carotid, and peripheral vessels. Plasma Hcy can be considered a marker of methionine metabolic efficiency, mainly affected by dietary intake of vitamins, especially folate, vitamin B_6, and B_{12}, as well as by genetic mutations of key metabolic enzymes and renal elimination.

1.1. Metabolism of Methionine

Hcy is 'a non-protein-forming' sulfuric amino acid that can be metabolized via transsulfuration pathway to form cystathionine, or through a remethylation pathway to form methionine (**Fig. 1**). Large amounts of methionine are activated by ATP-dependent methionine adenosil transferase to S-adenosil methionine (SAM) *(1)*. This compound is highly energetic because it is produced by hydrolysis of three phosphodiesteric links of ATP. From demethylation of SAM, S-adenosil homocysteine (SAH) is formed, which is rapidly transformed to Hcy and adenosine. Cystathionine-β-synthase (CBS) catalyzes the condensation of Hcy and serine to form cystathionine, utilizing pyridoxal phosphate (vitamin B_6) as a cofactor. Cystathionine is further catabolized to cysteine and α-ketobutyrate.

Remethylation of Hcy can be accomplished by alternate pathways in humans: In one pathway, betaine acts as the methyl donor and is transformed to dimethylglycine via the betaine-homocysteine methyltransferase *(2)*. This pathway occurs only in liver cells. In the second pathway, the enzyme $N^{5,10}$ methylenetetrahydrofolate reductase (MTHFR) catalyzes the conversion of $N^{5,10}$-methylenetetrahydrofolate to N^5-methyltetrahydrofolate; N^5-methyltetrahydrofolate is the methyl donor, and

From: *Methods in Molecular Medicine, vol. 52: Atherosclerosis: Experimental Methods and Protocols*
Edited by: A. F. Drew © Humana Press Inc., Totowa, NJ

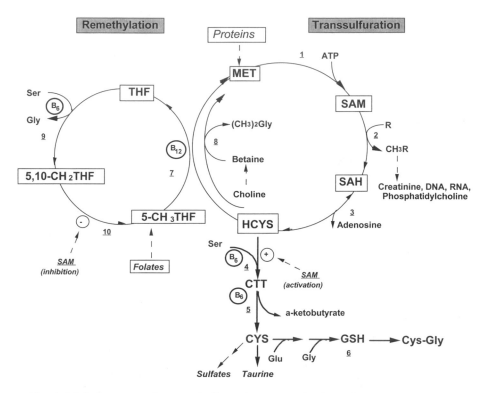

Fig. 1. Main homocysteine metabolic pathways. Activation of MET by methionine S-adenosyltransferase in the presence of ATP **(1)**; SAM demethylation in the presence of an acceptor R into S-adenosylhomocysteine (SAH) and R-CH3 **(2);** SAH is hydrolyzed into homocysteine (HCY) and adenosine by S-adenosylhomocysteine hydrolase **(3)**; condensation of serine (Ser) with HCY to produce cystathionine (CTT) in an irreversible reaction catalyzed by the pyridoxal-5'-phosphate (PLP)-containing enzyme, cystathionine β-synthase (CBS) **(4)**; CTT is hydrolized by a second PLP-containing enzyme, γ-cystathionase, to form cysteine (CYS) and α-ketobutyrate **(5)**; synthesis of glutathione (GSH) by condensation of CYS with glutamic acid (Glu) and glycine (Gly) **(6)**; demethylation of N^5-methyltetrahydrofolate (5-CH$_3$THF) into THF and HCY remethylation into MET by the MET synthase, dependent on the vitamin B_{12}-derived methylcobalamine **(7)**, whereas the reaction with betaine is confined mainly to the liver and is vitamin B_{12} independent **(8)**; the synthesis of $N^{5,10}$-methylene (5,10-CH$_2$THF) with Ser through the action of pyridoxal-5'-phosphate–dependent serine hydroxymethyltransferase **(9)**; reduction of 5,10-CH$_2$THF into 5-CH$_3$THF catalyzed by $N^{5,10}$-methylene THF reductase **(10)**.

cobalamin (vitamin B_{12}) acts as a cofactor; remethylation to methionine is catalyzed by N^5-methyltetrahydrofolate-homocysteine methyltransferase (methionine synthase). This enzyme is widely distributed; inherited deficiencies in enzymes necessary for Hcy remethylation can result in elevated blood levels of Hcy.

One of the major regulators of methionine metabolism is SAM, an allosteric activator of CBS *(3,4)* in the transsulfuration pathway, and an allosteric inhibitor of MTHFR activity *(5,6)*. This highly coordinated regulation helps remethylation of Hcy in low tissue concentration of methionine, while in high concentration the transsulfuration pathway allows the catabolism of surplus Hcy by conversion to other thiols *(3,7)*. Vitamin B_6 is required for an optimal transsulfuration, while vitamin B_2, B_{12} and folates are necessary for an efficient remethylation of Hcy to methionine.

This methionine cycle plays an important role in regulating several cellular functions. In fact, methionine metabolism provides SAM, the most predominant methyl donor in the human body (within cells), which provides its methyl group to more than 100 transmethylation reactions, including DNA, RNA, phospholipids, and necessary intermediates in polyamine synthesis. The remethylation of Hcy to form methionine is essential for folate cycling. Finally, the methionine cycle, feeding the transsulfuration pathway, leads to the synthesis of cysteine and glutathione (GSH), the latter representing the main cellular soluble thiol that acts as scavenger nucleophile, protecting cells against hypoxia, toxicity, many carcinogens, and mutagenicity or transformation by radiation.

1.2. Different Forms of Hcy in Human Plasma — The Redox Thiol Status

Hcy has been found to exist in plasma in several forms. Protein-bound *(8)* (disulfide-linked) Hcy accounts for 70–80% of the total pool, mainly bound to albumin *(9–11)*. Only a small amount (1–4%) of reduced Hcy is present, while the free oxidized fraction (about 30%) is represented by the dimer homocystine and mainly by mixed disulfides with cysteine *(12–15)*. Normal total plasma Hcy concentrations range in the normal population from 5–15 μM in the fasting state. In the transsulfuration pathway, Hcy is metabolized to GSH (**Fig. 1**) via cysteine. The GSH breakdown catalyzed by γ-glutamyltranspeptidase, forms cysteinylglycine, which, together with cysteine, Hcy, and GSH, represents the main aminothiol pool circulating in plasma and metabolically associated. These aminothiols and their interrelationship include a definite entity indicated as plasma redox-thiol status *(16)*.

The presence of reduced Hcy and the dynamic relation that exists among Hcy, cysteine, and related compounds in plasma suggest that plasma concentration and protein binding of aminothiols are mutually regulated. This regulation allows optimal amounts of these compounds for cellular function and exerts cell protection against toxic concentrations of Hcy and disulfides.

Hyperhomocysteinemia is responsible for variation in redox state of aminothiols *(17)* and may also have implications for the use of plasma Hcy in laboratory diagnosis. Experimental *(18,19)* and clinical studies *(11)* suggest that Hcy bound with plasma proteins shows some peculiar features, character-ized by transient reduction in protein-bound cysteine and cysteinylglycine during transient hyperhomocysteinemia (as during methionine loading). Bind-ing of the Hcy seems to be saturable, the maximal binding capacity being about 140 µmol/L *(11)*, and is associated with decreases in protein-bound cysteine and cysteinylglycine, indicating displacement of cysteine from its binding sites *(20)*. These findings indicate that proteins, preferentially interacting with Hcy, may buffer moderate fluctuations of circulating reduced Hcy and exert a protection of endothelial cells against transient increases of Hcy. However, when the binding capacity of Hcy approaches saturation, the free oxidized form and, in particular, the reduced Hcy increase exponentially as function of total Hcy (tHcy).

A positive linear relationship between the reduced/total Hcy ratio and plasma concentrations of the aminothiol forms has been found *(20)*. Unbalance among the different species of aminothiols may cause pathophysiological consequences. Dynamic states among aminothiols have been observed in either chronic hyperhomocysteinemia caused by cobalamin deficiency *(21)* or hyperhomocystinuria *(22)* or transient hyperhomocysteinemia postmethionine load (PML) *(23)*. Changes in the equilibrium among aminothiols also have been observed in hyperhomocysteinemic patients with vascular diseases *(17,24)* in which a decreased ratio of reduced/total Hcy has been documented.

These observations and the fast variation in redox equilibrium of thiols, which can occur in a few minutes *(25)*, indicates that the redox status of aminothiols may affect other sulfhydryl groups, including those of essential enzymes for their function or of structural proteins.

The vascular damage that occurs in hyperhomocysteinemic patients may be caused by a cascade effect elicited by the above-mentioned mechanisms.

1.3. Short Clinical and Methodological Accounts

Carson and Neill *(26)* and Gerritsen et al. *(27)* first described the clinical observation of homocystinuria as the first metabolic mistake of methionine associated with abnormal urinary excretion of homocystine and Hcy. In homocystinuric subjects, ectopia lentis, skeletal deformities, mental retarda-tion, thromboembolism, and severe, premature atherosclerosis are observed. High urinary concentrations of this aminothiol were assayed with a simple chemical analysis *(28)*, and in 1955 a method for Hcy determination in biologi-cal tissues became available, by conversion of Hcy to thiolactone, measured by spectrophotometric method *(29)*.

In 1964 Mudd et al. recognized the first genetic basis for homocystinuria, the inherited deficiency of CBS *(30)*. In 1969 McCully made the clinical observation linking elevated plasma Hcy concentration with vascular diseases *(31)*. He described autopsy evidence of extensive arterial thrombosis and atherosclerosis in two children with high plasma Hcy concentrations and homocystinuria.

In the middle 70s, the introduction of second generation of amino acid analyzers made possible the determination of free Hcy in the acid-soluble fraction of plasma *(32,33)*.

The initial clinical studies supporting the relationship between mild plasma hyperhomocysteinemia and increased cardiovascular risk were based on this methodological approach *(34–37)*.

During the last 25 yr the progress in research dealing with Hcy has been greatly facilitated by the introduction of new and optimized techniques that involve chromatographic methods with (a) postcolumn derivatization with ninidrine *(38–40)* and S-pyridinium derivatives *(17,41,42)*; (b) precolumn derivatization with adenosine *(10)*, N-methyl-N-(tert-butyldimethylsilyl) trifluoroacetamide *(43)*, o-phthaldialdehyde *(44)*, monobromobimane *(13, 45–49)*, and halogenated sulfonyl benzofurazanes *(12, 50–59)*; (c) without derivatization with an electrochemical detector *(19, 60–64)*. Recently, completely automatic immunoenzymatic methods have been developed *(65–67)*. All of the aforementioned methods have been employed for tHcy assay in an increasing amount of biological samples in more than 100 epidemiological or clinical studies; however, only the chromatographic methods have been able to assay, in addition to Hcy, the other thiols present in plasma or in urine and to measure the reduced, free oxidized or protein-bound species *(13,40,47)*.

At present, while much methodological effort has been directed toward the achievement of fully automatic, specific, and sensitive methods, growing interest has been raised in the correlation between different methods developed in different laboratories or with commercially available kits *(68,69)*. Unfortunately, the tested interlaboratory variability has been shown to be too high for correct interpretation concerning the risk for development or progression of cardiovascular disease in a patient *(70)*.

1.4. Hyperhomocysteinemia and Atherogenesis

Since McCully *(31)* first observed that mild to moderately high levels of Hcy could be associated with increased cardiovascular risk, and the pioneering study of Wilcken and Wilcken *(34)* showed that abnormal Hcy concentration after methionine loading could identify patients with coronary artery disease, a number of epidemiological and clinical studies have addressed the importance of moderate hyperhomocysteinemia as an independent risk factor for myocardial infarction, stroke, peripheral vascular disease, and total mortality *(9,15,36–38,71–94)*.

Although the precise molecular mechanisms and the relation between hyperhomocysteinemia and atherogenesis are still undetermined, several pieces of epidemiological evidence suggest that Hcy is atherogenic and not simply a marker of increased vascular risk. Hcy seems to play an important role in endothelial vascular dysfunction through different mechanism involving smooth muscle cell proliferation *(95)*, platelet activation, and leukocyte plugging *(96–102)*. Hcy auto-oxidation has been shown to facilitate the oxidation of low-density lipoproteins *(103,104)* and alter the normal antithrombotic phenotype of the endothelium by enhancing the activities of factor XII *(105)* and factor V *(106,107)* and depressing the activation of protein C *(108)*. Hcy inhibits the expression of thrombomodulin cofactor activity *(109)*; induces the expression of tissue factor *(110)*; suppresses the expression of heparan sulfate *(110)*, of antithrombin III, and von Willebrand factor *(110,111)*; all of these effects facilitate the formation of thrombin and create a prothrombotic environment.

Hcy is rapidly auto-oxidized when added to plasma, forming homocystine, mixed disulfides and Hcy thiolactone *(17)*. In physiological conditions, Hcy in the presence of O_2 reacts with nitric oxide (NO), to form S-nitroso-Hcy. The production of S-nitroso-Hcy inhibits the formation of hydrogen peroxide *(112)* and platelet aggregation; furthermore, S-nitroso-Hcy is also a potent vasodilator *(113)*.

Hcy promotes lipid peroxidation, which may decrease the expression of endothelial NO synthase, reducing the bioavailability of NO for vascular dilation *(104,114,115)*.

The expression of GSH peroxidase (Gpx), the key enzyme in the intracellular anti-oxidant defense, is suppressed by high concentrations of plasma Hcy but not cysteine, even in much higher concentrations of the latter in the endothelial cells *(116)*. As previously mentioned, Hcy is the only thiol able to form a cyclic compound by auto-oxidation: Hcy-thiolactone. The cyclic thioester, which can be formed in conditions of hyperhomocysteinemia, has been shown to react with primary amines, forming with an amide linkage, a homocystamide protein adduct *(117)*. It has been reported that Hcy-thiolactone is capable of modifying low-density lipoprotein to a form able to generate foam cells *(118)*, which, in turn, promote reactive oxygen species, including superoxide anion and hydrogen peroxide *(119)*. These data indicate that auto-oxidation of Hcy produces cytotoxic effects that may play a causal role in the genesis of thrombosis and atherosclerosis.

1.5. Principles for the Determination of tHcy and Other Thiols

In a clinical setting, it is useful not only to assess tHcy level in fasting blood samples, but also after a methionine loading test, in which the metabolism is stressed by oral administration of methionine (0.1 g L-methionine/kg body wt or 3.8 g/m² surface area).

PML tHcy concentrations are preferentially determined at peak levels (4–8 h) after injection of methionine. This test, which was originally designed to discriminate heterozygotes for CBS deficiency from healthy individuals *(120,121)*, improves the ability to distinguish between normal individuals and subjects with mild abnormalities of the Hcy metabolism *(121,122–127)*.

Hyperhomocysteinemia, in most studies defined as a tHcy concentration above the 80th–90th percentile of the control group, in the fasting state, is supposed to reflect abnormalities in Hcy remethylation, whereas an abnormal Hcy increase upon PML is considered to reflect defects in Hcy transsulfuration. Because of the existence of a cellular Hcy export mechanism in fasting state, plasma normally contains a small amount of tHcy, averaging 10 µM *(128)*. The increases in reference values for Hcy above fasting levels in PML have been less extensively studied. It is worthwhile for each laboratory to determine its own values in a normal population with standardized vitamin intake, to assess the upper limits of tHcy both in fasting and PML.

The principles of procedures for tHcy determination that may be applied to measurement of other thiols, such as cysteine, GSH, and cysteinylglycine, described in the following paragraphs, include sample collection and storage, reduction of oxidized forms of Hcy, the next derivatization of free sulfhydryl groups, and the HPLC assay by means of an isocratic method.

2. Materials

Homocystine standard, Tri-n-butylphosphine (TBP), dimethylformamide, ammonium-7- fluorobenzo-2-oxa-1,3-diazole-4-sulfonate (SBD-F), potassium dihydrogenphosphate, acetonitrile (CH_3CN), sodium hydroxide (NaOH), boric acid, ethylendiaminotetracetic acid sodium salts (EDTA), trichloroacetic acid (TCA), sodium chloride (NaCl), physiological solution (NaCl 0,14M) were purchased from Fluka (Sigma - Aldrich, Milan, Italy).

2.1. Plasma Sample Reduction and Derivatization

1. Reducing solution: 50 µL TBP in 450 µL dimethylformamide. This reagent is stable at 4°C for 2–3 d.
2. Precipitating solution: 10 g TCA and 0.0372 g EDTA dissolved in 100 mL distilled water. Solution is stored at room temperature.
3. 1.55 M NaOH: 6.2 g NaOH dissolved in 100 mL distilled water. Solution is stored at room temperature.
4. 1 M borate buffer: 100 mL oversaturated boric acid solution (61.83g/L), 0.15 mg EDTA, adjust pH to 11 with 5 M NaOH (200 g/L). Solution is stored at room temperature.
5. Derivatizing solution: 10 mg SBD-F dissolved in 1 mL borate buffer 0.125 M (7.73 g/L boric acid), adjust pH to 9.5 with 5 M NaOH. Solution must be stored at 4°C in the dark.

2.2. Analysis

1. Mobile phase: 13.61 g potassium dihydrogen phosphate in 1 L distilled water. Discard 90 mL of this solution and replace with 90 mL CH_3CN. Adjust pH to 2.1

with concentrated orthophosphoric acid and filter using Millipore membrane filters (pore size 0.22 μm). Use at room temperature but store at 4°C.

2. Washing solution: 700 mL CH$_3$CN in 300 mL distilled water.
3. Hcy standard solution (Hcystd) 300 μM homocysteine solution (corresponding to 600 μM Hcy solution) is employed as stock solution.
4. Working solution of Hcy is prepared by dissolving 4 mg Hcystd in 5 mL methanol then adding 45 mL 0.1 M HCl.

2.3. Apparatus

A Pro Star 240 HPLC Solvent Delivery Module coupled to a Pro Star 410 HPLC Autosampler (Varian, Inc., Walnut Creek California USA) was fitted with a Supelcosil Discovery LC-18 analytical column (250 mm × 4.6 mm I.D. Supelco, Sigma - Aldrich). Fluorescence intensities were measured using a Pro Star 360 Fluorimetric Detector coupled to a Star Chromatography Workstation (Varian).

3. Methods
3.1. Preanalytical Steps
3.1.1. Sample Collection

1. After overnight fasting, collect blood samples (up to 500 μL) into evacuated tubes containing EDTA, and gently mix (*see* **Notes 1** and **2**).
2. Separate plasma immediately by centrifugation at 1500–3000g for 5 min.
3. Store plasma samples at –20°C until tHcy analysis.

3.1.2. Sample Preparation

Plasma sample reduction and derivatization.

1. Mix plasma sample (100 μL) with 10 μL reducing solution (*see* **Note 3**) and incubate at 4°C for 30 min.
2. Add 100 μL precipitating solution, mix, and centrifuge at 5000–10000g for 15 or 5 min, respectively, to remove proteins.
3. Mix the clear supernatant (100 μL) with 10 μL 1.55 M NaOH and 100 μL borate buffer (1 M) and 10 μL of derivatizing solution (*see* **Note 4**).
4. Heat the final reaction mixture at 60°C for 60 min.
5. Cool at 4°C for 15 min before HPLC analysis with fluorescence detection. The adducts are stable for 1 d at room temperature, in the dark, and for several mo at –20°C.

Calibration

Either a physiological solution or pooled plasma with low levels of Hcy may be used to create the standard curve for calibration (*see* **Notes 7** and **8**).

1. Add 50 μL stock solution to 450 μL physiological solution or pooled plasma (v/v 1:10) to obtain the first point of the calibration curve (corresponding to 60 μM Hcystd).

2. Make the following dilutions (30, 15, 7.5, 3.75 μM) to obtain data for the remaining curve points.
3. Perform reduction and derivatization as described above for plasma samples (*see* **Note 5**).

3.2. Analytical Steps

3.2.1. High-Performance Liquid Chromatography (HPLC)

1. Condition the analytical column with mobile phase at a flow rate of 1 mL/min.
2. Set the excitation (Ex) and emission (Em) wavelengths on a fluorometric detector at 385 and 515 nm, respectively, for optimal response of the derivatives.
3. Inject 5–20 μL plasma samples or standards (*see* **Note 6**) into the analytical column.
4. Run at a flow rate of 1 mL/min at room temperature for 5–10 min.
5. The column can be used for up to 20 injections.
6. Wash the column for 10 min at a flow rate of 1 mL/min and leave the solution in the column for storage.
7. Obtain HPLC chromatograms: (a) blank sample; (b) standard mix; (c) low level of Hcy plasma sample; (d) high level of Hcy plasma sample (**Fig. 2**).

3.3. Statistical Analysis

Hcy sample concentration is obtained from peak area (or height) and automatically calculated by the software. Sample concentration is obtained from the peak area or the height of the calibration curve points (linear regression with least square estimation) (*see* **Notes 9–11**; **Fig. 3**). It is necessary to subtract the peak area of pooled plasma containing Hcy from each standard curve point (**Fig. 3**). Alternately, linear regression can be calculated manually using **Table 1**.

$$\text{Linear Regression} = y = bx + a \qquad (1)$$

where y = dependent variable value [concentration of Hcystd (μM)]
  x = independent variable value (tHcy chromatogram peak area or height)
  a = intercept
  b = slope

$$b = \frac{\Sigma x_i y_i - (\Sigma x_i)(\Sigma y_i)/n}{\Sigma x_i^2 - (\Sigma x_i)^2/n}$$

where n = sum cases

$$b = \frac{4513.35 - (107.95 \times 116.25)/5}{(4252.16 - 11653/5)} = 1.04 \quad (2)$$

$a = Y - bX$
$a = 23.25 - (1.04 \times 21.59) = 0.73 \qquad (3)$

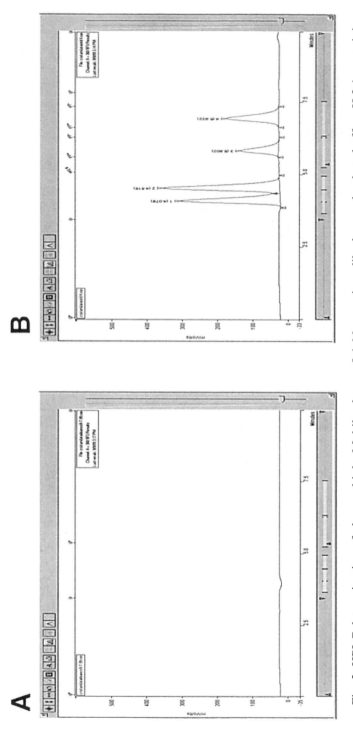

Fig. 2. HPLC determination of plasma thiols. Mobile phase = 0.1 M potassium dihydrogenphophate buffer pH 2.1, containing 80 mL/L acetonitrile. The analysis was carried out on Discovery column (250 × 4.6 m I. D., 5 µm) at flow rate of 1 mL/min. Excitation wavelength = 385 nm, emission wavelength = 515 nm. Peaks from left to right: (*1*) cysteine; (*2*) cysteinylglycine; (*3*) homocysteine; (*4*) glutathione. Chromatograms: (**A**) blank; (**B**) standards;

(continued)

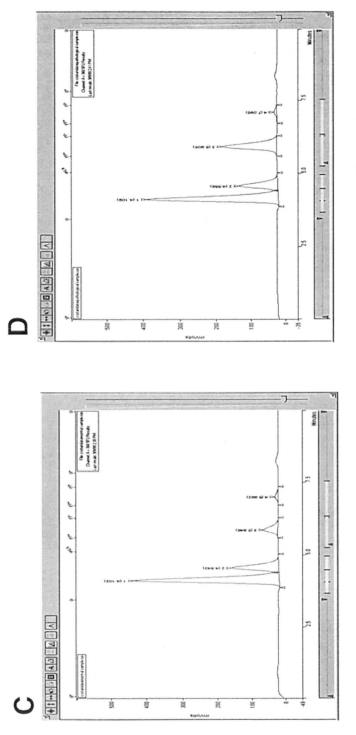

Fig. 2 (*continued from opposite page*); (**C**) sample with low Hcy level; (**D**) sample with high Hcy level.

87

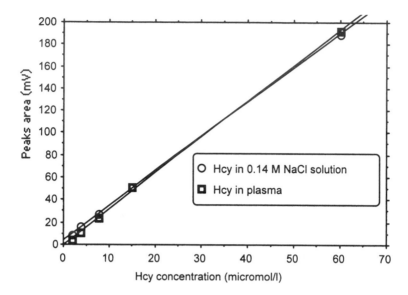

Fig. 3. Linear regression analysis performed by addition of Hcy increasing concentration. (1-60 μM) to a 0.14 M NaCl solution, pH 7.2 (O),or to a plasma. (□).

Table 1
Standard Concentrations and Relative Areas of Hcystd

N	Concentration (yi)	Area (xi)	yi2	xi2	yixi
1	60	56.37	3600.00	3177.58	3382.20
2	30	28.83	900.00	831.17	864.90
3	15	14.37	225.00	206.50	215.55
4	75	5.14	56.25	26.42	38.55
5	3.75	3.24	14.06	10.50	12.15
Total	116.25	107.95	4795.31	4252.16	4513.35

inserting values from (2) and (3) into equation 1, we obtain:

$$y = 1.04 \, x + 0.73 \qquad (4)$$

Plasma Hcy sample concentration is obtained by inserting in (4) Hcy peak area instead of independent variable x.

To evaluate the relation between the two variables (dependent and independent) the correlation coefficient (R) is calculated.

$$R = \frac{\Sigma xiyi - (\Sigma xi)(\Sigma yi)/n}{[\,(\Sigma xi^2 - (\Sigma xi)^2/n)\,(\Sigma yi^2 - (\Sigma yi)^2/n)\,]^{1/2}} \qquad (5)$$

This value can range from −1 to +1; R = 0 represents the independence between two variables.

Using areas and concentrations from **Table 1**:

$$R = \frac{4513.35 - (107.95 \times 116.25)/5}{[(4252.16 - 107.95/5)\ (4795.31 - 116.25/5)]^{1/2}} = \mathbf{0.99}$$

4. Notes

4.1. Sample Collection and Storage

1. Blood collection and processing are the most important and delicate phases of the preanalytical steps. Several studies *(48,129)* show the importance of collecting blood in prechilled EDTA-containing tubes followed by immediate centrifugation. Under these conditions, the separation of plasma and blood cells will prevent false-positive results that otherwise may reflect the intracellular erythrocyte Hcy synthesis and release *(43,128–131)*. This process is slowed when blood samples are left on ice. Plasma kept at 4°C does not show increased Hcy for 4 h. Sodium and lithium fluoride *(131)* added as stabilizer for Hcy, in evacuated tubes containing heparin as an anticoagulant, are inadequate *(132)*. Others suggest that acidified citrate at pH 4.3 can be considered a whole-blood preservative because it inhibits the rise in Hcy over time to a degree similar to that obtained by storage on crushed ice *(133)*. However, the authors noted a difference (up to 10%) between the mean baseline concentration of tHcy measured in EDTA-treated blood that was stored at 0°C, and tHcy concentrations in blood taken in acidic citrate that was stored at room temperature. A recent report *(127)* proposes a specially prepared blood collecting system, in which the blood sample is lysed by adding Nonidet P4O/EDTA/citric acid solution to inhibit Hcy generating and converting enzymes at the time of venipuncture. The authors, who stabilize Hcy concentration for 48 h at room temperature and without correction for hematocrit, found Hcy lysate values that are correlated (the square/correlation coefficient > 0.9) with plasma EDTA Hcy values. However, they found Hcy concentrations in lysed blood lower than in plasma and concluded that it will be necessary to perform prospective studies in a larger patient population *(134)*. For all these reasons, we believe that storage of the blood sample on wet ice at 2–4°C in the refrigerator after venipuncture, along with rapid centrifugation and separation of the plasma, is the only currently available means of providing accurate tHcy measurements.
2. There is no problem in stabilizing plasma samples because the tHcy in these biological fluids is stable for at least 4 d at room temperature, for several weeks at 4°C, and for years at −20°C *(129)*.

4.2. Reduction of Sulfhydryl Groups (-SH)

3. At present there is no reagent able to reduce disulfur bridges in sulfhydryl groups without complications. Moreover, the selection of reductant depends on the

separation and detection system used. Sulfhydryl-containing reducing agents such as dithioerythritol, dithiothreitol, and mercaptoethanol form adducts with thiol-specific reagents and therefore may consume derivatization reagent and interfere with the chromatographic elution of other thiols; sodium borohydride forms gas during the reaction, creating practical problems. TBP, the reductant chosen for this method, neither reacts with thiol-specific reagents nor forms gas during reaction; however, it is an irritant and toxic because of N, N-dimethyl formamide. Instead of TBP, it is sufficient to use a newer phosphine reagent, tris(2-carboxylethyl)phosphine, that is stable and soluble in aqueous solution *(134)*. The sulfhydryl group formed during the reduction step can be reoxidized before derivatization or detection, and variable reoxidation is a source of spurious results; thiol oxidation is catalyzed by many transition metals; inclusion of EDTA in the reaction mixture chelates divalent metals and inhibits oxidation.

4.3. Derivatization with SBD-F

4. At present, there is no universally accepted derivative reagent, but the procedure using SBD-F for measuring the concentration of Hcy in aqueous solution is an attractive possibility, because of the high selectivity of the fluorogen for sulfhydryl groups, and because SBD-F itself and its hydrolysis products do not provide peaks in the chromatographs. SBD-F is less reactive than 7-fluoro-2,1,3-benzoxadiazole-4-sulfonamide (ABD-F) and requires more drastic condition (pH 9.5 at 60°C for 1 h instead of pH 8–9.5 at 50°C for 10 min for ABD-F); furthermore, it is not reactive toward amines *(135)*, whereas ABD-F derivatizes amines, giving low fluorescence yields *(136)*. Like halogeno-sulfonylbenzofurazans, among the fluorogenic reagents available, bimanes are specific for sulfhydryl groups and produce a highly fluorescent thioether. One drawback is represented by the reagent itself: The hydrolysis products and the impurities are fluorescent, and these materials give rise to several reagent peaks that may interfere with Hcy determination.

5. All fluorescent adducts are light sensitive, and this behavior is different among different thiols. For this reason, it is important to keep samples in the dark after derivatization, allowing the Hcy-SBD adducts to be stable for 1 d at room temperature or for several days at 4°C, or for months at –20°C. SBD-derivatives remain stable for 3 d at room temperature, using 0.4 M orthophosphoric acid *(58)*. The stability of the Hcy-SBD adducts, and the very high resolution of chromatographic separation without interfering peaks, give these reagents the advantage.

4.4. Calibration Curves in Physiological/Plasma Solution

6. For a reliable comparison of measured plasma Hcy concentrations from different laboratories, use of the same accepted calibrator for Hcy is recommended. Because of the high purity of commercially available homocystine, its chemical stability, and its ready conversion to Hcy with reductants, this compound appears to be the most appropriate to calibrate Hcy assays.

7. During preparation of the calibration curves, it has been observed that addition of thiols to buffer or to physiological solution yielded 20% less fluorescence than when the same amounts were added to plasma *(44,51,53)*. This has been attributed to the presence of the plasma proteins, ionic strength, or other species affecting the derivation step, and for these reasons use of plasma-based calibrators is recommended.

8. Because the method reported here shows no differences in the calibration slopes between physiological solution and plasma, it is simpler and equally effective to dilute Hcystd (calibrators) in physiological solution. This is probably due to the high ionic strength of borate buffer (1 *M*) used in the present method; in fact, lowering the borate buffer molarity increases the difference between the two calibration curve slopes. The same phenomenon occurs when the proteins in the plasma sample are precipitated by less concentrated (1%) TCA, instead of TCA at 10% (data not shown). Therefore, the calibration slopes for Hcy diluted in two different matrices are indistinguishable from each other when borate buffer (1 *M*) and TCA 10% are used **(Fig. 3)**.

4.5. Validation Studies

9. The linearity of the method has been evaluated by addition of increasing concentrations of Hcystd (1–120 μM) to physiological solution. A linear regression analysis yielded y= ax+b (r=1), where x is the peak area and y the concentration of SBD-Hcy (fluorescence intensity vs thiol concentration μmol/L).

10. The absolute detection limit is related to the fluorimetric detector performance. In our laboratory, the absolute detection limit, determined as three times the baseline noise level, was 20 pmol for Hcy. The performance of the assay system was monitored by including control samples. These samples were spiked with known concentrations of Hcy. Blank runs (containing no thiol compounds) gave no peaks under the same chromatographic conditions **(Fig. 2A)**.

11. Intra-assay precision was calculated by performing 10 different extractions of pooled plasma samples on the same day. The coefficient of variation [C.V. (%)] was 1.2 for Hcy. Inter-assay precision was calculated using the results from 10 separate determinations obtained within a 1-mo period; the C.V. was 2.8 for tHcy.

12. The recovery test was performed adding known Hcy concentrations (ranging from 7–70 μM) to the same plasma sample (n=10); analytical recovery, calculated as recovery % = 100× (tHcy + Hcystd)–(tHcy/Hcystd), was ~100%.

4.6. HPLC of tHcy with or without Internal Standard

13. The question "with or without" internal standard (I.S.) for the determination of plasma thiols rises from two main considerations: (1) the rate of oxidation of various thiols is different, and (2) the light sensitivity of the SBD-adducts is different. For these reasons, some authors believe that a sulfhydryl compound used as I.S. may have a different behavior with respect to Hcy, altering the analytical result *(134–137)*. In a previous study *(56)* three sulfhydryl compounds, α-

mercaptopropionylglycine (MPG), 2-mercaptoethylamine (ME), and N-acetylcysteine (NAC), were evaluated to determine whether the use of an I.S. could improve precision. To elute these I.S., we had to apply different chromatographic conditions that lengthen the analysis by up to 4 to 5 times with respect to the isocratic condition without I.S. (data not shown). The intra-assay precision of a single I.S., tested on 10 replicates for each, was 3.7, 4.5, and 2.5% for MPE, NAC and ME, respectively. The C.V. of plasma tHcy using MPE, NAC, and ME as internal recovery standards (10 replicates of each I.S.) was higher than without: 6.5, 5.1, and 4.5 for tHcy + MPE, tHcy +NAC, and tHcy+ME, respectively. These results indicate that the present method with I.S. is less reproducible than the one without I.S.

4.7. Correlation with Other HPLC and Immunoenzymatic Methods

14. The method without I.S. was applied in two different laboratories on two different HPLC systems equipped with different fluorescence detectors. The results obtained on 50 assays showed a good agreement (r=0.998). Moreover, 50 samples with low and high tHcy concentrations were tested with a different HPLC (Bio-Rad Labs) and immunoenzymatic methods. The correlation coefficient was 0.997 and 0.995, respectively.

4.8. Measurement of Plasma tHcy

15. This method has been tested in different HPLC systems; SBD-tHcy measurement generally does not require sensitive fluorometric detectors. If one of these detectors is used, a small amount of sample has to be injected. If the intra-assay C.V. is less than 1% it will be possible to inject up to 1 µL of sample. These conditions allow less frequent washing of columns (10 times less), increasing column life. Since this method is devoid of I.S. a calibration curve (or almost two points of this) and two controls at different levels of Hcy concentration (10–30 µ*M*) should be repeated every analytical session. It is also important to acquire a control population without risk factors or previous vascular diseases to obtain the reference range. On 163 normal volunteers, blood withdrawals for Hcy have been performed, as described in **Subheadings 3.1.1.** and **4.1.** An incremental curve and a subsequent decrease in tHcy concentration have been determined PML, with replicates withdrawals on 20 subjects. Several samples showed maximal tHcy concentration at 8 h, but for the sake of simplicity the fourth h PML has been chosen. Mean reference values before and PML are 11 µ*M* and 30 µ*M*, respectively. The percentile values for fasting and PML are represented in **Table 2**.

4.9. Micromethods for Newborns

16. The present method, used routinely for tHcy determination in adults, can be modified to process very small amounts of newborn plasma samples. A blood sample from heel capillary circulation is collected generally in the fourth day of life,

Table 2
Fasting and PML Hcy Mean Reference Values

Volunteers	N	10th% μM	25th% μM	50th% μM	75th% μM	90th% μM	97th% μM
Fasting	163	6.52	7.46	9.23	10.69	12.34	22
PML	163	15.86	18.27	22.4	27.39	33	50

using a heparinized capillary glass tube, and centrifuged. Sample collection: 10 µL of plasma samples (instead of 100 µL in adults) is added to 90 µL physiological solution and 10 µL of reducing solution (incubation at 4°C for 30 min). After incubation, proteins are removed by precipitation adding 100 µL precipitating solution, mixed and centrifuged at 5000–10000*g* for 15 or 5 min, respectively. The clear supernatant (100 µL) is mixed with 10 µL 1.55 M NaOH , 100 µL borate buffer (1M), and then derivatized by adding 10 µL derivatizing solution. This final reaction mixture is heated at 60°C for 60 min, then cooled at 4°C for 15 min before HPLC analysis with fluorescence detection at room temperature. 50 µL stock solution (**Subheading 3.1.2.**) is added to 1450 µL physiological solution to obtain the first point of calibration curve (corresponding to 20 µ*M* Hcystd); the following curve points (10, 5, 2.5, 1.25 µ*M*) are obtained making dilutions (v/v) with physiological solution. The calibration curve is subjected to reduction and derivatization as described for plasma samples.

This method shows linearity in a range from 1 to 10 µL plasma samples. If plasma volume is less than 10 µL, it is possible to use the same calibration curve by making up the volume with physiological solution; sample is processed as described above and finally injected using volumes inversely related to the starting plasma volumes. For instance, if the fluorometric detector sensitivity allows injection of 5 µL SBD-adduct in normal conditions (10 µL plasma), 50 µL will be injected if 1 µL plasma is the starting sample volume (2 µL plasma injection of 25 µL, etc). Intra-assay and inter-assay precision is 4.5% and 7.2%, respectively. The recovery test is performed using known Hcy concentrations ranging from 1 to 30 µ*M* to the same plasma sample (n = 10); analytical recovery is 95%. The mean value obtained from heel capillary circulation of 768 newborns collected in the fourth day of life is 4.98 ± 2.63 µ*M* (range 0.7–17.85 µ*M*). The percentile values are: 25th = 3.13, 50th = 4.43, 75th = 6.21, and 97th = 11.98 µ*M*.

References

1. Finkelstein, J. D. and Martin, J. J. (1986) Methionine metabolism in mammals. Adaptation to methionine excess. *J. Biol. Chem.* **261,**1582–1587.
2. Skiba, W. E., Taylor, M. P., Wells, M. S., Mangum, J. H., and Award, W. M., (1982) Human hepatic methionine biosynthesis. Purification and characterization of betaine: homocysteine S-methyltransferase. *J. Biol. Chem.* **257,** 14944–14948.

3. Finkelstein, J. D. and Martin J. J. (1984) Methionine metabolism in mammals. Distribution of homocysteine between competing pathways. *J. Biol. Chem.* **259,** 9508–9513.

4. Finkelstein, J. D., Kyle, W. E., Martin, J. J., and Pick, A. (1975) Activation of cystathionine synthase by adenosylmethionine and adenosylethionine. *Biochem. Byophys. Res. Commun.* **66,** 81–87.

5. Kutzbach, C. and Stokstad, E. L. R. (1971) Mammalian methylenetetrahydrofolate reductase. Partial purification, proprieties, and inhibition by S-adenosylmethionine. *Biochim. Biophys. Acta.* **250,** 459–477.

6. Jencks, D. A. and Matthews, R. G. (1987) Allosteric inhibition of methylenetetra-hydrofolate reductase by adenosylmethionine. Effects of adenosylmethionine and NADPH on the equilibrium between active and inactive forms of the enzyme and on the kinetics of approach to equilibrium. *J. Biol. Chem.* **2625,** 2485–2493.

7. Selhub, J. and Miller, J. W. (1992) The pathogenesis of homocysteinemia: interruption of the coordinate regulation by S-adenosylmethionine of the remethylation and transsulfuration of homocysteine. *Am. J. Clin. Nutr.* **55,** 131–138.

8. Kang, S. S., Wong, P. W. K., and Beker, N. (1979) Protein-bound homocysteine in normal subjects and in patients with homocystinuria. *Pediatr. Res.* **13,** 1141–1143.

9. Araki, A., Sako, Y., Fukushima, Y., Matsumoto, M., Asada, T., and Kita, T. (1989) Plasma sulfhydryl-containing amino acids in patients with cerebral infarction and in hypertensive subjects. *Atherosclerosis* **79,** 139–146.

10. Refsum, H., Hellands, S., and Ueland, P. M. (1985) Radioenzymic determination of homocysteine in plasma and urine. *Clin. Chem.* **31,** 624–628.

11. Wiley, V. C., Dudman, N. P. B., and Wilcken, D. E. L. (1988) Interrelations between plasma free and protein-bound homocysteine and cysteine in homocystinuria. *Metabolism* **37,** 191–195.

12. Araki, A. and Sako, Y. (1987) Determination of free and total homocysteine in human plasma by high-performance liquid chromatography with fluorescence detection. *J. Chromatogr.* **422,** 43–52.

13. Mansoor, M. A., Svardal, A. M., and Ueland, P. M. (1992) Determination of the in vivo redox status of cysteine, cysteinylglycine, homocysteine and glutathione in human plasma. *Anal. Biochem.* **200,** 218–229.

14. Mansoor, M. A., Svardal, A. M., Schneede, J., and Ueland, P. M. (1992) Dynamic relation between reduced, oxidized and protein-bound homocysteine and other thiol components in plasma during methionine loading in healthy men. *Clin. Chem.* **38,** 1316–1321.

15. Murphy-Chutorian, D. R., Wexman, M. P., Grieco, A. J., Heininger, J. A. B., Glassman, E., Gaull, G. E., Ng, S. K., Feit, F., Wexman, K., and Fox, A. C. (1985) Methionine intolerance: A possible risk factor for coronary artery disease. *J. Am. Coll. Cardiol.* **6,** 725–730.

16. Ueland, P. M. (1995) Homocysteine species as component of plasma redox thiol status. *Clin. Chem.* **41,** 340–342.

17. Andersson, A., Lindgren, A., and Hultberg, B. (1995) Effect of thiol oxidation and thiol export from erythrocytes on determination of redox status of homocysteine and other thiols in plasmas from healthy subjects and patients with cerebral infarction. *Clin. Chem.* **41,** 361–366.

18. Smolin, L. A. and Benevenga, N. J. (1982) Accumulation of homocyst(e)ine in vitamin B-6 deficiency: A model for the study of cystathionine beta-synthase deficiency. *J. Nutr.* **112,** 1264–1272.

19. Smolin, L. A. and Benevenga, N. J. (1984) The use of cysteine in the removal of protein-bound homocysteine. *Am. J. Clin. Nutr.* **39,** 730–737.

20. Ueland, P. M., Mansoor, A. M., Guttormsen, A. B., Muller, F., Aukrust, P., Refsum, H., and Svardal, M. (1996) Reduced, oxidized and protein-bound forms of homocysteine and other aminothiols in plasma comprise the redox thiol status. A possible element of the extracellular antioxidant defense system. *J. Nutr.* **126,** 1281S–1284S.

21. Mansoor, M., Ueland, P. M., and Svardal, A. M. (1994) Redox status and protein binding of plasma homocysteine and other aminothiols in patients with hyperhomocysteinemia due to cobalamin deficiency. *Am. J. Clin. Nutr.* **59,** 631–635.

22. Mansoor, M.A., Ueland, P. M., Aarsland, A., and Svardal, A. M. (1993) Redox status and protein binding of plasma homocysteine and other aminothiols in patients with homocystinuria. *Metabolism* **42,** 1481–1485.

23. Ueland, P. M. and Refsum, H. (1989) Plasma homocysteine, a risk factor for vascular disease: plasma levels in healt disease, and drug therapy. *J. Lab. Clin. Med.* **114,** 473–502.

24. Mansoor, M. A., Bergmark, C., Svardal, A. M., Lonning, P. E., and Ueland, P. M. (1995) Redox status and protein binding of plasma homocysteine and other aminothiols in patients with early-onset peripheral vascular disease. *Arterioscler. Thromb. Vasc. Biol.* **15,** 232–240.

25. Mansoor, M. A., Guttormsen, A. B., Fiskerstrand, T., Refsum, H., Ueland, P. M., and Svardal, A. M. (1993) Redox status and protein-binding of plasma aminothiols during the transient hyperhomocysteinemia that follows homocysteine administration. *Clin. Chem.* **39,** 980 985.

26. Carson, N. A. J. and Neill, D. W. (1962) Metabolic abnormalities detected in a survay of mentally backward individuals in Northern Ireland. *Arch. Dis. Child.* **37,** 505–513.

27. Gerritsen, T., Vaugn, J. G., and Waisman, H. A. (1962) The identification of homocystine in the urine. *Biochem. Biophys. Res. Commun.* **9,** 493–496.

28. Wannmacker, C. M. D., Wejner, M., Giuliani, R., and Filo, C. S. D. (1982) An improved specific laboratory test for homocystinuria. *Clin. Chim. Acta.* **125,** 367–369.

29. Raker, E. (1955) Glutathione-homocysteine transhydrogenase. *J. Biol. Chem.* **217,** 367–374.

30. Mudd, S. H., Finkelstein, J. D., Irreverre, F., and Laster, L. (1964) Homocystinuria an enzymatic defect. *Science* **143,** 1443–1445.

31. McCully, K. S. (1969) Vascular pathology of homocysteinemia: Implications for the pathogenesis of arteriosclerosis. *Am. J. Pathol.* **56,** 111–128.

32. Gupta, V. J. and Wilcken, D. E. L. (1978) The detection of cysteine-homocysteine mixed disulfide in plasma of normal fasting man. *Eur. J. Clin. Invest.* **8,** 205–207.

33. Wilcken, D. E. L. and Gupta, V. J. (1979) Cysteine-homocysteine mixed disulfide: differing plasma concentrations in normal men and women. *Clin. Sci.* **57,** 211–215.

34. Wilcken, D. E. and Wilcken, B. (1976) The pathogenesis of coronary artery disease. A possible role for methionine metabolism. *J. Clin. Invest.* **57,** 1079–1082.

35. Kang, S. S., Wong, P. W. K., and Curley, K. (1982) The effect of D-penicillamine on protein-bound homocyst(e)ine in homocystinurics. *Pediatr. Res.* **116,** 370–372.

36. Wilcken, D. E., Reddy, S. G., and Gupta, V. J. (1983) Homocysteinemia, ischemic heart disease, and the carrier state for homocystinuria. *Metabolism* **32,** 363–370.

37. Brattstrom, L. E., Hardebo, J. E., and Hultberg, B. L. (1984) Moderate homocysteinemia-a possible risk factor for arteriosclerotic cerebrovascular disease. *Stroke* **15,** 1012–1016.

38. Clarke, R., Daly, L., Robinson, K., Naughten, E., Cahalane, S., Fowler, B., and Graham, I. (1991) Hyperhomocysteinemia: an independent risk factor for vascular disease. *N. Engl. J. Med.* **324,** 1149–1155.

39. Andersson, A., Brattstrom, L., Israelsson, B., Isaksson, A., Hamfelt, A., and Hultberg, B. (1992) Plasma homocysteine before and after methionine loading with regard to age, gender, and menopausal status. *Eur. J. Clin. Invest.* **22,** 79–87.

40. Candito, M., Bedoucha, P., Mahagne, M. H., Scavini, G., and Chatel, M. (1997) Total plasma homocysteine determination by liquid chromatography before and after methionine loading. Results in cerebrovascular disease. *J. Chromatogr. Biomed. Appl.* **692,** 213–216.

41. Andersson, A., Isaksson, A., Brattstrom, L., and Hultberg, B. (1993) Homocysteine and other thiols determined in plasma by HPLC and thiol-specific postcolumn derivatization. *Clin. Chem.* **39,** 1590–1597.

42. Kaniowska, E., Chwatko, G., Glowacki, R., Kubalczyk, P., and Bald E. (1998) Urinary excretion measurement of cysteine and homocysteine in the form of their S-pyridinium derivatives by high-performance liquid chromatography with ultraviolet detection. *J. Chromatogr. A.* **798,** 27–35.

43. Stabler, S. P., Marcell, P. D., Podell, E. R., and Allen, R. H. (1987) Quantitation of total homocysteine, total cysteine and methionine in normal serum and urine using capillary gas chromatography mass-spectrometry. *Anal. Biochem.* **162,** 185–196.

44. Fermo, I., Arcelloni, C., De Vecchi, E., Vigano, S., and Paroni, R. (1992) High-performance liquid chromatographic method with fluorescence detection for the determination of total homocyst(e)ine in plasma. *J. Chromatogr.* **593,** 171–176.

45. Fahey, R. C., Newton, G. L., Dorian, R., and Kosower, E. M. (1981) Analysis of biological thiols: Quantitative determination of thiols at the picomole level based upon derivatization with monobromobimanes and separation by cation-exchange chromatography. *Anal. Biochem.* **111,** 57–65.

46. Velury, S. and Howell, S. B. (1988) Measurement of plasma thiols after derivatization with monobromobimane. *J. Chromatogr.* **424,** 141–146.

47. Jacobsen, D. W., Gatautis, V. J., and Green, R. (1989) Determination of plasma homocysteine by high-performance liquid chromatography with fluorescence detection. *Anal. Biochem.* **178**, 208–214.
48. Refsum, H., Ueland, P. M., and Svardal, A. M. (1989) Fully automated fluorescence assay for determining total homocysteine in plasma. *Clin. Chem.* **35**, 1921–1927.
49. Pastore, A., Massoud, R., Motti, C., Lo Russo, A., Fucci, G., Cortese, C., and Federici, G. (1998) Fully automated assay for total homocysteine, cysteine, cysteinylglycine, glutathione, cysteamine, and 2-mercaptopropionylglycine in plasma and urine. *Clin. Chem.* **44**, 825–832.
50. Ubbink, J. B., Vermaak, W. J. H., and Bissbort, S. (1991) Rapid high-performance liquid chromatographic assay for total homocysteine levels in human serum. *J. Chromatogr.* **565**, 441–446.
51. Durand, P., Fortin, L. J., Lussier-Cacan, S., Davignon, J., and Blanche, D. (1996) Hyperhomocysteinemia induced by folic acid deficiency and methionine load-applications of a modified HPLC method. *Clin. Chim. Acta.* **252**, 83–93.
52. Dudman, N. P. B., Guo, X. W., Crooks, R., Xie, L., and Silberberg, J. S. (1996) Assay of plasma homocysteine: Light sensitivity of the fluorescent 7-benzo-2-oxa-1,3-diazole-4-sulfonic acid derivative, and use of appropriate calibrators. *Clin. Chem.* **42**, 2028–2032.
53. Kuo, K., Still, R., Cale, S., and McDowell, I. (1997) Standardization (external and internal) of HPLC assay for plasma homocysteine. *Clin. Chem.* **43**, 1653–1655.
54. Feussner, A., Rolinski, B., Weiss, N., Deufel, T., Wolfram, G., and Roscher, A. A. (1997) Determination of total homocysteine in human plasma by isocratic high-performance liquid chromatography. *Eur. J. Clin. Chem. Clin. Biochem.* **35**, 687–691.
55. Reddy, N. M. and Behnke, C. (1997) A rapid and simple assay to determine total homocysteine and other thiols in pediatric samples by high pressure liquid chromatography and fluorescence detection. *J. Liquid Chrom. Rel. Technol.* **20**, 1391–1408.
56. Accinni, R., Campolo, J., Bartesaghi, S., De leo, G., Lucarelli, C., Cursano, C. F., and Parodi, O. (1998) High-performance liquid chromatographic determination of total plasma homocysteine with or without internal standards. *J. Chromatogr. A.* **828**, 397–400.
57. Fermo, I., Arcelloni, C., Mazzola, G., D'Angelo, A., and Paroni, R. (1998) High-performance liquid chromatographic method for measuring total plasma homocysteine levels. *J. Chromatogr. Biomed. Appl.* **719**, 31–36.
58. Rizzo, V., Montalbetti, L., Valli, M., Bosoni,T., Scoglio, E., and Moratti, R. (1998) Study of factors affecting the determination of total plasma 7-fluorobenzo-2-oxa-1,3-diazole-4-sulfonate (SBD)-thiol derivatives by liquid chromatography. *J. Chromatogr. Biomed. Appl.* **706**, 209–215.
59. Pfeiffer, C., Huff, D. L., and Gunter, E. W. (1999). Rapid and accurate HPLC assay for plasma total homocysteine and cysteine in a clinical laboratory setting. *Clin. Chem.* **45**, 290–292.
60. Swift, M. E. and Schultz, T. D. (1986) Relationship of vitamins B-6 and B-12 to homocysteine levels: Risk for coronary heart disease. *Nutr. Rep. Int.* **34**, 1–4.

61. Malinow, M. R., Kang, S. S., Taylor, L. M., Wong, P. W. K., Coull, B., Inahara, T., et al. (1989) Prevalence of hyperhomocyst(e)inemia in patients with peripheral arterial occlusive disease. *Circulation* **79,** 1180–1188.

62. Harvey, P. R. C., Ilson, R. G., and Strasberg, S. M. (1989). The simultaneous determination of oxidized and reduced glutathione in liver tissue by ion-pairing reverse phase high performance liquid chromatography with a coulometric electrochemical detector. *Clin. Chim. Acta.* **180,** 203–212.

63. Martin, S. C., Hilton, A. C., Bartlett, W. A., and Jones, A. B. (1998) Plasma total homocysteine measurement by ion-paired reversed-phase HPLC with electrochemical detection. *Biomed. Chromatogr.* **12,** 1–2.

64. Martin, S. C., Tsakas-Ampatzis, I., Barlett, A., and Jones, A. F. (1999) Measurement of plasma total homocysteine by HPLC with colorimetric detection. *Clin. Chem.* **45,** 150–152.

65. Sundrehagen, E. (1993). Homocysteine assay. Pat. Appl. PCT/Gb93/00138.

66. Shipchandler, M. T. and Moore, E. G.(1995). Rapid, fully automated measurement of plasma homocysteine with the Abbot IMx analyzer. *Clin. Chem.* **41,** 991–994.

67. Frantzen, F., Faaren, A. L., Alfheim, I., and Nordhei, A. K. (1998). Enzymes conversion immunoassay for determining total homocysteine in plasma or serum. *Clin. Chem.* **44,** 311–316.

68. Dias, V. C., Bamforth, F. J., Tesanovic, M., Hyndman, M., Parsons, H. G., and Cembronwski, G. S. (1994) Evaluation and intermethod comparison of the Biorad high performance liquid chromatographic method for plasma total homocysteine. *Clin. Chem.* **44,** 2199–2201.

69. Pfeiffer, C. M., Twite, D., Shih, J., Holets-McCormack, S. R., and Gunter, E. W. (1999) Method comparison for total plasma homocysteine between the Abbott IMx analyzer and an HPLC assay with internal standardization. *Clin. Chem.* **45,** 152–153.

70. Eliason, S. C. (1999) Interlaboratory variability for total homocysteine analysis in plasma. *Clin. Chem.* **45,** 315–316.

71. Malinow, M. R. (1994) Homocyst(e)ine and arterial occlusive disease. *J. Intern. Med.* **236,** 603–617.

72. Boushey, C. J., Beresford, S. A., Omenn, G. S., and Motulsky, A. G. (1995) A quantitative assessment of plasma homocysteine as a risk factor for vascular disease. Probable benefits of increasing folic acid intakes. *JAMA* **274,** 1049–1057.

73. Malinow, M. R. (1996) Plasma homocyst(e)ine: A risk factor for arterial occlusive disease. *J. Nutr.* **126,** 1238S–1243S.

74. Nygard, O., Nordrehaug, J. E., Refsum, H., Ueland, P. M., Farstad, M., and Vollset, S. E. (1997) Plasma homocysteine levels and mortality in patients with coronary artery disease. *N. Engl. J. Med.* **337,** 230–236.

75. Mayer, E. L., Jacobsen, D. W., and Robinson, K. (1996) Homocysteine and coronary atherosclerosis. *J. Am. Coll. Cardiol.* **27,** 517–527.

76. Verhoef, P., Stampfer, M. J., Buring, J. E., Gaziano, J. M., Allen, R. H., Stabler, S. P., Reynolds, R. D., Kok, F. J., Hennekens, C. H., and Willett, W. C. (1996) Homocysteine metabolism and risk of myocardial infarction: Relation with vitamins B6, B12, and folate. *Am. J. Epidemiol.* **143,** 845–859.

77. Kang, S. S, Wong, P. W., Cook, H. Y., Norusis, M., and Messer, J. V. (1986) Protein-bound homocyst(e)ine. A possible risk factor for coronary artery disease. *J. Clin. Invest.* **77,** 1482–1486.

78. Malinow, M. R., Nieto, F. J., Kruger, W. D.,Duell, P. B., Hess, D. L., Gluckman, R.. A., Block, P. C., Holzgang, C. R., Anderson, P. H., Seltzer, D., Upson, B., and Lin, Q. R. (1997) The effects of folic acid supplementation on plasma total homocysteine are modulated by multivitamin use and the methylenetetrahydrofolate reductase genotype. *Arterioscler. Thromb.* **17,** 1157–1162.

79. Dudman, N. P. B., Wilcken, D. E., Wang, J., Lynch, J. F., Macey, D., and Lundberg, P. (1993) Disordered methionine/homocysteine metabolism in premature vascular disease. Its occurrence, cofactor therapy, and enzymology. *Arterioscler. Thromb.* **13,** 1253–1260.

80. Pancharuniti, N., Lewis, C. A., Sauberlich, H. E., Perkins, L. L., Go, R. C., Alvarez, J. O., Macaluso, M., Acton, R. T., Copeland, R. B., and Cousins, A. L. (1994) Plasma homocyst(e)ine, folate, and vitamin B-12 con–centrations and risk for early-onset coronary artery disease. *Am. J. Clin. Nutr.* **59,** 940–948.

81. Malinow, M. R., Sexton, G., Averbuch, M., Grossman, M., Wilson, D., and Upson, B. (1990) Homocyst(e)inemia in daily practice. *Coron. Artery. Dis.* **1,** 215–220.

82. von Eckardstein, A., Malinow, M. R., Upson, B., Heinrich, J., Schulte, H., Schonfeld, R., Kohler, E., and Assmann, G. (1994) Effects of age, lipoproteins, and hemostatic parameters on the role of homocyst(e)inemia as a cardiovascular risk factor in men. *Arterioscler. Thromb.* **14,** 460–464.

83. Stampfer, M. J., Malinow, M. R., Willett, W. C., Newcomer, L. M., Upson, B., Ullmann, D., Tishler, P. V., and Hennekens, C. H. (1992) A prospective study of plasma homocyst(c)inc and risk of myocardial infarction in US physicians. JAMA **268,** 877–881.

84. Genest, J. J. Jr., McNamara, J. R., Salem, D. N., Wilson, P. W., Schaefer, E. J., and Malinow, M. R. (1990) Plasma homocyst(e)ine levels in men with prema–ture coronary artery disease. *J. Am. Coll. Cardiol.* **16,** 1114–1119.

85. Wu, L.L., Wu, J., Hunt, S. C., James, B. C., Vincent, G. M., Williams, R. R., and Hopkins, P. N. (1994) Plasma homocyst(e)ine as a risk factor for early familial coronary artery disease. *Clin. Chem.* **40,** 552–561.

86. Israelsson, B., Brattstrom, L. E., and Hultberg, B. L. (1988) Homocysteine and myocardial infarction. *Atherosclerosis* **71,** 227–233.

87. Graham, I. (1994) Interactions between homocysteinemia and conventional risk factors in vascular disease (abstract). *Eur. Heart. J.* **15,** 530.

88. Arnesen, E., Refsum, H., Bonaa, K. H., Ueland, P. M., Forde, O. H., and Nordrehaug, J. E. (1995) Serum total homocysteine and coronary heart disease. *Int. J. Epidemiol.* **24,** 704–709.

89. Coull, B. M., Malinow, M. R., Beamer, N., Sexton, G., Nordt, F., and de Garmo, P. (1990) Elevated plasma homocyst(e)ine concentration as a possible independent risk factor for stroke. *Stroke* **21,** 572–576.

90. Brattstrom, L., Israelsson, B., Norrving, B., Bergqvist, D., Thorne, J., Hultberg, B., and Hamfelt, A. (1990) Impaired homocysteine metabolism in early-onset cerebral and peripheral occlusive arterial disease. Effects of pyridoxine and folic acid treatment. *Atherosclerosis* **81,** 51–60.

91. Brattstrom, L., Lindgren, A., Israelsson, B., Malinow, M. R., Norrving, B., Upson, B., Hamfelt, A. (1992) Hyperhomocysteinemia in stroke: Prevalence, cause, and relationships to type of stroke and stroke risk factors. *Eur. J. Clin. Invest.* **22,** 214–221.

92. Lindgren, A., Brattstrom, L., Norrving, B., Hultberg, B., Andersson, A., Johansson, B. B. (1995) Plasma homocysteine in the acute and convalescent phases after stroke. *Stroke* **26,** 795–800.

93. Bergmark, C., Mansoor, M. A., Swedenborg, J., de Faire, U., Svardal, A. M., and Ueland, P. M. (1993) Hyperhomocysteinemia in patients operated for lower extremity ischaemia below the age of 50-effect of smoking and extent of disease. *Eur. J. Vasc. Surg.* **7,** 391–396.

94. Molgaard, J., Malinow, M. R., Lassvik, C., Holm, A. C., Upson, B., and Olsson, A. G. (1992) Hyperhomocyst(e)inemia: An independent risk factor for intermittent claudication. *J. Intern. Med.* **231,** 273–279.

95. Tsai, J. C., Perrella, M. A., Yoshizumi, M., Hsieh, C. M., Haber, E., Schlegel, R., and Lee, M. E. (1994) Promotion of vascular smooth muscle cell growth by homocysteine: A link to atherosclerosis. *Proc. Natl. Acad. Sci. USA* **91,** 6369–6373.

96. Harker, L. A., Slichter, S. J., Scott, C. R., and Ross, R. (1974) Homocystinemia. Vascular injury and arterial thrombosis. *N. Engl. J. Med.* **291,** 537–543.

97. Harker, L. A, Ross, R., Slichter, S. J., and Scott, C. R. (1976) Homocystine-induced arteriosclerosis. The role of endothelial cell injury and platelet response in its genesis. *J. Clin. Invest.* **58,** 731–741.

98. McDonald, L., Bray, C., Field, C., Love, F., and Davies, B. (1964) Homocystinuria, thrombosis and the blood-platelets. *Lancet* **1,** 745–746.

99. DiMinno, G., Davi, G., Margaglione, M., Cirillo, F., Grandone, E., Ciabattoni, G., Catalano, I., Strisciuglio, P, Andria, G., Patrono, C., and Mancini, M. (1993) Abnormally high thromboxane biosynthesis in homozygous homocystinuria. Evidence for platelet involvement and probucol-sensitive mechanism. *J. Clin. Invest.* **92,** 1400–1406.

100. Uhlemann, E. R.,TenPas, J., Lucky, A. W., Schulman, J. D., Mudd, S. H., and Shulman, N. R. (1976) Platelet survival and morphology in homocystinuria due to cystathionine synthase deficiency. *N. Engl. J. Med.* **295,** 1283–1286.

101. Hill-Zobel, R. L., Pyeritz, R. E., Scheffel, U., Malpica, O., Engin, S., Camargo, E., Abbott, M., Guilarte, T. R., Hill, J., McIntyre, P. A., Murphy, E. A., and Tsan, M. F. (1982) Kinetics and distribution of [111]Indium-labeled platelets in patients with homocystinuria. *N. Engl. J. Med.* **307,** 781–786.

102. Graeber, J., Slott, J. H., Ulane, R. E., Schulman, J. D., and Stuart, M. J. (1982) Effect of homocysteine and homocystine on platelet and vascular arachidonic acid metabolism. *Pediatr. Res.* **16,** 490–493.

103. Hirano, K., Ogihara, T., and Miki, M. (1994) Homocysteine induces iron-catalyzed lipid peroxidation of low-density lipoprotein that is prevented by α-tocopherol. *Free. Radic. Res.* **21,** 267–276.

104. Blom, H. J., Boers, G. H., Demacker, P. N., Hak-Lemmers, H. L., Te Poele-Pothoff, M. T., and Trijbels, J. M. (1995) Lipid peroxidation and susceptibility of low-density lipoprotein to in vitro oxidation in hyperhomocysteinemia. *Eur. J. Clin. Invest.* **25,** 149–154.

105. Ratnoff, O. D. (1968) Activation of Haghnam factor by L-Homocystine. *Science* **162,** 1007–1009.

106. Hilden, M., Brandt, N. J., Nilsson, I. M., and Schonheyder, F. (1974) Investigations of coagulation and fibrinolysis in homocystinuria. *Acta. Med. Scand.* **195,** 533–535.

107. Rodgers, G. M. and Kane, W. H. (1986) Activation of endogenous factor V by a homocysteine-induced vascular endothelial cell activator. *Clin. Invest.* **77,** 1909–1916.

108. Rodgers, G. M. and Conn, M. T. (1990) Homocysteine, an atherogenic stimulus, reduces protein C activation by arterial and venous endothelial cells. *Blood* **75,** 895–901.

109. Hayashi, T., Honda, G., and Suzuki, K. (1992) An atherogenic stimulus homocysteine inhibits cofactor activity of thrombomodulin and enhances thrombomodulin expression in human umbilical vein endothelial cells. *Blood* **79,** 2930–2936.

110. Nishinaga, M., Ozawa, T., and Shimada, K. (1993) Homocysteine, a thrombogenic agent, suppresses anticoagulant heparan sulfate expression in cultured porcine aortic endothelial cells. *J. Clin. Invest.* **92,** 1381–1386.

111. Fryer, R. H., Wilson, B. D., Gubler, D. B., Fitzgerald, L. A., and Rodgers, G. M. (1993) Homocysteine, a risk factor for premature vascular disease and thrombosis, induces tissue factor activity in endothelial cells. *Arterioscler Thromb.* **13,** 1327–1333.

112. Stamler, J. S., Osborne, J. A., Jaraki, O., Rabbani, L. E., Mullins, M., Singel, D., and Loscalzo, J. (1993) Adverse vascular effects of homocysteine are modulated by endothelium- derived relaxing factor and related oxides of nitrogen. *J. Clin. Invest.* **91,** 308–318.

113. Stamler, J. S., Simon, D. I., Osborne, J. A., Mullins, M. E., Jaraki, O., Michel, T., Singel, D. J., and Loscalzo, J. (1992) S-nitrosylation of proteins with nitric oxide: Synthesis and characterization of biologically active compounds. *Proc. Natl. Acad. Sci. USA* **89,** 444–448.

114. Chin, J. H., Azhar, S., and Hoffman, B. B. (1992) Inactivation of endothelial derived relaxing factor by oxidized lipoproteins. *J. Clin. Invest.* **89,** 10–18.

115. Liao, J. K, Shin, W. S., Lee, W. Y., and Clark, S. L. (1995) Oxidized low-density lipoprotein decreases the expression of endothelial nitric oxide synthase. *J. Biol. Chem.* **270,** 319–324.

116. Upchurch, G. R. Jr., Welch, G. N., Fabian, A. J., Freedman, J. E., Jhonson, J. L., Keaney, J. F., and Loscalzo, J. (1997) Hcy decreases bioavailable NO by mechanism involving glutathione peroxidase. *J. Biol. Chem.* **272,** 17012–17017.

117. Benesch, R. and Benesch, R. E. (1956) Formation of peptide bonds by aminolysis of homocysteine thiolactone. *J. Am. Chem. Soc.* **78,** 1597–1599.

118. Naruszewicz, M., Mirkiewicz, A. J., Olszewski, J., and McCully, K. S. (1994) Thiolation of low-density lipoprotein by homocysteine thiolactone causes increased aggregation and altered interaction with cultured macrophages. *Nutr. Metab. Cardiovasc. Dis.* **4,** 70–77.

119. Welch, G. N. and Loscalzo, J. (1998) Homocysteine and atherothrombosis. *N. Engl. J. Med.* **338,** 1042–1050.

120. Fowler, B., Sardharwalla, I. B., and Robins, A. J. (1971) The detection of heterozygotes for homocystinuria by oral loading with ʟ-methionine. *Biochem. J.* **122,** 23–24.

121. Boers, G. H., Fowler, B., Smals, A. G., Trijbels, F. J., Leermakers, A. I., Kleijer, W. J., and Kloppenborg, P. W. (1985) Improved identification of heterozygotes for homocystinuria due to cystathionine synthase deficiency by the combination of methionine loading and enzyme determination in cultured fibroblasts. *Hum. Genet.* **69,** 164–169.

122. Falcon, C. R., Cattaneo, M., Panzeri, D., Martinelli, I., and Mannucci, P. M. (1994) High prevalence of hyperhomocyst(e)inemia in patients with juvenile venous thrombosis. *Arterioscler. Thromb.* **14,** 1080–1083.

123. Mudd, S. H., Levy, H. L., and Skovby, F. (1995) Disorders of transulfuration, in *The Metabolic and Molecular Bases of Inherited Disease.* (Scriver, C. R., Beaudet, A. L., Sly, W. S., Valle, D., Stanbury, J. B., Wyngarden, J. B., and Fredrickson, D. S., eds.), McGraw-Hill, New York, pp. 1279–1327.

124. Fermo, I., Viganò-D'Angelo, S., Paroni, R., Mazzola, G., Calori, G., and D'Angelo, A. (1995) Prevalence of moderate hyperhomocysteinemia in patients with early-onset venous and arterial occlusive disease. *Ann. Int. Med.* **123,** 747–753.

125. Cattaneo, M., Martinelli, I., and Mannucci, P. M. (1996) Hyperhomocysteinemia as a risk factor for deep-vein thrombosis. *N. Engl. J. Med.* **335,** 974–975.

126. Graham, I. M., Daly, L. E., Refsum, H. M., Robinson, K., Brattstrom, L. E., Ueland, P. M., et al. (1997) Plasma homocystine as a risk factor for vascular disease. The European Concerted Action Project. JAMA **277,** 1775–1781.

127. Probs, R., Brandl, R., Blumke, M., and Neumeier, D. (1998) Stabilization of homocysteine concentration in whole blood. *Clin. Chem.* **44,** 1567–1569.

128. Ueland, P. M., Refsum, H., Stabler, S. P., Malinow, M. R., Andersson, A., and Allen, R. H., (1993). Total homocysteine in plasma or serum: Methods and applications. *Clin. Chem.* **39,** 1764–1773.

129. Fiskerstrand, T., Refsum, H., Kvalheim, G., and Ueland, P. M. (1993) Homocysteine and other thiols in plasma and urine: Automated determination and sample stability. *Clin. Chem.* **39,** 263–270.

130. Andersson, A., Isaksson, A., and Hultberg, B. (1992). Homocysteine export from erythrocytes and its implication for plasma sampling. *Clin. Chem.* **38,** 1311–1315.

131. Moller, J. and Rasmussen, K. (1995). Homocysteine in plasma: Stabilization of blood samples with fluoride. *Clin. Chem.* **41,** 758–759.

132. Hucghes, M. P., Carlon, T. H., McLaughlin, M. K., and Bankson, D. D. (1998). Addition of sodium fluoride to whole blood does not stabilize plasma homocysteine but produces dilution effects on plasma constituents and hematocrit. *Clin. Chem.* **44,** 2204–2206.

133. Willems, H. P. J., Bos, G. M. J., Gerrits, W. B. J., den Heijer, M., Vloet S., and Blom, H. J. (1998) Acid citrate stabilized blood samples for assay of total homocysteine. *Clin. Chem.* **44,** 342–345.

134. Gilfix, B. M., Blank, D. W., and Rosenblatt, D. S. (1997) Novel reductant for determination of total plasma homocysteine. *Clin. Chem.* **43,** 687–688.

135. Imai, K. (1987) Derivatization in liquid chromatography. *Adv. Chromatogr.* **27,** 215–245.

136. Imai, K., Uzu, S., and Toyo'oka, T. (1990) Fluorogenic reagents, having benzofurazan structure, in liquid chromatography. *J. Pharm. Biomed. Anal.* **7,** 1395–1403.

137. Munday, R. (1989) Toxicity of thiols and disulfides: involvement of free-radical species. *Free Radic. Biol. Med.* **7,** 659–673.

9

Assay for Serum Glycated Lipoproteins

Akira Tanaka

1. Introduction

Modified low density lipoprotein (LDL) is considered to be a risk factor for the development and progression of atherosclerosis *(1–3)*. Glycated LDL and oxidized LDL are the only modified lipoproteins that exist naturally in the human body, but oxidized LDL does not exist in the circulation because of the presence of many antioxidizing agents *(4)*. LDL cannot be oxidized until it has entered the arterial wall from the circulation. The only modified LDL that exists in the circulation is glycated LDL. It has been shown to be more easily oxidized than native LDL *(5–7)*. These findings indicate that the glycation of LDL may be the initial step in the development of atherosclerosis.

Glucose binds nonenzymatically to LDL to form glycated LDL *(8,9)*. Glycation enhances the uptake of LDL by macrophages in the arterial wall *(2,10)*. The increased uptake of glycated LDL increases the formation of foam cells. Their accumulation in the arterial wall leads to the formation of arterial atherosclerotic lesions *(5)*.

Glucose binds nonenzymatically to LDL to form a Schiff base. This base then undergoes Amadori rearrangement to become a ketoamine, which subsequently becomes 1-deoxfructosyl-LDL *(8)*. In alkaline solution, the cis-diol arrangement that this compound contains binds reversibly to boronate to form a complex *(11,12)*. Boronate affinity chromatography can therefore be used to separate glycated from nonglycated proteins.

We developed an automated analytical system for glycated lipoproteins using high-performance liquid chromatography (HPLC) with an affinity boronate column and a gel permeation column *(13)*. The system consists of three processes (*see* **Fig. 1.**). In the first, serum proteins are resolved into glycated proteins and nonglycated proteins by affinity chromatography with

From: *Methods in Molecular Medicine, vol. 52: Atherosclerosis: Experimental Methods and Protocols*
Edited by: A. F. Drew © Humana Press Inc., Totowa, NJ

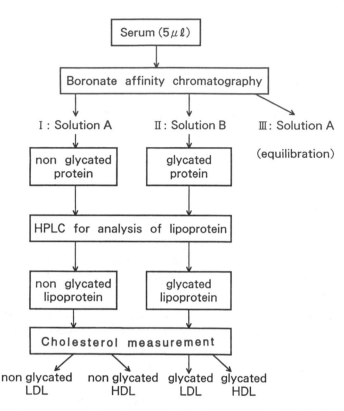

Fig. 1. Flow chart summarizing the procedure for automated analysis of glycated lipoproteins.

the boronate column. In the second, glycated proteins and nonglycated proteins are separately resolved into glycated and non-glycated lipoproteins (LDL and high-density lipoprotein [HDL]) with the gel permeation column *(14)*. In the last, the cholesterol content of glycated and non-glycated lipoproteins (LDL and HDL) is measured enzymatically *(14)*. These three processes are automatically regulated by a system controller. This system can measure glycated lipoproteins (glycated LDL and glycated HDL) in a small sample of serum (5 mL) and in a short time (40 min/sample). The method can be used clinically because of the large number of samples it can measure. (*see* **Fig. 2.**)

2. Materials

2.1. Instruments

1. Degasser (SD-8023, Tosoh Co.).
2. Pumps.
   a. Pump-1 (CCPM-II, Tosoh Co.): The pump for solution A and solution B, which are used for resolving serum proteins into glycated and nonglycated proteins.

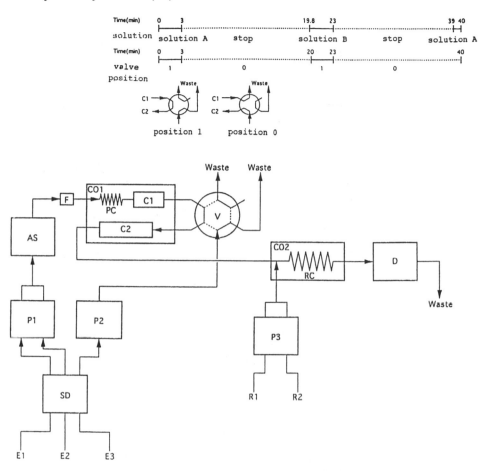

Fig. 2. The automated analytical system for glycated lipoproteins. E1, Solution A for analysis of nonglycated protein; E2, Solution B for analysis of glycated protein; E3, Solution for analysis of lipoprotein (TSK eluent LP-1); R1, R2, Reagent for measuring cholesterol; SD, Degasser; P1, P2, P3, pump; AS, Autosampler; F, Filter; CO1, Column oven; PC, Preheating coil; C1, Column (TSK gel boronate-5PW, 4.6×10 mm); C2, Column (TSK gel Lipopropak, 7.5×3000 mm); V, Switching-valve unit; CO2, Reactor; RC, Reactive coil (0.4 mmI.D.×7.5 m); D, Detector (A550).

 b. Pump-2 (CCPS, Tosoh Co.): The pump for TSK eluent LP-1 (Tosoh Co.) , which is used for resolving serum proteins into serum lipoproteins.

 c. Pump-3 (CCPM-II, Tosoh Co.): The pump for the agent for measuring cholesterol.

3. Autosampler (AS-8020, Tosoh Co.): Serum sample is automatically injected into the boronate column with the autosampler.

4. Line-Filter (Filter-K,Tosoh Co.): This is set between the Pump-1 and the boronate column.

5. Column:
   a. TSK gel Boronate-5PW (4.6×10 mm, Tosoh Co.): This column separates the glycated protein (bound fraction) from the nonglycated protein (unbound fraction).
   b. Lipopropak (7.5×300 mm, Tosoh Co.): This column resolves the glycated protein and the nonglycated protein into each lipoprotein class.
6. Column Oven (CO-8020-C,Tosoh Co.): The column oven keeps analytical temperature, in which serum proteins are resolved into glycated and nonglycated proteins by use of the boronate column, to be 20°C. The size of preheating coil is 0.2 mm x 2 m.
7. Reactor (CO-8020-C,Tosoh Co.): The mixture of reagent for measuring cholesterol and each lipoprotein is incubated in the reactor at 45°C. The size of reacting coil is 0.4 mm I.D.× 7.5 m.
8. Switching-valve unit (VC-8020,Tosoh Co.): The effluent from the boronate column is continously injected into Lipopropak by use of the switching-valve unit, which is controlled by the system controller.
9. Detector (UV-8020,Tosoh Co.): The mixture of agent for measuring cholesterol and each lipoprotein is incubated in the reactor at 45°C and then passes through the detector, being monitored continuously at A 550.
10. System controller (SC-8020,Tosoh Co.): The switching-valve unit and the flow of solution A and B are controlled by the system controller according to the analytical program. HPLC cholesterol pattern of each lipoprotein is shown separately for the glycated and nonglycated lipoprotein on the monitor of the system controller, and the area under curve of each lipoprotein (LDL or HDL) is calculated automatically by the system controller.

2.2. Solutions

1. Solution A: 50 mM glycine, 0.2 M MgCl$_2$, 0.05% NaN3, pH 7.6. Solution A is used to acquire nonglycated protein (unbound fraction) and to equilibrate the TSK gel Boronate-5PW. The flow rate of solution A is 0.6 mL/min.
2. Solution B: 50 mM glycine, 0.2 M MgCl$_2$, 0.2 M sorbitol, 0.05% NaN3, pH 7.6; (Tosoh Co.). Solution B is used to acquire glycated protein (bound fraction).The flow rate of solution B is 0.6 mL/min.
3. TSK eluent LP-1 (Tosoh Co.): The Lipopropak resolves the glycated protein or the nonglycated protein into each lipoprotein. The eluent was TSK eluent LP-1 and its flow rate is 0.6 mL/min.
4. Reagent for measuring cholesterol (Detaminar L TC, Kyowa Medics; *see* **Note 1**): Flow rate of R-1 is 0.225 mL/min and flow rate of R-2 is 0.075 mL/min.

3. Methods

3.1. Resolution of Sserum Proteins into Glycated Proteins and Nonglycated Proteins (see Note 1)

1. Inject at least 30 μL (5 μL + dead space volume) of serum sample into the boronate column with autosampler to separate the glycated protein (bound

fraction) from the nonglycated protein (unbound fraction). Use the following conditions for separating glycated protein from non-glycated protein:

   a. Flow rate of the eluent (solution A and B) is 0.6 mL/min and the analytical temperature is 20°C (*see* **Note 2**).

   b. Pump-1 is used to keep the flow rate of eluent constant, and the column oven is used to keep the analytical temperature constant.

2. Nonglycated protein (unbound fraction) is collected from time 0 to 3.0 min. The flow of solution A is stopped from 3.0 to 19.8 min.

3. Glycated protein (bound fraction) is collected from 19.8 to 23.0 min. The flow of solution B is stopped from 23.0 to 39.0 min. From 39.0 to 40.0 min, solution A is used to equilibrate the column. This process is regulated by the system controller. Solution A and B pass through the degasser before the boronate column.

3.2. Resolution of Protein into LDL and HDL with the Gel Permeation Column

1. The effluents from the boronate column, glycated protein or nonglycated protein, are separately and continuously injected into Lipopropak (the gel permeation column), by use of the switching-valve unit, to resolve both samples into each lipoprotein (LDL or HDL). The switching-valve unit is controlled by the system controller according to the analytical program.

2. The conditions for resolving glycated protein or nonglycated protein into each lipoprotein by use of Lipopropak are as follows:

   a. The eluent is TSK eluent LP-1, and its flow rate is 0.6 mL/min.

   b. The analytical temperature is 20°C (*see* **Note 2**).

3. Pump-2 is used to keep the flow rate of eluent constant, and the column oven is used to keep the analytical temperature constant.

3.3. Measurement of the Cholesterol Content of Glycated and Nonglycated Lipoproteins (LDL and HDL)

1. The reagent for measuring cholesterol is added continuously to the effluents (glycated lipoproteins or nonglycated lipoproteins) from Lipopropak by pump-3.

2. The mixture is incubated in the reactor (the size of reacting coil: 0.4 mm I.D. × 7.5 m) at 45°C and passed through the detector, being monitored continuously at a wavelength of 550nm. The flow rate of the reagent for measuring cholesterol is 0.3 mL/min (R-1: 0.225 mL/min; R-2: 0.075 mL/min).

3. The HPLC cholesterol pattern of each lipoprotein is shown separately for the glycated and nonglycated lipoprotein on the monitor of the system controller, and the area under curve of each lipoprotein (LDL or HDL) is calculated automatically by the system controller. Glycated LDL and glycated HDL are presented as a percentage of the areas of total LDL and total HDL, respectively (*see* **Notes 3** and **4**).

4. The following formulas are used:

   a. Glycated LDL (%) = [(area of glycated LDL) / (area of glycated LDL + area of nonglycated LDL)] × 100.
   b. Glycated HDL (%) = [(area of glycated HDL) / (area of glycated HDL + area of nonglycated HDL)] × 100.

4. Notes

1. During the assay, the bottle of reagent for measuring cholesterol (R-1 and R-2) should be placed in ice water.
2. The most important thing in this assay is to maintain a constant analytical temperature, in which serum protein is resolved into glycated protein and nonglycated protein by the boronate column. The higher the analytical temperature, the greater is the amount of glycated protein *(13)*. The higher the analytical temperature, the greater is the nonspecific binding by the boronate column. In this system, the boronate column is placed in the column oven at a constant temperature.
3. Recovery by the boronate column is calculated *(13)*: The area under the curve monitored at absorbance 550 nm by the detector, without the boronate column, is defined as 100 %. The percentage of the sum of the areas of LDL and HDL in the bound fraction and the areas of LDL and HDL in the unbound fraction has been calculated for two healthy controls and six diabetic patients. The recovery was 92.1 ± 1.2%. The coefficient of variation (CV) for intra-assay of glycated LDL and glycated HDL is 4.1% and 3.3%, respectively.
4. The mean values of glycated LDL in 30 healthy controls and 177 diabetic patients are 28.7 ± 5.2% and 40.2 ± 14.7%, respectively. Correspondingly, the mean values of glycated HDL in 30 healthy controls and 177 diabetic patients are 5.2 ± 1.4% and 14.9 ± 6.8%, respectively. Levels of both glycated LDL and glycated HDL in diabetic patients are significantly higher than those in healthy controls (both, $p < 0.0001$, Mann-Whitney U test) *(15)*.

References

1. Lyons, T. J. (1991) Oxidized low density lipoproteins—A role in the pathogenesis of atherosclerosis in diabetes? *Diabet. Med.* **8,** 411–419.
2. Makita, T., Tanaka, A., Nakajima, K., Nakano, T., and Numano, N. (1999) Importance of glycation in acceleration of low density lipoprotein (LDL) uptake into macrophages in patients with diabetes mellitus. *Int. Angiol.* **18,** 149–153.
3. Makita, T., Tanaka, A., and Numano, F.(1999) Effect of glycated low density lipoprotein on smooth muscle cell proliferation. *Int. Angiol.*, in press.
4. Colaco, C. A. L. S. and Roser, B. J.(1994) Atherosclerosis and glycation. *BioAssays* **16,** 145–147.
5. Lyon, T. J. (1992) Lipoprotein glycation and its metabolic consequences. *Diabetes* **41,** 67–73.
6. Wolff, S. P. and Dean, R. T.(1987) Glucose autoxidation and protein modification;the potential role of autoxidative glycation in diabetes mellitus. *Biochem. J.* **245,** 243–250.

7. Mullarkey, C. J., Edelstein, D., and Brownlee, M. (1990) Free radical generation by early glycation products; a mechanism for accelerated atherogenesis in diabetes. *Biochem. Biophys. Res. Commun.* **173,** 932–939.

8. Gonen, B., Baenziger, J., Schonfeld, G., Jacobson, D., and Farrar, P. (1981) Nonenzymatic glycosylation of low density lipoproteins in vitro. Effects on cell-interactive properties. *Diabetes* **30,** 875–878.

9. Schleicher, E., Deufel, T., and Wieland, O. H. (1981) Non-enzymatic glycosylation of human serum lipoproteins. *FEBS Lett.* **129,** 1–4.

10. Lopes-Virella, M. F. R., Klein, R. L., Lyons, T. J., Stevenson, H. C., and Witzum, J. L. (1988) Glycosylation of low-density lipoprotein enhances cholesteryl ester synthesis in human monocyte-derived macrophages. *Diabetes* **37,** 550–557.

11. Gould, B. J., Hall, M., and Cook, J. G. H. (1984) A sensitive method for the measurement of glycosylated plasma proteins using affinity chromatography. *Ann. Clin. Biochem.* **21,** 16–21.

12. Dhima, K., Ito, N., Abe, F., Hirota, M., Yano, M., Yamamoto, Y., Uchida, T., and Noguchi, K. (1988) High performance liquid chromatography assay of serum glycated albumin. *Diabetology* **31,** 327–631.

13. Tanaka, A.,Yui, K.,Tomie, N., Baba, T., Tamura, M., Makita, T., Numano, F., Nakatani, S., and Kato, Y. (1997) New assay for glycated lipoproteins by high-performance liquid chromatography. *Ann. N.Y. Acad. Sci.* **811,** 385–394.

14. Okazaki, M., Sasamoto, K., Muramatsu, T., and Hosaki, S. (1997) Analysis of plasma lipoproteins by gel permeation chromatography, in *Handbook of Lipoprotein Testing.* (Rifai, N., ed.), AACC press, Washington, DC, pp. 531–548.

15. Numano, F., Tanaka, A., Makita, T., and Kishi, Y. (1997) Glycated lipoprotein and atherosclerosis. *Ann. N.Y. Acad. Sci.* **811,** 100–114.

10

Lipoprotein(a) Quantitation

Michael Bender and Werner Gross

1. Introduction

Lipoprotein(a) (Lp[a]) was first discovered in 1963, by Kare Berg, as a variant of the beta-lipoproteins. Many years later, Lp(a) has been identified as an independent risk factor for the development of coronary heart disease (*1*). During the last two decades the structure and composition of Lp(a) has been investigated using different physicochemical and biochemical methods (*2,3*). These studies revealed that Lp(a) resembles the cholesterol-rich low-density lipoprotein (LDL) particle, except for an additional glycoprotein called apolipoprotein(a) (apo[a]), which is mainly produced in the liver. Apo(a) is covalently linked via a disulfide bridge to apolipoprotein B-100, the major protein constituent of LDL. In contrast to apolipoprotein B-100, which is important for the structure of the lipoprotein particle, it is supposed that apo(a) is loosely adhered to the surface of the particle.

In 1987, the cDNA sequence of human apo(a) was published (*4*). It was shown that the apo(a) sequence is highly homologous (78–100%) to elements of plasminogen. Apo(a) contains an inactive protease domain and multiple secondary structure elements, known as kringles, which consist of 77–79 amino acids, stabilized by three disulfide bridges. Of the five plasminogen-kringles, only kringles-IV and -V are found in apo(a). The number of kringle-IV domains in apo(a) can vary between 12 and 51. Therefore, the molecular weight of apo(a) can vary between 350 kDa and 800 kDa. This structural variation is attributed to more than 30 different *apo(a)* alleles, thus leading to apo(a) isoforms that may be identified by pulse-field DNA-electrophoresis (*5*) or SDS-protein electrophoresis in agarose (*6*). Additionally, apo(a) is highly glycosylated (carbohydrate content about 20–30% of the protein mass) (*2*) (*See* **Table 1**).

From: *Methods in Molecular Medicine, vol. 52: Atherosclerosis: Experimental Methods and Protocols*
Edited by: A. F. Drew © Humana Press Inc., Totowa, NJ

Table 1
Characteristics of Lipoprotein(a) and Apolipoprotein(a)

Lp(a) particle diameter	≈ 25 nm
Lp(a) density range	1.05 –1.09 kg/L
Lp(a) molecular weight	$3.8 – 4.2 \times 10^6$ Dalton
Apo(a) molecular weight	350 – 800 kDa
Plasma level	≈ 0 – 3000 mg/L
Lp(a) heterogeneity	Apo(a) size polymorphism (34 different isoforms), differences in the lipid moiety

The plasma concentration of Lp(a) varies considerably from almost zero to more than 1 g/L, and the distribution in Caucasians is highly skewed to low values *(7)*. Less-skewed distributions are found in African-Americans, and different Asian ethnic groups have higher median values *(8)*. Lp(a) exhibits a very high degree of inheritability, as determined in a study of twins *(9)*. The apo(a) size has been found to be inversely correlated to the individual plasma concentration of total Lp(a) *(8)*. The Lp(a) level has been found to be remarkably constant in young healthy individuals. Diet changes and drugs that change LDL levels have only a negligible effect on Lp(a) *(10)*. The risk of myocardial infarction increases rapidly above the threshold level for Lp(a) concentration of 300 mg/L *(11)*.

Methods for the detection and quantification of Lp(a) in liquor cerebrospinalis *(12)*, arterial walls *(13)*, and atherosclerotic plaques *(14)* have been described. The strong intra-individual and inter-individual heterogeneity of Lp(a) in plasma complicates the development of comparable assays and agreement about international recommendations for standardization and measurement. First, there are apo(a) isoforms with different molecular weights; therefore, it is common to give the apo(a) isoform in terms of the number of kringle-IV units. Second, most individuals are heterozygous for apo(a), thus expressing two isoforms and consequently bringing out different Lp(a) particles. The discrimination and preparation of these different particles is difficult *(15,16)*. Third, the lipid moiety and the carbohydrate moiety of Lp(a) particles vary intra-individually and inter-individually. Fourth, the catabolism of Lp(a) may produce particles with smaller immunoreactive fragments of apo(a) *(17)*.

For Lp(a) quantitation in the clinical laboratory, several different methods have been developed, and some of them are commercially available *(18)*. With the exception of one method, which determines Lp(a) by its cholesterol content *(19)*, all are based on immunological procedures directed toward the protein moiety. Many difficulties in Lp(a) determination result from the lack of primary or secondary standard material and an appropriate reference method. Therefore, the calibration of the immunological assays with different Lp(a) control sera leads to a bias deviation of 50-100%. In 1998, for the first time, preliminary results of an international project for standardization of Lp(a) measurements were published to overcome these problems *(20)*.

For the measurement of Lp(a), we recommend two procedures: an immunoradiometric assay (IRMA) and an electroimmunoassay (EIA). Both methods are easy to perform and have sufficient accuracy, as described in several method evaluations *(21–24)*. In some countries, usage of IRMA is restricted because special permission is required to work with radioactivity.

The IRMA uses two monoclonal anti-apo(a) antibodies against different apo(a) epitopes. One antibody is labeled with ^{125}I, the other one is coupled to Sepharose™ particles. In a one-step sandwich technique, the Sepharose™-^{125}I-antibody-Lp(a)-complex is separated by low-speed centrifugation, and the samples are then analyzed in a g-counter.

For the EIA or rocket-immunoelectrophoresis *(25)*, the samples are electrophoresed in an agarose gel containing a monospecific polyclonal antibody against apo(a). Driven by electrical forces, the samples move through the gel until the antigen concentration has been diluted to form a precipitation front. The precipitation lines are rocket shaped, and either the length or the area of the rockets may be used for quantification. The EIA is an easy method to measure Lp(a) concentration *(11,26)*, and a special advantage is that the precipitates are visible. Optical control is not only possible, but is also recommended *(27)*. Another important advantage of the EIA is the relative insensitivity to Lp(a) heterogeneity *(28)*. Although the technique can easily be established in the laboratory, we strongly recommend commercially available kits because of better inter-assay precision at the beginning *(26)*. Both of these methods are described in this chapter (*see* **Fig. 1.**).

2. Materials

1. Lp(a) immunoradiometric assay (Mercodia, Uppsala, Sweden).
2. Gamma-counter (Beckman 5500, Palo Alto, CA).
3. 5 mL tubes (Sarstedt, Nümbrecht, Germany).
4. Counter tubes (NEN Dupont, Dreieich, Germany).
5. Vortex
6. Magnetic stirrer.
7. Laboratory centrifuge.
8. Electroimmunodiffusion Lp(a) kit (Immuno AG, Heidelberg, Germany, Cat. no. 8514005).
9. Rapidophor electrophoresis equipment: electrophoresis chamber, 3 plastic gel holder, power supply, (Immuno AG, Heidelberg, Germany).
10. Optical gel analyzer (Behring AG, Marburg, Germany).
11. 0.9% NaCl solution.

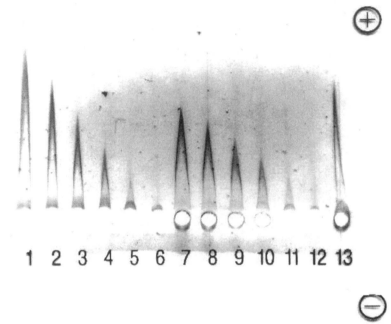

Fig. 1. An electroimmunoassay (Electroimmunodiffusion Lp(a), Immuno AG) with isolated lipoprotein(a) in different concentrations (lanes 1–6), lipoprotein(a) standard material included in the test in different concentrations (lanes 7–12), and a plasma probe (lane 13).

3. Methods
3.1. Preanalytical Considerations

In contrast to other lipid parameters, Lp(a) concentration hardly changes over time and is not directly related to the individual's nutrition status. Elevated Lp(a) levels were found in combination with other acute-phase proteins, during pregnancy, and in postmenopausal women *(18)*. Diseases of the kidney, such as nephrotic syndrome and end-stage renal disease, are also correlated with higher Lp(a) levels *(29)*.

Standardized sampling is an important factor for high preanalytical precision. As proposed by the European Atherosclerosis Society (EAS), this includes fasting for 12–14 h, the same body position for taking blood, short congestion (<1min), the same type of sample (either serum or plasma), the same anticoagulants (preferably EDTA), immediate processing, and storage at 0°–4°C. Nevertheless, the biological variability for Lp(a) is about 10% for values >150 mg/L and about 15% for values ≤150 mg/L *(30)*. Taken together, the analytical and the biological variability result in a total intra-individual variability for Lp(a) of about 20%.

3.2. Lp(a) Control Materials

Presently, there is no internationally accepted reference material for Lp(a) available. Most commercial calibrators are lyophilized sera or plasma samples, which can be used for only a short time after reconstitution. The results of long-term storage experiments with Lp(a) plasma samples show that the concentrations decrease depending on the storage conditions *(31)*. Many methodical comparisons clearly show that the assay calibrators are often not compatible with other methods *(20–24)*. The isolation of pure Lp(a) as a primary standard is laborious *(32)* and is only partially helpful for immunological determination as it cannot overcome Lp(a) heterogeneity. Therefore, it is recommended to use the calibrators included with the assays.

3.3. Immunoradiometric Assay (IRMA) to Measure Lp(a) in Plasma

Each IRMA kit contains six lyophilized apo(a) standards (0.4; 1; 2; 5; 10; 20 u/L), 5.5 mL anti-apo(a)-tagged with iodine 125 ($\approx$ 28 µg), 5.5 mL anti-apo(a)-Sepharose™, two lyophilized Lp(a) controls (low and high), 5 mL pretreatment solution (buffer improving the epitope exposure of Lp(a) particles), 220 mL diluent buffer solution (containing BSA and Tween for stabilization of the Lp(a)-antibody-complexes), and two phosphate buffer tablets.

1. The total radioactivity of the antibody labeled with radioactive iodine (^{125}I) in the IRMA kit is determined by pipeting 50 µL of anti-apo(a) solution tagged with iodine 125 into a counter tube and by measuring the γ-counts for 1 min (counts per minute, cpm). The count rate should be higher than 30 000 cpm (*see* **Note 1**).
2. Collect up to 80 plasma samples for one test series and store at least 200 µL of each selected sample at −25°C (*see* **Note 2**).
3. At least 1 h prior to analysis, reconstitute the apo(a) standards 0.4; 1; 2; 5; 10; and 20 µ/L and the controls (low and high) with 500 µL ddH$_2$O at room temperature. Dissolve the two phosphate buffer tablets in 200 mL ddH$_2$O using a magnetic stirrer.
4. Thaw the plasma samples at room temperature and vortex thoroughly. The accurately detectable Lp(a) concentration range is 12 mg/L to 590 mg/L. If in the first series the Lp(a) levels of the samples are higher than the highest standard, the analysis has to be repeated with appropriately diluted samples.
5. Pipet 50 µL of the plasma samples and 50 µL pretreatment solution into 5-mL tubes, mix, and incubate for 1 h at room temperature. Prepare the two controls (low and high) in the same manner (*see* **Note 3**).
6. To stabilize the antibody-Lp(a)-complexes add 2 mL phosphate buffer solution into each tube and mix.
7. The standards in the following step are performed in duplicate (*see* **Note 4**). Pipet carefully at the bottom of the counter tubes 50 µL of the standards and 50 µL of the samples, respectively. Add 50 µL anti-apo(a) tagged with iodine 125 and 50 µL anti-apo(a)-Sepharose™ into each tube (*see* **Note 5**).
8. Fasten the counter tubes in a rack and shake vigorously for 1 h.

9. Centrifuge the counter tubes for 10 min at 1500*g* and fasten the counter tubes again in the rack.

10. Decant the counter tubes immediately in one movement and place them upside down for 30 s on absorbent paper. Transfer the counter tube rack — still upside down — onto a further dry absorbent paper and tap the counter tubes a couple of times on the absorbent paper to get rid of residual drops.

11. Close the counter tubes and count the radioactivity-(^{125}I) for 1 min (cpm) by means of a γ-counter.

12. Plot the count rates (cpm) of the standards against their concentration and calculate the Lp(a) concentration of the samples by linear regression (*see* **Note 6**). The concentrations of the standards must be multiplied by the dilution factor of 42 and by an additional factor of 0.7 to obtain the results in mg/L (*see* **Note 7**).

3.4. Electroimmunoassay (EIA) to Measure Lp(a) in Plasma

Each EIA kit contains three anti-apo(a) agarose gels fixed on transparent gelfoils (each with 13 sample wells), a lyophilized Lp(a) standard, 20 mL Tris-borate electrophoresis buffer, 100 mL protein staining solution (45% v/v ethanol, 45% v/v water, 10% v/v acetic acid, 0.4 mmol/L amidoblack), 100 mL protein destaining solution (45% v/v ethanol, 45% v/v water, 10% v/v acetic acid), and dry absorbent paper.

1. At least 1 h prior to analysis, reconstitute the Lp(a) standard with 500 μL ddH$_2$O water at room temperature. Dilute the electrophoresis buffer solution with 580 mL bidistilled water.

2. Dilute the Lp(a) standard 1:2 and 1:5 with the electrophoresis buffer solution (*see* **Note 8**).

3. Pour the buffer solution into the electrophoretic buffer chambers (*see* **Note 9**).

4. The first three wells of the gel are for the Lp(a) standard solutions (undiluted, 1:2, and 1:5, respectively) to establish the reference curve. If in the first series the Lp(a) levels of the samples are higher than the undiluted standard, the analysis has to be repeated with appropriately diluted samples. 5 μL of each sample are pipetted into the wells (*see* **Note 10**).

5. The gel is fixed in the plastic holder and placed in the electrophoresis chamber. The polarity of the gel has to be checked. Connect the plug in and set the conditions for the run: 180 min with Rapidophor electronic or 60V/30mA/180min with a common power supply.

6. After the electrophoresis is completed, the gel is washed for 30 min in isotonic saline. Thereafter, the wet gel is covered with a sheet of moistened paper and two sheets of dry absorbent paper and compressed for 5–10 min with a weight. Then the gel is washed again for 10 min in isotonic saline, and the pressing procedure is repeated. The gel is then completely dried on the foil, either with hot air or at a maximum temperature of 90°C in an oven (*see* **Note 11**).

7. Immerse the foil 2 min in protein staining solution. Then place the foil in protein destaining solution for 5 min and renew the solution for a further 5 min. Finally, the foil is dried completely.

8. For analysis, assess the quality of the formed rockets. To determine Lp(a) concentrations, plot the length of the rockets against the corresponding standard concentrations and calculate the Lp(a) concentrations of the samples by linear regression (*see* **Note 12**).

4. Notes

1. The total radioactivity in the delivered IRMA kits can vary, depending on the date after ^{125}I-labeling and the time of storage. We found that values less than 30 000 cpm lead to imprecise reference curves and therefore the kit should not be used.
2. It is preferable to use the IRMA test kit within one run, because standard solutions may change over time and radioactivity decreases rapidly. The half-life of ^{125}I is 60 d.
3. The Lp(a) concentrations of the included controls (low and high) are not indicated. The average values of the last 5 yr are 125 mg/L and 399 mg/L for the two controls (low and high, respectively).
4. To identify inaccurate results caused by improper handling, it is recommended to use the standards in duplicate. The determination of samples in duplicate in routine analysis is not always carried out, since economic factors often have to be considered *(33)*.
5. The total volume of 150 µL is not sufficient to cover the bottom of the counter tube completely. However, an additional transfer step is saved, and the low intraassay precision ($\approx$3%) indicates that sufficient mixing occurs and the antibody-antigen reaction is very reproducible.
6. The coefficient of regression for the six standard solutions is usually better than 0.999. However, the slope is variable and depends on the total radioactivity (*see* **Note 1**). Although plots of the standard concentrations in log scale are recommended, we prefer the linear analysis because it facilitates the calculations and diminishes the risk of analytical errors. The difference between the results from linear and logarithmic analysis is usually less than 10 mg/L.
7. The results obtained in this assay are given in µ/L] and must therefore be converted to mg Lp(a)/L. The conversion factor of 0.7 is an empirical value, which was included in the test some years ago. The necessity for this factor was demonstrated in a publication comparing several methods *(21)*.
8. The original dilution 1:10 (about 50 mg Lp(a)/L) as recommended is too low to produce sharp rockets, and the determined value is out of linearity. Therefore, the exactly measurable Lp(a) concentration range of this method lies between 100 mg/L and 700 mg/L.
9. The buffer solution can be used three times when the polarity of the electrode-cassette is changed after each run.
10. After long storage of the gels the wells could be too flat to hold 5 µL, and part of the pipeted solution overflows. Therefore, we suggest in those cases the volume reduction to 4 µL.
11. The washing procedure is important for getting sharp precipitation lines.
12. For the optical determination of the rocket length it is preferable to use an optical analyzer (e.g., from Behring) for immunodiffusion plates. However, modern

digital analysis on the computer screen is probably as accurate as the former. Although digital analysis enables quantification of the rocket areas, we prefer analysis of the rocket length, as irregularities of the rocket shapes could increase the imprecision for the area quantification.

References

1. Dahlen, P. H. and Stenlund, H. (1997) Lp(a) lipoprotein is a major risk factor for cardiovascular disease: Pathogenic mechanisms and clinical significance. *Clin. Genet.* **52,** 272–280.
2. Marcovina, S. M. and Morrisett, J. D. (1995) Structure and metabolism of lipoprotein(a). *Curr. Opin. Lipidol.* **6,** 136–145.
3. Fless, G. M. and Santiago, J. Y. (1997) Molecular weight determination of lipoprotein(a) in solutions containing either NaBr or D_2O: Relevance to the number of apolipoprotein(a) subunits in Lp(a). *Biochemistry* **36,** 233–238.
4. McLean, J. W., Tomlinson, J. E., Kuang, W., Eaton, D. L., Chen, E. Y., Fless, G. M., Scanu, A. M., and Lawn, R. M. (1987) cDNA sequence of human apolipoprotein(a) is homologous to plasminogen. *Nature* **330,** 132–137.
5. Lackner, C., Cohen, J. C., and Hobbs, H. H. (1993) Molecular definition of the extreme size polymorphism in apolipoprotein(a). *Hum. Mol. Genet.* **2,** 933–940.
6. Marcovina, S. M., Zhang, Z. H., Gaur, V. P., and Albers, J. J. (1993) Identification of 34 apolipoprotein(a) isoforms: Differential expression of apolipoprotein(a) alleles between American blacks and whites. *Biochem. Biophys. Res. Commun.* **191,** 1192–1196.
7. Dahlen, G. H. (1994) Lp(a) lipoprotein in cardiovascular disease. *Atherosclerosis* **108,** 111–126.
8. Utermann, G. (1989) The mysteries of lipoprotein(a). *Science* **246,** 904–910.
9. Austin, M. A., Sandholzer, C., Selby, J. V., Newman, B., and Utermann, G. (1992) Lipoprotein(a) in women twins: Heritability and relationship to apolipoprotein(a) phenotypes. *Am. J. Hum. Genet.* **51,** 829–840.
10. Angelin, B. (1997) Therapy for lowering lipoprotein(a) levels. *Curr. Opin. Lipidol.* **8,** 337–341.
11. Kostner, G. M., Avogaro, P., Cazzolato, G., Marth, E., Bittolo-Bon, G., and Quinci, G. B. (1981) Lipoprotein(a) and the risk for myocardial infarction. *Atherosclerosis* **38,** 51–61.
12. Gaillard, O., Meillet, D., Gervais, A., Delattre, J., Galli, J., and Schuller, E. (1994) Lipoprotein(a) in cerebrospinal fluid measured by highly sensitive time-resolved immunofluorimetric assay. *Clin. Chem.* **40,** 1975–1976.
13. Rath, M., Niendorf, A., Reblin, T., Dietel, M., Krebber, H., and Beisiegel, U. (1989) Detection and quantitation of lipoprotein(a) in the arterial wall of 107 coronary bypass patients. *Arteriosclerosis* **9,** 579–592.
14. Gaubatz, J. W., Mital, P., and Morrisett, J. D. (1996) Electrophoretic methods for quantitation of lipoprotein(a). *Methods Enzymol.* **263,** 218–237.

15. Hervio, L., Girard-Globa, A., Durlach, V., and Angles-Cano, E. (1996) The antifibrinolytic effect of lipoprotein(a) in heterozygous subjects is modulated by the relative concentration of each of the apolipoprotein(a) isoforms and their affinity for fibrin. *Eur. J. Clin. Invest.* **26,** 411–417.

16. März, W., Beckmann, A., Scharnagl, H., Siekmeier, R., Mondorf, U., Held, I., Schneider, W., Preissner, K. T., Curtiss, L. K., Groß, W., and Hüttinger, M. (1993) Heterogenous lipoprotein(a) size isoforms differ by their interaction with the LDL receptor and the LRP/α_2-macroglobulin receptor. *FEBS Lett.* **325,** 271–275.

17. Scanu, A. M. and Edelstein, C. (1997) Learning about the structure and biology of human lipoprotein(a) through dissection by enzymes of the elastase family: Facts and speculations. *J. Lipid Res.* **38,** 2193–2206.

18. Lippi, G. and Guidi, G. (1998) Standardization and clinical management of lipoprotein(a) measurements. *Clin. Chem. Lab. Med.* **36,** 5–16.

19. Seman, L. J., Jenner, J. L., McNamara, J. R., and Schaefer, E. J. (1994) Quantification of Lp(a) in plasma by assaying cholesterol in lectin bound plasma fraction. *Clin. Chem.* **40,** 400–403.

20. Tate, J. R., Rifai, N., Berg, K., Couderc, R., Dati, F., Kostner, G. M., Sakurabayashi, I., and Steinmetz, A. (1998) International federation of clinical chemistry standardization project for the measurement of lipoprotein(a). Phase 1. Evaluation of the analytical perfomance of lipoprotein(a) assay systems and commercial calibrators. *Clin. Chem.* **44,** 1629–1640.

21. März, W., Siekmeier, R., Gross, W., and Kostner, G. M. (1993) Determination of lipoprotein(a): Evaluation of three methods. *Eur. J. Clin. Chem. Clin. Biochem.* **31,** 295–302.

22. März, W., Siekmeier, R., Groß, E., and Groß, W. (1993) Determination of lipoprotein(a): Enzyme immunoassay and immunoradiometric assay compared. *Clin. Chim. Acta* **214,** 153–163.

23. Bender, M. and Groß, W. (1999) Comparison of a kinetic nephelometry with an immunoradiometric assay for the determination of lipoprotein(a). *J. Lab. Med.* **23,** 85–90.

24. Siekmeier, R., März, W., Scharnagl, H., Nauck, M., Mayer, H., Wieland, H., Groß, W., and Seiffert, U. B. (1996) Determination of lipoprotein(a): Comparison of a novel latex enhanced immunoturbidimetric assay and an immunoradiometric assay. *J. Lab. Med.* **20,** 294–298.

25. Laurell, C. B. and McKay, E. J. (1981) Electroimmunoassay. *Methods Enzymol.* **73,** 339–369.

26. März, W. and Groß, W. (1983) Quantification of human serum lipoprotein Lp(a): Zone immunoelectrophoresis assay, a new sensitive method as compared to electroimmunoassay. *Clin. Chim. Acta* **134,** 265–279.

27. Groß, W. and März, W. (1999) Application of electrophoretic techniques to the diagnosis of disorders of lipoprotein metabolism. Examples at the levels of lipoproteins and apolipoproteins. *Anal. Chim. Acta* **383,** 169–184.

28. Kostner, G. M. (1992) Standardization of lipoprotein(a) assays. *Clin. Chim. Acta* **211,** 191–194.

29. Wanner, C., Greiber, S., Krämer-Guth, A., Heinloth, A., and Galle, J. (1997) Lipids and progression of renal disease: Role of modified low density lipoprotein and lipoprotein(a). *Kidney Int.* **52,** S102–S106.
30. Marcovina, S. M., Gaur, V. P., and Albers, J. J. (1994) Biological variability of cholesterol, LDL-, HDL-cholesterol, Lp(a) and apolipoproteins A-I and B. *Clin. Chem.* **40,** 574–578.
31. Kronenberg, F., Lobentanz, E. M., König, P., Utermann, G., and Dieplinger, H. (1994) Effect of sample storage on the measurement of Lp(a), apoB and apoA-IV, total and HDL cholesterol and trigylcerides. *J. Lipid Res.* **35,** 1318–1328.
32. Groß, E., März, W., Siekmeier, R., Scharrer, I., and Groß, W. (1993) Isolation of lipoprotein(a) using the regenerate of a dextran sulfate cellulose LDL apheresis system. *Protein Expr. Purif.* **5,** 112–117.
33. Sadler, W. A. and Smith, M. H. (1990) Use and abuse of imprecision profiles: Some pitfalls illustrated by computing and plotting confidence intervals. *Clin. Chem.* **36,** 1346–1350.

11

Isolation and Characterization of Glycosaminoglycans from Human Atheromatous Vessels

Eleni Papakonstantinou, Michael Roth, and George Karakiulakis

1. Introduction

The complex cascade of events leading to the formation of atheromatous plaques depends on the interaction between several cell types, growth factors, cytokines, and molecules of the extracellular matrix (ECM) *(1)*. Among different molecules of the ECM involved in atherogenesis, the glycosaminoglycans (GAGs) have been reported to contribute to key events leading to the formation of atherosclerotic lesions *(2)*. GAGs are linear acidic polysaccharides of variable length and composition, which occur either in free form or attached to a protein core to form proteoglycans *(3)*. On the basis of their composition, GAGs are grouped into four major categories: hyaluronic acid, heparin and heparan sulfate, chondroitin and dermatan sulfates, and keratan sulfate. ECM GAGs provide structural links between fibrous and cellular elements, contribute to viscoelastic properties, regulate permeability and retention of plasma components within the matrix *(2,4)*, inhibit vascular cell growth *(5)*, affect hemostasis and platelet aggregation *(6)*, and interact with lipoproteins *(7)* and various growth factors *(8,9)*.

Regarding atherosclerosis, it has been shown that specific GAGs such as dermatan sulfate and chondroitin sulfates A and C increase during early fibrous plaque formation in the tunica media of human coronary arteries and aortas *(10–12)*. Hyaluronic acid (HA), a commonly expressed GAG, appears to be of particular interest, since tissues enriched in HA may undergo expansion because of the ability of this molecule to bind large amounts of water, thus creating a loose, hydrated micro environment that facilitates cell migration, a critical event in atherogenesis *(1)* and arterial development *(13)*. In this context,

From: *Methods in Molecular Medicine, vol. 52: Atherosclerosis: Experimental Methods and Protocols*
Edited by: A. F. Drew © Humana Press Inc., Totowa, NJ

it has been reported that HA is secreted by vascular smooth muscle cells (VSMC) *(14)*; HA-synthesizing enzymes increase during VSMC proliferation *(15)*; and HA decreases in the tunica media of atherosclerotic vessels *(10,11,16)*. More recently, we have shown that VSMC, under conditions of induced proliferation, similar to those involved in atherosclerosis, secrete a 340-kDa HA *(17)* that inhibits VSMC proliferation and enhances their migration through an artificial basement membrane *(18)*. Furthermore, human atheromatous aortas distinctly express HA of 340 kDa *(19)*. The abundance of this molecule in the tunica media as compared with the low levels in the tunica intima and atherosclerotic plaque correlates with its function as a negative control element of VSMC proliferation and a positive control element of VSMC migration during the development of atherosclerotic lesions *(19)*.

The ability of GAGs to mediate key events in the progression of atherogenesis may offer alternative targets for pharmacological intervention to regulate GAG homeostasis in human atheromatous vessels and thus prevent and/or treat atherosclerosis.

In this chapter, we describe the methodology for the isolation, purification, and characterization of GAGs from human atheromatous vessels.

2. Materials

2.1. Homogenization of Tissue Specimens

1. 100 mM Tris-HCl, pH 8.0.

2.2. Isolation and Purification of Total GAGs

2.2.1. Lipid Extraction

1. Chloroform.
2. Methanol.
3. Ethanol.

2.2.2. Protein Digestion

1. 100 mM Tris-HCl, pH 8.0, containing 1 mM CaCl$_2$.
2. Pronase (protease from *Streptomyces griseus*), 30 mg/mL, dissolved in the above buffer and preincubated for 30 min at 60°C to eliminate any glycosidase activity (store at –20°C for up to 15 d).

2.2.3. DNA Digestion

1. 1 M NaCl.
2. 1 M MgCl$_2$.

3. DNase I (EC 3.1.21.1) 20,000 U/mL dissolved in ddH$_2$O.
4. 0.1 M CaCl$_2$.
5. Pronase prepared as in **Subheading 2.2.2.**

2.2.4. β-elimination

1. 5 M NaOH.
2. 1 M NaBH$_4$ dissolved in 0.1 *M* NaOH. Make fresh as required just before adding to the samples.
3. Acetic acid 50% (v/v).

2.2.5. Purification of Total GAGs

1. Sephadex G-25 fine (e.g., Pharmacia).
2. Glass column (0.75 cm × 110 cm, optimally).
3. 10 m*M* pyridine acetate buffer, pH 5.0 (store at room temperature).

2.2.6. Determination of Uronic Acids

1. 0.025 *M* sodium tetra borate solution in sulfuric acid (store at room temperature).
2. 0.125% carbazol solution in ethanol (make fresh as required and use it as a suspension).
3. Glucuronic acid 1 mg/ml in ddH$_2$O (store at –20°C).

2.3. Fractionation of Total GAGs

2.3.1. Fractionation by Size Exclusion Chromatography

1. Superose 6 (e.g., Pharmacia).
2. Glass column (0.75 cm × 95 cm, optimally).
3. 50 m*M* pyridine acetate, pH 5.0.

2.3.2. Fractionation by High-Pressure Liquid Chromatography (HPLC)

1. Bio-gel TSK 40XL gel filtration column (300 mm × 7.8 mm, optimally), for HPLC.
2. MXGL 0035 precolumn (40 mm × 7.8 mm, optimally).
3. 7 m*M* Tris-HCl, pH 7.4, containing 200 m*M* NaCl.
4. UV/VIS monitor (e.g., Bio Rad, model 1706).
5. Refractive index monitor (e.g., Bio Rad, model 1755).

2.3.3. Fractionation by Anion-Exchange Chromatography

1. DEAE Sephacel (e.g., Pharmacia).
2. Glass column (1.25 cm × 10 cm, optimally).

3. 0.1 M pyridine and 0.47 M HCOOH, pH 3.0.
4. 2 M NaCl.
5. Bio-gel MA7P anion exchange column (50 mm × 7.8 mm, optimally) for HPLC equipped with a Carbo-C cartridge precolumn.
6. 10 mM phosphate buffer, pH 6.0.
7. 100 mM phosphate buffer, pH 6.0.

2.3.4. Electrophoresis on Cellulose Acetate Membranes

1. 100 mM pyridine/470 mM formic acid, pH 3.0 (store at 4°C and use for up to 10 electrophoreses).
2. 0.1 M barium acetate buffer, pH 8.0 (make fresh as required).
3. Cellulose acetate membranes. Store at 4°C and equilibrate in electrophoresis buffer (**items 1** or **2** above) for 10–15 min before use, at room temperature.
4. Electrophoresis chamber (Bioblock Scientific).
5. Staining solution: 0.2% (w/v) alcian blue (Fluka) in 0.1% (v/v) acetic acid (filter to remove undissolved particles and store at room temperature). Staining solution may be used several times.
6. Destaining solution: 0.1% (v/v) acetic acid.

2.3.5. Polyacrylamide Gel Electrophoresis (PAGE)

1. Glass plates (e.g., 0.8 mm × 12 cm × 12 cm).
2. 30% (w/v) acrylamide containing 0.8% (w/v) N,N-methylene-bis-acrylamide.
3. 10-fold concentrated solution of a buffer composed of 0.9 M Tris-HCL base, 0.9 M boric acid, and 24 mM EDTA, pH 8.3.
4. 10% (w/v) ammonium persulfate.
5. TEMED.
6. Staining solution: 0.5% (w/v) alcian blue dissolved in 25% (v/v) isopropyl alcohol and 1% (v/v) acetic acid (filter to remove undissolved particles and store at room temperature). Staining solution may be used several times.
7. Destaining solution: 25% (v/v) isopropyl alcohol and 1% (v/v) acetic acid.

2.4. Chemical and Structure Analysis of the Fractionated GAGs

2.4.1. Carbohydrate Analysis by Gas Chromatography

1. 0.625 M HCl in methanol.
2. Absolute methyl acetate.
3. Absolute t-butyl alcohol.
4. Nitrogen gas.
5. Dry methanol.
6. Pyridine.
7. Acetic anhydride.

8. Silylation reagent Sylon TP (possible source: Supelco).
9. Hexane.
10. Silica glass column (12.5 m × 0.2 mm, optimally) coated with 0.33 mm methyl-silicon gum (e.g., Hewlett-Packard).
11. Gas chromatographer (e.g., Hewlett-Packard gas chromatographer 7620 A), equipped with a 5970 Mass selective detector.

2.4.2. Sulfate Determination

1. 6.25 M HCl.
2. 4 M HCl.
3. Ethanol.
4. 0.5 M acetate buffer, pH 4.0, containing 60 µg/mL sodium sulfate.
5. 0.5 M acetate buffer, pH 4.0, containing 10 mg/mL barium chloranilate. Prepare barium chloranilate by mixing 1 L of 0.1% aqueous chloranilic acid with 1 L of 5% aqueous barium chloride and permitting the mixture to stand overnight at room temperature. Wash the aged precipitate with water until the supernatant liquid is free of chloride ions, the presence of which is determined by the white precipitate formed following addition of $AgNO_3$. Remove water by centrifuging the precipitate three times with ethyl alcohol and once with diethyl ether and drying for 1 h at 60°C in a vacuum oven (store at room temperature).
6. 0.5 M acetate buffer, pH 4.0.

2.4.3. Treatment of the Purified Glycans with GAG-Degrading Enzymes

1. 0.1 M Tris-HCl buffer, pH 7.0, containing 1 mM $CaCl_2$ and 0.1 M NaCl.
2. Heparin lyase I (EC 4.2.2.7, *Flavobacterium heparinum*, possible source: Seikagaku).
3. Heparan sulfate lyase (EC 4.2.2.8, *Flavobacterium heparinum*, possible source: Seikagaku).
4. 0.1 M Tris-HCl buffer, pH 8.0, containing 0.05 M sodium acetate.
5. Chondroitin ABC lyase (EC 4.2.2.4, *Proteus vulgaris*, possible source: Seikagaku).
6. 0.1 M Tris-HCl buffer, pH 7.4.
7. Chondroitin B lyase (EC 4.2.2.5, *Flavobacterium heparinum*, possible source: Seikagaku).
8. 50 mM Tris-HCl buffer, pH 7.4.
9. Keratan sulfate 1,4-β-D-galactanohydrolase (EC 3.2.10.3, *Pseudomonas* sp., possible source: Seikagaku).
10. 0.02 M Sodium acetate, buffered with acetic acid to pH 6.0, containing 0.15 M NaCl.
11. Hyaluronate lyase (EC 4.2.2.1, *Streptomyces hyalurolyticus*, possible source: Seikagaku).

3. Methods

3.1. Tissue Specimens

Postmortem biopsies of human aortas or other arteries must be obtained at autopsy within 6 h following death by accident, from individuals whose medical history must be free from diseases, such as hypertension and diabetes. The internal mammary artery may serve as a useful control tissue specimen, since it exhibits a low incidence of atherosclerosis, and therefore it is considered the best choice for coronary revascularization.

Specimens of the wall of the aorta, of coronary arteries with distinct atheromatous lesions, or of internal mammary arteries may also be obtained following surgical dissection from patients undergoing coronary artery bypass grafting. Small vessels (e.g., coronary arteries) are used whole. In large vessels (e.g., aortas) the atheromatous plaque may be dissected away and the vessels can be separated in their respective layers: tunica intima (endothelium and subendothelial layer), tunica media, and tunica adventitia.

Irrespective of origin, homogenize tissue specimens for 10-s bursts with 30-s intervals, at 4°C to avoid overheating, at a concentration of 2 g tissue per 15 mL of 100 mM Tris-HCl buffer, pH 8.0 (*see* **Note 1**).

3.2. Isolation and Purification of Total GAGs

3.2.1. Lipid Extraction

1. To the homogenized tissue specimens, add 4 vol of a 1:2 mixture of chloroform/ methanol (v/v) and leave for 2 h at room temperature, or at 4°C overnight (*see* **Note 2**).
2. Centrifuge at 1000–3000g for 20 min, at 4°C; discard the supernatant and add 5–10 mL ethanol to remove the remaining organic solvents.
3. Centrifuge again as above, discard the supernatant, and dry the resulting pellet at 40°C for about 4 h, or more if required.

3.2.2. Protein Digestion

1. Weigh the dried pellets and resuspend in 100 mM Tris-HCl buffer, pH 8.0, containing 1 mM CaCl$_2$ (approximately 2 mL buffer per 30 mg dry defatted tissue).
2. Add 50 µL of 30 mg/mL Pronase. Incubate for 72 h at 60°C, by adding equal amounts of Pronase at 24-h intervals (*see* **Note 3**).

3.2.3. DNA Digestion

1. Add NaCl and MgCl$_2$ to the solution to achieve a final concentration of 150 mM and 10 mM, respectively.
2. Add 30 µL 20,000 U/mL DNase I dissolved in ddH$_2$O and incubate for 18 h at 37°C.

3. Adjust the CaCl$_2$ concentration to 1 mM and stop the reaction by adding 50 μL of 30 mg/mL Pronase, dissolved as above, and incubate the mixture at 60°C for 24 h.

3.2.4. β-Elimination

1. Titrate the samples with 5 M NaOH to pH 10.0–11.0 and incubate in the presence of 1 M NaBH$_4$ (dissolved in 0.1 M NaOH) at 43°C overnight, under nitrogen.
2. Neutralize the samples with 0.2 vol 50% (v/v) acetic acid, on ice, to avoid overheating of the samples (*see* **Note 4**).

3.2.5. Purification of Total GAGs

1. Separate GAGs from Pronase and DNase digestion products by gel filtration on a Sephadex G-25 fine column (0.75 cm × 110 cm, optimally), by elution with 10 mM pyridine acetate buffer, pH 5.0.
2. Collect 2 mL fractions at an optimal flow rate of 0.66–1.75 mL/min.
3. Identify the fractions containing GAGs by measuring their uronic acid content, as described in **Subheading 3.2.6.**
4. Pool the fractions containing uronic acids, lyophilize, and dissolve in ddH$_2$O.
5. The purification of the glycans from the digestion products by gel filtration on Sephadex G-25 column should yield a single peak of glycans, with a recovery rate of approximately 90% (*see* **Note 5**).

3.2.6. Determination of Uronic Acids

1. Take an aliquot from the samples to be tested and bring volume up to 250 μL with ddH$_2$O.
2. Add 1.25 mL of cold 0.025 M sodium tetra borate solution in sulfuric acid, vortex, and boil for 10 min.
3. Cool at room temperature and then add 50 μL of 0.125% carbazole solution in ethanol.
4. Vortex and boil for 15 min.
5. Cool at room temperature and read the absorbance at 530 nm.
6. Prepare a standard curve by treating 1–15 μg of glucuronic acid through all above described steps.
7. Estimate the uronic acid concentration in each fraction, employing the standard curve (*see* **Note 6**).

3.3. Fractionation of Total GAGs

3.3.1. Fractionation by Size Exclusion Chromatography

Size fractionation of total GAGs (minimum 1–2 mg uronic acids) can be achieved by size exclusion chromatography on a Superose 6 column (0.75 cm × 95 cm, optimally).

1. Apply lyophilized GAG samples (dissolved in 1–5 mL ddH$_2$O) on the column and elute with 50 mM pyridine acetate, pH 5.0.
2. Collect fractions (1–2 mL) at an optimal flow rate of 0.8 mL/min and determine those containing uronic acids as described in **Subheading 3.2.6.**
3. Display the results in a graphic form (uronic acid content vs fraction number), pool the fractions containing fractionated GAGs of similar size according to graphic representation, lyophilize, dissolve in ddH$_2$O, and store at 4°C (*see* **Note 7**).

3.3.2. Fractionation by High–Pressure Liquid Chromatography (HPLC)

For small quantities of total GAGs (less than 1 mg uronic acids) isolated and purified from vessels, size fractionation can be achieved by HPLC. A suitable column for HPLC analysis of GAGs could be a Bio-gel TSK 40XL gel filtration column (300 mm × 7.8 mm, optimally), equipped with an MXGL 0035 precolumn (40 mm × 7.8 mm, optimally).

1. Elute GAGs with 7 mM Tris-HCl, pH 7.4, containing 200 mM NaCl, at an optimal flow rate of 0.3 mL/min and collect fractions every 30 s.
2. During HPLC gel-filtration analyses, monitor the absorbance at 206 nm using a UV/VIS monitor and a refractive index monitor.
3. Pool fractions containing the fractionated GAGs of similar size according to graphic representation of UV and refractive index.
4. Dialyze pooled fractions against large quantities of ddH$_2$O, lyophilize, dissolve in ddH$_2$O, and determine their uronic acid content as described in **Subheading 3.2.6.** Store at 4°C (*see* **Note 8**).

3.3.3. Fractionation by Anion-Exchange Chromatography

Ion-exchange chromatography of the purified total GAGs (minimum 0.5 mg uronic acids) can be performed using a DEAE Sephacel anion-exchange column (1.25 cm × 10 cm).

1. Equilibrate column with a buffer containing 0.1 M pyridine and 0.47 M HCOOH, pH 3.0, and elute GAG sample with a continuous NaCl gradient (0–1 M) followed by a single-step increase of the NaCl concentration to 2 M.
2. Maintain a constant flow rate of 0.5 mL/min with the help of a peristaltic pump and collect fractions of 1.5 mL.
3. Determine the GAG-containing fractions as described in **Subheading 3.2.6.**
4. Display the results in a graphic form (uronic acid content vs fraction number) and pool the fractions containing fractionated GAGs of similar ionic charge according to graphic representation.
5. Dialyze pooled fractions against large quantities of ddH$_2$O, lyophilize, dissolve in ddH$_2$O, and store at 4°C (yield approximately 85%).

For small quantities of total GAGs (less than 0.5 µg uronic acids) ion-exchange chromatography can also be performed by HPLC using a Bio-gel MA7P anion-exchange column (50 mm × 7.8 mm, optimally) equipped with a Carbo-C cartridge precolumn.

1. Equilibrate the column with 10 mM phosphate buffer, pH 6.0, and elute GAGs with a gradient of 10 mM to 100 mM phosphate buffer, pH 6.0, at an optimal flow rate of 1.2 mL/min.
2. Collect fractions every 30 s and monitor the absorbance at 206 nm, using a UV/VIS monitor and a refractive index monitor.
3. Pool GAG-containing fractions according to graphic representation of UV and refractive index.
4. Dialyze pooled fractions against large quantities of ddH$_2$O, lyophilize, dissolve in ddH$_2$O, and store at 4°C (*see* **Note 8**).

3.3.4. Electrophoresis on Cellulose Acetate Membranes

1. Apply 1–4 µL GAG solution containing about 1–4 µg uronic acids at the origin (10 mm from the cathode side) of a cellulose acetate membrane.
2. Carry out electrophoresis in 100 mM pyridine/470 mM formic acid, pH 3.0, under 7 mA constant current, at room temperature, for 1 h. Alternatively, cellulose acetate electrophoresis can be conducted in 0.1 M barium acetate, pH 8.0, under 5 mA constant current, at room temperature, for 4 h.
3. After electrophoresis, stain the cellulose acetate membranes with 0.2% (w/v) alcian blue in 0.1% (v/v) acetic acid for 10 min and destain with 0.1% (v/v) acetic acid for about 20 min (*see* **Note 9**).

3.3.5. Polyacrylamide Gel Electrophoresis (PAGE)

1. Prepare linear gradient 4–20% polyacrylamide gels, using a stock solution of 30% (w/v) acrylamide, 0.8% (w/v) N,N-methylene-bis-acrylamide, and a 10-fold concentrated solution of a buffer composed of 0.9 M Tris base, 0.9 M boric acid, and 24 mM EDTA, pH 8.3. Polymerize the gels by adding 32 µL of 10% (w/v) ammonium persulfate and 3.2 µL tetramethylethylenediamine/16 mL acrylamide-Tris-borate-EDTA solution.
2. Prefocus the gels at room temperature for 1/2 h at 200 V with Tris-borate-EDTA as running buffer, using a fan ventilator for cooling.
3. Prepare an amount of total GAGs (6–10 µg uronic acids) in a twofold concentrated solution of running buffer, also containing 30% glycerol and trace amounts of phenol red.
4. Carry out PAGE at 300 V at room temperature for about 4 h, using a fan ventilator for cooling.

5. Terminate electrophoresis when the tracking dye reaches about 1 cm above the end of the gel.
6. Stain the gels with a solution of 0.5% (w/v) alcian blue dissolved in 25% (v/v) isopropyl alcohol and 1% (v/v) acetic acid for 12 h. Use the same solution without the dye for destaining (*see* **Note 10**).

3.4. Chemical and Structure Analysis of the Fractionated GAGs

3.4.1. Carbohydrate Analysis by Gas Chromatography

1. Dry GAG samples (25–30 µg uronic acids) in a speed vacuum system, dissolve pellets in 80 µL of 0.625 M HCl in methanol, and then add 20 µL absolute methyl acetate.
2. Incubate samples for 17 h at 70°C.
3. Add 20 µL absolute t-butyl alcohol and evaporate under a stream of nitrogen gas, at room temperature.
4. Add 100 µL dry methanol, 10 µL pyridine, and 10 µL acetic anhydride, successively, with intermediate mixing to re-*N*-acetylate the amino sugars.
5. Leave solutions at room temperature for 15 min and subsequently evaporate to dryness, initially under a nitrogen stream and then by vacuum.
6. After thorough drying, add 40 µL of the silylation reagent Sylon TP, vortex, and leave for 1 h at room temperature.
7. Re-evaporate the derivatized samples under a nitrogen stream, dissolve immediately in 50 µL hexane and centrifuge at 4000*g* for 5 min.
8. Determine the sugar composition in 40 µL aliquots of the supernatant on a silica glass column (12.5 m × 0.2 mm, optimally) coated with 0.33 µM methyl-silicon gum in a gas chromatographer, equipped with a 5970 Mass selective detector. Use a glycan molecule (e.g., inositol) known to be absent in the biological material under investigation, as internal standard.

3.4.2. Sulfate Determination

1. Clean all glassware twice with 6.25 *M* HCl for 5 min each time, rinse with ddH$_2$O, and then dry in an oven at 100°C.
2. Dry GAG samples (10–20 µg uronic acids) and hydrolyze by adding 300 µL of 4 *M* HCl and drying in a vacuum oven for 4 h at 100°C.
3. Add 300 µL ddH$_2$O, dry samples again as above, and redissolve in 50 µL ddH$_2$O.
4. Add 200 µL ethanol, vortex, and then add 25 µL 0.5 *M* acetate buffer, pH 4.0, containing 60 µg/mL sodium sulfate.
5. Vortex, add 25 µL of 0.5 *M* acetate buffer, pH 4.0, containing 10 mg/mL barium chloranilate, and mix 10 times by vortexing at 1-min intervals.
6. Centrifuge at 3000*g* for 10 min, dilute 200-µL aliquots of the supernatant with 800 µL of 0.5 *M* acetate buffer, pH 4.0, and measure the absorption of the liberated chloranilic acid at 327.5 nm (*see* **Note 11**).

3.4.3. Enzymatic Characterization of GAGs

3.4.3.1. TREATMENT OF THE PURIFIED GLYCANS WITH GAG-DEGRADING ENZYMES

Treat dried GAGs (10 µg uronic acids) in a final volume of 10 µL as follows:

a. Treatment with heparinase: dissolve samples in 0.1 M Tris-HCl buffer, pH 7.0, containing 1 mM CaCl$_2$ and 0.1 M NaCl, and add 5 × 10^{-3} U heparin lyase. Incubate at 35°C for 15 h.
b. Treatment with heparitinase: Dissolve samples as above and add 5 × 10^{-3} U heparan sulfate lyase. Incubate at 43°C for 16 h.
c. Treatment with chondroitinase ABC: Dissolve samples in 0.1 M Tris-HCl buffer, pH 8.0, containing 0.05 M sodium acetate, and add 5 × 10^{-3} U chondroitin ABC lyase. Incubate at 37°C for 16 h.
d. Treatment with chondroitinase B: Dissolve samples in 0.1 M Tris-HCl buffer, pH 7.4, and add 0.2 U chondroitin B lyase. Incubate at 37°C for 16 h.
e. Treatment with keratanase: Dissolve samples in 50 mM Tris-HCl buffer, pH 7.4, and add 0.1 U keratan sulfate 1,4-β-D-galactanohydrolase. Incubate at 37°C for 5 h.
f. Treatment with hyaluronidase: Dissolve samples in 0.02 M sodium acetate, buffered with acetic acid to pH 6.0, containing 0.15 M NaCl, and add 5 U hyaluronate lyase. Incubate at 60°C for 14 h.

Substrates incubated separately with the respective buffers should serve as controls (*see* **Note 12**).

3.4.3.2. EVALUATION OF ENZYMATIC DIGESTION WITH GAG-DEGRADING ENZYMES

Evaluate enzymatic digestion of the purified glycans with GAG-degrading enzymes by either electrophoresis on cellulose acetate membranes (*see* **Subheading 3.3.4.**) and/or PAGE (*see* **Subheading 3.3.5.**) and quantitate by scanning densitometry. Alternatively, digestion can be quantitated by HPLC as described in **Subheading 3.3.2.** by monitoring the absorbance at 232 nm.

4. Notes

1. Tissue specimens (**Subheading 3.1.**): Homogenization of large-vessel tissue specimens is quite laborious because of the elasticity of the vessel wall. Cutting the specimens with a razor blade into small pieces (2–3 mm^3) and sonication will aid homogenization considerably.
2. Lipid extraction (**Subheading 3.2.1.**): The ratio of chloroform/methanol should be 1:2, otherwise, two separated layers will appear. Should this happen, add a further 1–2 mL methanol to the mixture and mix by shaking.
3. Protein digestion (**Subheading 3.2.2.**): The intervals between consecutive additions of Pronase, at the recommended enzyme/substrate ratio, should not be less than 22 h, which is the time required for complete autodigestion of Pronase.
4. β-elimination (**Subheading 3.2.4.**): The pH of the samples should not be less than 10.0, otherwise tubes may explode because of the excess production of H$_2$. Neutralization with acetic acid should be performed in a fume hood.

5. Purification of total GAGs (**Subheading 3.2.5.**): When handling small quantities of GAGs, instead of gel filtration, extracted GAGs can be precipitated by adding 4 vol of ethanol in the presence of 0.1 vol 3 M CH$_3$COONa, at –20°C for 16 h. In this case, recover total GAGs by centrifugation at 2,000g for 20 min, dissolve pellet in ddH$_2$O (optimal GAG concentration 1 mg/mL), and store at 4°C (yield approximately 85%).

6. Determination of uronic acids (**Subheading 3.2.6.**): Contamination of the samples by dust or chlorinated tap water may give a green color following the addition of the sulfuric acid reagent, because of formation of oxidants. To account for oxidant interference, subtract the absorption of sample at 920 nm from that at 530 nm, since the optical densities of the contaminant at these points are almost equivalent *(20)*.

7. Fractionation by size-exclusion chromatography (**Subheading 3.3.1.**): The apparent molecular weight of the fractionated GAGs could be estimated using as molecular-weight markers GAGs of known molecular size. Commercially available GAGs do not usually have a precisely defined molecular mass because of size polydispersity of the molecules. To determine the exact molecular size of any GAG molecule, sedimentation equilibrium and sedimentation velocity analyses must be performed in an analytical ultracentrifuge (e.g., Beckman Model E), which must be equipped with Rayleigh interference and Schlieren optics. In either case, an interference-double-sector cell 12 mm Epon-filled-charcoal and an An-D rotor should be used. For this type of analysis, dissolve dried GAG samples in 7 mM Tris-HCl, containing 200 mM NaCl, pH 7.4. For sedimentation equilibrium analysis, a range of speeds from 4800 to 8000 rpm should be used. The speed can be adapted for different molecular masses and concentrations. When samples with molecular masses smaller than 5×10^3 are to be analyzed, speeds of 34,000 and 44,000 rpm should be used, according to the "midpoint mode" method of Yphantis *(21)*. The initial concentration of glycans with molecular masses smaller than 5×10^3 can be determined in a separate run in a synthetic-boundary capillary type. Sedimentation velocity analysis should be performed at 34,000 and 40,000 rpm using interference optics. All runs must be performed at 20°C. The molecular weights may be calculated using a linear regression computer program to obtain the best linear fit of concentration versus r^2 (r = radial distance) *(22)*.

8. Fractionation by high-pressure liquid chromatography (**Subheading 3.3.2.**) and fractionation by anion-exchange chromatography (**Subheading 3.3.3.**): Instead of using dialysis, GAGs can be precipitated from the pooled fractions by adding a mixture of ethanol and CH$_3$COONa, as described in **Note 5**.

9. Electrophoresis on cellulose acetate membranes (**Subheading 3.3.4.**): Perform electrophoresis on cellulose acetate membranes initially using 100 mM pyridine/470 mM formic acid, pH 3.0, and repeat using 0.1 M barium acetate, pH 8.0. This is necessary since hyaluronic acid can be separated from dermatan sulfate only in pyridine/formic acid buffer, whereas dermatan sulfate can be separated from heparan sulfate only in barium acetate buffer *(23)*. Destaining period of cellulose acetate membranes should be judged accordingly to obtain optimal contrast.

10. PAGE (**Subheading 3.3.5.**): GAGs usually migrate on PAGE as broad bands because of the size polydispersity of the molecules. Thus, determination of the

exact molecular mass can be achieved only as described in **Note 7**. However, an average molecular mass can be estimated by PAGE using as molecular weight markers GAGs of known molecular size *(24)*. Destaining period of gels should be judged accordingly to obtain optimal contrast.

11. Sulfate determination (**Subheading 3.4.2.**): The benzidine method also can be used for the determination of sulfate. This method has the advantage over the barium chloranilate method in that it is more sensitive (sensitivity: minimum 25 μg of SO_4^{2-} ion/mL) and can be used in the presence of small amounts of bivalent cations, such as PO_4^{3-} and Mg^{2+} present in biological tissues. However, if one is deterred by the toxicity of benzidine, the barium chloranilate method offers the advantage of rapidity and convenience, and it also can be used in the presence of PO_4^{3-} ions. Furthermore, the sensitivity of this method is increased by addition of small amounts of SO_4^{2-} ions *(25)*.

12. Enzymatic characterization of GAGs (**Subheading 3.4.3.**): Incubation times and enzyme concentrations used should be those required for the complete degradation of their respective standard substrates. This should be estimated in a preliminary investigation, whereby the standard GAGs (10 μg) chondroitin sulfate A, chondroitin sulfate B, chondroitin sulfate C, hyaluronic acid, keratan sulfate, heparan sulfate, and heparin are treated with all mentioned GAG-degrading enzymes, following appropriate incubation conditions.

References

1. Ross, R. (1993) The pathogenesis of atherosclerosis: A perspective for the 1990s. *Nature* **362,** 801–809.
2. Wight, T. N. (1989) Cell biology of arterial proteoglycans. *Atherosclerosis* **9,** 1–20.
3. Kjelleås, L. and Lindahl, U. (1991) Proteoglycans: Structures and Interactions. *Annu. Rev. Biochem.* **60,** 443–475.
4. Wight, T. N. (1985) Proteoglycans in pathological conditions: Atherosclerosis *Fed. Proc.* **44,** 381–385.
5. Fritze, L. M. S., Reilly C. F., and Rosenberg, R. D. (1985) An antiproliferative heparan sulfate species produced by post confluent smooth muscle cells. *J. Cell Biol.* **100,** 1041–1049.
6. Vijayagopal, P., Radhakrishnamurty, B., Srinivasan, S. R., and Berenson, G. S. (1980) Studies of biological properties of proteoglycans from bovine aorta. *Lab. Invest.* **42,** 190–196.
7. Iverius, P. H. (1972) The interaction between human plasma lipoproteins and connective tissue glycosaminoglycans. *J. Biol. Chem.* **247,** 2607–2613.
8. Ruoslahti, E. and Yamaguchi, Y. (1991) Proteoglycans as modulators of growth factor activities. *Cell* **64,** 867–869.
9. Penc, S. F., Pomahac, B., Winkler, T., Dorschner, R. A., Eriksson, E., Herndon, M., and Gallo, R. L. (1998) Dermatan sulfate released after injury is a potent promoter of fibroblast growth factor-2 functions. *J. Biol. Chem.* **273,** 28116–28121.
10. Tammi, M., Sepala, P. O., Lehtonen, A., and Mottonen, M. (1978) Connective tissue components in normal and atherosclerotic human coronary arteries. *Atherosclerosis* **29,** 191–194.

11. Yla-Herttuala, S., Sumuvuori, H., Karkola, K., Mottonen, M., and Nikkari, T. (1986) Glycosaminoglycans in normal and atherosclerotic human coronary arteries. *Lab. Invest.* **54,** 402–407.
12. Hollmann, J., Schmidt, A., von Bassewitz, D.-B., and Buddecke, E. (1989) Relationship of sulphated glycosaminoglycans and cholesterol content in normal and atherosclerotic human aorta. *Arteriosclerosis* **9,** 154–158.
13. Rooney, P. and Kumar, S. (1993) Inverse relationship between hyaluronan and collagens in development and angiogenesis. *Differentiation* **54,** 1–9.
14. Ross, R. (1971) The smooth muscle cells: II. Growth of smooth muscle cells in culture and formation of elastic fibers. *J. Cell Biol.* **50,** 172–186.
15. Hollmann, J., Thiel, J., Schmidt, A., and Buddecke, E. (1986) Increased activities of chondroitin sulfate synthesizing enzymes during proliferation of arterial smooth muscle cells. *Exp. Cell Res.* **167,** 484–494.
16. Klynstra, F. B., Botchen, C. J. F., and Van Der Laan, E. J. (1967) Distribution and composition of acid mucopolysaccharides in normal and atherosclerotic human aortas. *J. Atheroscler. Res.* **7,** 301–309.
17. Papakonstantinou, E., Karakiulakis, G., Roth, M., and Block, L. H. (1995) Platelet-derived growth factor stimulates the secretion of hyaluronic acid by proliferating human vascular smooth muscle cells. *Proc. Natl. Acad. Sci. USA* **92,** 9881–9885.
18. Papakonstantinou, E., Karakiulakis, G., Eickelberg, O., Perruchoud, A. P., Block, L. H., and Roth, M. (1998) A 340 kDa hyaluronic acid secreted by human vascular smooth muscle cells regulates their proliferation and migration. *Glycobiology* **8,** 821–830.
19. Papakonstantinou, E., Roth, M., Block, L. H., Mirtsou-Fidani, V., Argiriadis, P., and Karakiulakis, G. (1998) The differential distribution of hyaluronic acid in the layers of human atheromatic aortas is associated with vascular smooth muscle cell proliferation and migration. *Atherosclerosis* **138,** 79–89.
20. Bitter, T. and Muir, H. M. (1962) A modified uronic acid carbazol reaction. *Anal. Biochem.* **4,** 330–334.
21. Yphantis, D. A. (1960) Rapid determination of molecular weights of peptides and proteins. *Ann. NY Acad. Sci.* **88,** 586.
22. Papakonstantinou, E. and Misevic, G. (1993) Isolation and characterization of a new class of acidic glycans implicated in sea urchin embryonal cell adhesion. *J. Cell. Biochem.* **53,** 98–113.
23. Hata, R. and Nagai, Y. (1972) A rapid and micro method for separation of acidic glycosaminoglycans by two-dimensional electrophoresis. *Anal. Biochem.* **45,** 462–468.
24. Papakonstantinou, E., Karakiulakis, G., Aletras, A., and Misevic, G. (1994) A novel class of adhesion acidic glycans in sea urchin embryos. Isolation, characterization and immunological studies during early embryonal development. *Eur. J. Biochem.* **224,** 1067–1077.
25. Spencer, B. (1960) The ultra micro determination of inorganic sulphate. *Biochem. J.* **75,** 435–440.

12

Culture of Human Smooth Muscle Cells

Marisa A. Gallicchio

1. Introduction

The wall of a human artery consists of three distinct tunics. The tunica intima is lined by a layer of endothelial cells facing the lumen. Smooth muscle cells (SMCs) are the predominant cell type in the tunica media of arteries. They are surrounded by a basal lamina containing collagen IV, proteoglycans, glycosaminoglycans, glycoproteins, and extracellular matrix (ECM) molecules: collagens type 1, III, V, and VI, and elastin. The external tunica adventitia consists primarily of collagen fibers, elastic tissue, and fibroblasts. Because smooth muscle cells play a dominant role in the development of intimal hyperplasia during atherosclerosis, these cells have been studied extensively in vitro.

Smooth muscle cells have been cultured since 1913/14, when cells were described as elongated elements *(1,2)*. SMCs display two phenotypes in culture: contractile and synthetic. The function of the spindle-shaped, contractile SMCs in normal adult artery is to constrict and maintain vascular tension or tone in response to hormonal and hemodynamic stimuli. The synthetic, fibroblast-like phenotype synthesizes interstitial, extracellular matrix proteins (fibronectin, collagen types I and II, and tropoelastin), and growth factors, and is involved in migration, prolif-eration, and the maintenance of vessel integrity in response to mechanical injury *(3,4)*. Dedifferentiation from contractile to synthetic phenotypes occurs early in the development of human atheroma and may be necessary for the migration of SMCs to form a neointima following endothelial cell denudation and arterial injury *(5,6)*. Several laboratories have demonstrated that arterial SMC subpopulations with individual biochemical and phenotypic properties can be isolated from nor-mal arterial media *(7)*. Isolated cells maintained their characteristics in culture over several passages, indicating heterogeneity of arterial SMCs.

From: *Methods in Molecular Medicine, vol. 52: Atherosclerosis: Experimental Methods and Protocols*
Edited by: A. F. Drew © Humana Press Inc., Totowa, NJ

Two main methods of SMC isolation exist. The first is by enzyme dispersion of tissue, using collagenase and elastase to overcome the high collagen and elastin content of ECM *(3)*. SMC isolates obtained are morphologically in a well-differentiated, contractile state, resembling cells *in situ (4)*. These cells undergo a change in phenotype to the synthetic state within 1 or 2 passages, in the presence of serum, characterized by increased mitogenic activity and expression of intracellular organelles such as Golgi, ribosomes, rough endoplasmic reticulum, and mitochondria *(3)*. A detailed method for the isolation of cells with enzymes is reviewed elsewhere *(8)*. The second main method of SMC isolation, known as explant culture, is described in this chapter *(9)*. This involves isolation of cells migrating out from 5 mm^3 explants of arterial tissue in culture. Cells from explants undergo more population doublings, to migrate out from explants and proliferate throughout the culture dish, than cells isolated enzymatically. Because of this, cells from explants have been found to be less contractile *(3)*. Cell growth is maintained for repeated passages over several months until growth eventually slows and cells become senescent. A third method of SMC isolation from human atheromatous tissue also exists *(9)*.

Tissue culture allows cells to be studied under defined, controlled conditions for their proliferation in response to growth factors, migration, extracellular matrix synthesis, and lipoprotein metabolism and in the absence of variables such as blood pressure. Cultured SMCs allow studies on receptor binding, signal transduction pathways, protein phosphorylation, and proliferation to be made. Studies on hypertension may also be performed where cells isolated from spontaneously hypertensive rats proliferate faster than cells from normotensive rats *(10)*. Tissue culture also overcomes the problem of human tissue availability, since huge numbers of cells can be replicated from a small amount of tissue and stored until needed.

Heterogeneity in SMC isolates exists *(7)*. Such variability of isolated smooth muscle cells may be due to the organ from which the tissue is derived, the method of isolation (enzymatic vs explanted cells), passage number, enzymes used in isolation, growth media, and adhesive substrates. Several media are used to grow SMC, including Dulbecco's modification of Eagle's Minimal Essential Medium (DMEM), MEM (Eagle's Minimal Essential Medium), Medium 199 with Earle's or Hank's salt (M199), Ham F12 or DMEM:F12 in a 1:1 ratio. SMCs are normally grown in medium containing 5–10% bovine calf serum (BCS) on plastic. Cell attachment to plastic may be increased by coating with fibronectin, vitronectin, laminin, collagen, or lysine *(9,11)*.

Human tissues are available from vessels discarded after cardiac bypass surgery such as saphenous vein and internal mammary artery. Varicose veins, umbilical vein and artery, and vascularized pulmonary sections are also readily available.

Under the light microscope, SMCs appear flattened and spindle shaped with central oval nuclei and long cytoplasmic extensions (**Fig. 1A**). Confluent cells appear aligned in parallel so that the broad nuclear region of a cell lies adjacent to the thin cytoplasmic area of another, forming a "hill-and-valley" appearance. Unlike endothelial cells, SMCs do not show contact inhibition and will therefore grow as multilayers. SMCs are also characterized by the demonstration of contractile α-actin and desmin filaments in their cytoplasm (**Fig. 1B**). Smooth muscle α-actin expression persists in cells even after extensive passaging in culture. Contaminating fibroblasts either do not have contractile proteins or demonstrate background staining with anti α-actin antibodies that is irregularly arranged and not filamentous as seen in SMCs *(3,4,12)*. Cells in the synthetic state show decreased intensity of SMC-specific contractile proteins *(13)*. Other SMC-specific markers include myosin heavy chain and calponin, a protein that binds to thin filaments *(8)*.

SMCs are commercially available from several companies, including Clonetics (MD, USA), Promocell (Heidelberg, Germany) and Technoclone (Vienna, Austria). Rat SMC lines, such as A10 and A7R5, are also commercially available, but tend to display an altered phenotype *(14)*.

During tissue culture, cells are grown on a plastic surface in the presence of unknown growth factors present in serum, a situation that differs from the in vivo cellular environment. The lack of a normal three-dimensional architecture, cell-to-cell, cell-matrix, and hormonal interactions may result in the normal differentiated phenotype being lost during culture. Efforts are now being made toward inducing or maintaining differentiation of SMCs in vitro. This may be done by coculturing SMCs with endothelial cells. SMCs may also cultured on ECM proteins, such as laminin and fibronectin, which induce the also phenotypic modulation of cells *(15)*.

2. Materials

2.1. Isolation of Smooth Muscle Cells

1. Scalpel.
2. 10-cm diameter Petri dish.
3. Hank's Balanced Salt Solution (HBSS) may be bought as a solution (Sigma). To this, is added 50 U/mL penicillin (Sigma), 50 µg/mL streptomycin (Sigma), 0.25 µg/mL amphotericin B (Sigma), $0.01M$ HEPES and 0.35 g/L sodium bicarbonate buffer. Penicillin, streptomycin, and amphotericin solutions are aliquoted and stored at –20°C for up to 6 mo. Amphotericin is light sensitive and is thus stored in the dark. HBSS containing antibiotics and buffer is stored at 4°C in the dark for up to 1 mo.
4. Calcium- and magnesium-free (Ca^{2+} and Mg^{2+}) HBSS is prepared as for HBSS and stored in the dark at 4°C for up to 1 mo.

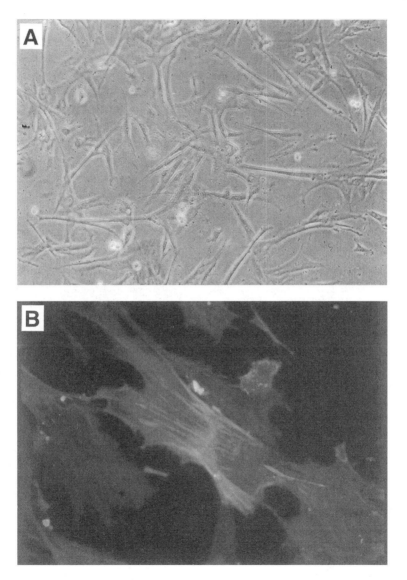

Fig. 1. Culture of human smooth muscle cells. **(A)** Spindle shaped human aortic smooth muscle cells (HASMC) photographed by phase microscopy (×100). **(B)** Human arotic smooth muscle cells stained fluorescently for α-actin (×250). (Courtesy of Professors J. Wojta and B. Binder, University of Vienna.)

5. Medium 199 (M199) with Earle's salts may be bought as a solution without glutamine or bicarbonate (Sigma). M199 working stock is made up by adding 50 U/mL penicillin, 50 µg/mL streptomycin, 0.25 µg/mL amphotericin B, 2 mM

L-glutamine, and 2.2 g/L sodium bicarbonate to liquid M199 medium. L-glutamine is aliquoted and stored at –20°C for up to 6 mo. Avoid freeze thawing aliquots of antibiotics and glutamine. M199 medium is stored at 4°C in the dark for up to 1 mo.

6. 10%(v/v) bovine calf serum (BCS)/M199 growth medium is prepared fresh using working stock M199 and stored at 4°C for up to 2 wk.

7. Serum is heat inactivated at 56°C for 30 min. to inactivate complement and destroy mycoplasma. Serum is supplied frozen and should be thawed overnight at 4°C, then completely thawed at 37°C before heat inactivation.

8. Serum starvation medium for experimental purposes is made up of M199 working stock plus either 0.5%(w/v) BSA or 5 µg/mL insulin, 5 µg/mL transferrin, and 5 ng/mL sodium selenite.

2.2. Characterization of Smooth Muscle Cells

1. Nunc culture chamber slides.
2. Fluorescence microscope with blue filter.
3. 10%(v/v)BCS/M199.
4. HBSS.
5. 1%(w/v) bovine serum albumin (BSA)/phosphate buffered saline (PBS) ph 7.4.
6. 3%(w/v) formalin/PBS pH 7.4.
7. Vectrashield (Vectashield or 50%(v/v) glycerol/PBS).
8. Acetone.
9. BCS.
10. Anti-human smooth muscle α actin (Boehringer Mannheim).
11. Anti-human desmin antibody.
12. Fluorescein (FITC) conjugated secondary antibodies (excitation/emission maxima 494/520nm; Boehringer Mannheim).

2.3. Passaging of Smooth Muscle Cells

1. 0.25%(w/v) trypsin/0.02%(w/v) EDTA in PBS.
2. Ca^{2+}- and Mg^{2+}-free HBSS.
3. 10%(v/v)BCS/M199.

2.4. Freezing Smooth Muscle Cells

1. 0.25%(w/v) trypsin/0.02%(w/v)EDTA in PBS.
2. Ca^{2+}- and Mg^{2+}-free HBSS.
3. 10%(v/v)BCS/M199.
4. 10%(v/v)dimethyl sulfoxide (DMSO)/10%(v/v)BCS/M199.
5. Cryotubes.
6. Nalgene freezer container.

2.5. Thawing Smooth Muscle Cells

1. 10%(v/v)BCS/M199.
2. 10-cm diameter Petri dish.
3. 50-mL sterile centrifuge tube.

3. Methods

3.1. Isolation of Smooth Muscle Cells

1. Cut blood vessel wall into 0.5-cm^3 pieces (*see* **Note 1**).
2. Scratch intersecting grooves into a Petri dish with a scalpel blade, and place tissue pieces on these with the flat, luminal surface face down (*see* **Note 2**).
3. Add just enough 10%(v/v)BCS/M199 to cover tissue pieces.
4. Incubate and change medium every 2 to 3 d (*see* **Note 3**).
5. When cells have migrated out, wash in Ca^{2+}- and Mg^{2+}-free HBSS (*see* **Note 4**).
6. Incubate in 1.5 mL prewarmed trypsin at 37°C for 5 min.
7. Forcefully resuspend cells from the plate in trypsin by aspirating with a disposable pipet.
8. Centrifuge 1500 rpm, 5 min.
9. Plate out in 10%(v/v)BCS/M199 in a Petri dish. This is called the first passage.

3.2 Characterization of Smooth Muscle Cells

1. Seed Nunc chamber slides with SMCs and grow to semiconfluence.
2. Aspirate medium and wash cells in HBSS.
3. Fix cells in acetone at −20°C for 8 min.
4. Wash cells in 1%(w/v)BSA/PBS.
5. Coat cells in bovine calf serum and incubate for 10 min at 37°C.
6. Aspirate serum.
7. Incubate cells at room temperature for 1 h with primary antibody diluted in 1%(w/v)BSA/PBS according to manufacturer's recommendations.
8. Wash cells in 1%(w/v)BSA/PBS.
9. Incubate cells at room temperature for 2 h with FITC labelled secondary antibody diluted in 1%(w/v)BSA/PBS according to manufacturer's recommendations.
10. Wash cells in 1%(w/v)BSA/PBS.
11. Fix cells in 3%(w/v)formalin/PBS for 10 min at room temperature.
12. Wash in water.
13. Mount in Vectashield.
14. View cells at 200× magnification under fluorescence.
15. Protect slides from light and store at 4°C.

3.3. Passaging Smooth Muscle Cells

1. Rinse confluent cells with prewarmed (37°C) Ca^{2+}- and Mg^{2+}-free HBSS.
2. Add 1.5 mL prewarmed trypsin to each 10-cm diameter Petri dish.

3. Let sit for 5 min at 37°C.
4. Free cells by forcefully pipeting trypsin up and down.
5. Add cell suspension to 5 mL 10%(v/v)BCS/M199.
6. Centrifuge 1500 rpm for 5 min.
7. Aspirate supernatant.
8. Resuspend pellet in 3 mL M199 growth medium.
9. Add 1 mL cell suspension to 3 Petri dishes each containing 7.5 mL M199 growth medium.

3.4. Freezing Smooth Muscle Cells

1. Rinse confluent 10 cm diameter Petri dish of SMC with prewarmed (37°C) Ca^{2+}- and Mg^{2+}- free HBSS.
2. Add 1.5 mL prewarmed trypsin to 10-cm diameter Petri dish of cells.
3. Let sit for 5 min at 37°C.
4. Free cells by forcefully pipeting trypsin up and down.
5. Add cell suspension to 5 mL 10%(v/v)BCS/M199.
6. Centrifuge at 1500 rpm for 5 min.
7. Aspirate supernatant.
8. Resuspend pellet in 1 mL cold (4°C) 10%(v/v)DMSO/20%(v/v)BCS/M199 (*see* **Note 13**).
9. Add to cryotube.
10. Store tube at –80°C overnight in Nalgene freezer container then place into liquid nitrogen (–196°C).

3.5. Thawing Smooth Muscle Cells

1. Take cryotube out of liquid nitrogen and quickly thaw in 37°C water bath.
2. Transfer cell suspension to a 50-mL tube.
3. Add 1 mL prewarmed 10%(v/v)BCS/M199 and wait 1 min.
4. Add 2 mL prewarmed 10%(v/v)BCS/M199 and wait 1 min.
5. Add 4 mL prewarmed 10%(v/v)BCS/M199 and wait 1 min.
6. Make up volume to 20 mL with prewarmed 10%(v/v)BCS/M199.
7. Centrifuge 1500 rpm for 5 min.
8. Aspirate supernatant.
9. Resuspend cells in 10%(v/v)BCS/M199 medium and dilute into three Petri dishes (*see* **Note 18**).
10. Change medium next day.

4. Notes
4.1. Isolation of Smooth Muscle Cells

1. Some investigators remove the intima and adventitia, leaving only the media for explant culture.

2. Tissue pieces must be firmly attached to the Petri dish if migration of cells out of the tissue piece is to occur. This can be achieved by air drying tissue pieces for 10 min after they have been placed onto the scratched Petri dish. Fill Petri dish with small amount (about 3 mL) of medium.

3. Cells start to migrate after explants have been in culture for 3 or 4 d. Depending on the overall number of explants per dish, cells may be passaged 10–14 d after explant culture. Explants derived from vessels, which have been digested by collagenase for endothelial cell isolation, do not yield as many smooth muscle cells as undigested blood vessels.

4. HEPES, used in buffering HBSS, is reported to be toxic to smooth muscle cells *(3)*.

5. Some investigators substitute amino acid D-valine for L-valine to decrease fibroblast growth as these cells cannot use the D dimer *(16)*.

6. Veins up to 24-h old and kept at 4°C will still yield cells.

7. Contaminating cobblestone-shaped endothelial cells may occasionally grow out of explants, but will not survive in culture for more than a few days.

8. Various batches and sources of sera may be tried to determine the optimal one. Iron-supplemented bovine calf serum (Hyclone Labs, Logan, UT, USA) is a cheap alternative to many sera. SMCs are generally not fastidious in serum growth requirements.

4.2. Characterization of Smooth Muscle Cells

9. Peroxidase-labeled secondary antibodies may be substituted for fluorescein-labeled antibodies.

10. When viewing cells, note the morphology of cells as well as the percentage of cells stained by fluorescent label to determine the purity of cultures.

11. If SMCs are left to grow as a very dense multilayer, stained actin and desmin filaments may not be individually distinguishable. Dense cell growth also prevents making distinctions among other cell types.

4.3. Passaging Smooth Muscle Cells

12. SMCs can be passaged at a dilution or split ratio of up to 1 in 10, depending on initial cell number. If in culture for too long, SMC multilayers form impenetrable sheets that cannot be dispersed by trypsin.

4.4. Freezing Smooth Muscle Cells

13. Cells must be resuspended in DMSO solution as a single-cell suspension. If cells are in clumps, the likelihood of these being viable upon thawing decreases.

14. Gloves should be worn while handling DMSO as it can easily penetrate skin, carrying toxic impurities with it.

15. Exposure to liquid nitrogen requires eye and hand protection. Face shields should preferably be worn, together with protective gloves.

4.5. Thawing Smooth Muscle Cells

16. When thawing cryotubes, wear eye protective goggles, as tubes are liable to explode after being kept in the liquid N_2 phase.
17. Cryotubes may be labeled on the outside and color coded on top for quick identification of vials.
18. Cells have been thawed and passaged or split 1:3.

References

1. Champey, C. (1913/14) Quelques resultats de la methode de culture des tissus. 1. Generalities. II Le muscle lisse (note preliminaire). *Arch. Zool. Exp. Gen.* **53,** 42–51.
2. Lewis, M. R. and Lewis, W. H. (1914) Mitochondria in tissue culture. *Science* **39,** 330–333.
3. Campbell, J. H. and Campbell, G. R. (1993) Culture techniques and their applications to studies of vascular smooth muscle. *Clin. Sci.* **85,** 501–513.
4. Chamley-Campbell, J., Campbell, G., and Ross, R. (1979) The smooth muscle cell in culture. *Physiol. Rev.* **59,** 1–61.
5. Babaev, V. R., Bobryshev, Y. V., Stenina, O. V., Tararak, E. M., and Gabbiani, G. (1990) Heterogeneity of smooth muscle cells in atheromatous plaque of human aorta. *Am. J. Pathol.* **136,** 1031–1042.
6. Okamoto, E., Imataka, K., Fujii, J., Nakahara, K., Nishimura, H., Yazaki, Y., and Nagai, R. (1992) Heterogeneity in smooth muscle cell population accumulating in the neointimas and the media of post-stenotic dilatation of rabbit carotid artery. *Biochem. Biophys. Res. Commun.* **185,** 459–464.
7. Frid, M. G., Dempsey, E. C., Durmowicz, A. G., and Stenmark, K. R. (1997) Smooth muscle cell heterogencity in pulmonary and systemic vessels. *Arterioscler. Thromb. Vasc. Biol.* **17,** 1203–1209.
8. Pauly, R. R., Bilato, C., Cheng, L., Monticone, R., and Crow, M. T. (1998) Vascular smooth muscle cell cultures. *Methods Cell Biol.* **52,** 133–154.
9. McMurray, H. F., Parrott, D. P., and Bowyer, D. E. (1991) A standardized method of culturing aortic explants, suitable for the study of factors affecting the phenotypic modulation, migration and proliferation of aortic smooth muscle cells. *Atherosclerosis* **86,** 227–337.
10. Pang, S. C. and Venance, S. L. (1992) Cultured smooth muscle approach in the study of hypertension. *Can. J. Physiol. Pharmacol.* **70,** 573–579.
11. Thyberg, J. (1996) Differentiation properties and proliferation of arterial smooth muscle cells in culture. *Int. Rev. Cytol.* **169,** 183–265
12. Gown, A. M., Vogel, A. W. A., Gordon, D., and Lu, P. L. (1985) A smooth muscle-specific monoclonal antibody recognizes smooth muscle actin isozymes. *J. Cell Biol.* **100,** 807–813.
13. Owens, G. K., Loeb, A., Gordon, D., and Thompson, M. M. (1986) Expression of smooth muscle-specific α-isoactin in cultured vascular smooth muscle cells: Relationship between growth and cytodifferentiation. *J. Cell Biol.* **102,** 343–352.

14. Kines, B. W. and Brandt, B. L. (1976) Characterisation of two putative smooth muscle cell lines from rat thoracic aorta. *Exp. Cell Res.* **98,** 349–366.
15. Hedin, U., Bottger, B. A., Forsbery, E., Johannsson, S., and Thyberg, J. (1988) Diverse effects of fibronectin and laminin on phenotypic properties of cultured arterial smooth muscle cells. *J. Cell Biol.* **107,** 307–319.
16. Gilbert, S. F. and Migeon, B. R. (1975) D-valine as a selective agent for normal human and rodent epithelial cells in culture. *Cell* **5,** 11–17.

13

Culture of Human Endothelial Cells

Marisa A. Gallicchio

1. Introduction

Endothelial cells line the luminal surface of all blood vessels in the body. The endothelial surface in adult humans is composed of approximately $1–6\times10^{13}$ cells and covers an area of 1–7 m^2. Endothelium serves many functions, including fluid and solute exchange through cell contraction, provision of an antithrombogenic surface through tissue plasminogen activator (tPA) and prostacyclin release, synthesis of angiogenic factors such as adenosine, allowance of leukocyte trafficking through adhesion molecule synthesis, presentation of antigens to the immune system, maintenance of vascular tone through nitric oxide and endothelin synthesis, and metabolism of circulating molecules through the release of enzymes such as lipoprotein lipase.

Endothelial cells (ECs) were first grown in 1922 as migrating outgrowths of cells from chicken liver sinusoid explants (1). Human endothelial cells from umbilical vein (HUVECs) were first isolated in the early 1970s (2,3). ECs have been harvested from many organ systems and from different species (4–9). Endothelial dysfunction is involved in the two big diseases of the Western world, atherosclerosis (EC of large vessels) and cancer (angiogenesis), as well as inflammation, immune disorders, transplant rejection, and angiogenesis in human biology.

The harvesting of ECs from large veins occurs by cannulating vessels and enzymatically removing cells with collagenase. The advantage is that yield is good, and cells are of high purity. The disadvantage is that collagenase may affect surface proteins. If blood vessels are large, cells may be scraped. However, cells may become mechanically damaged with poor yields.

From: *Methods in Molecular Medicine, vol. 52: Atherosclerosis: Experimental Methods and Protocols*
Edited by: A. F. Drew © Humana Press Inc., Totowa, NJ

There are also many published methods for the isolation of microvascular ECs. These include the isolation of microvessels, after collagenase digestion, using Percoll gradient separation, with subsequent growth of ECs out from microvessel explants. More recently, magnetic beads have been used in isolations. Tissue specimens are minced and enzymatically digested. ECs are specifically selected, using lectin- or antibody-covered beads and selective medium. However, this method does not preclude contamination by other cell types such as mesothelial cells *(10)*. An even more recent method of ECs isolation is the implantation of sponges containing angiogenic factors into organs to promote infiltration of ECs *(11)*.

A variety of media are used in the culture of ECs, including Medium 199 (M199), Dulbecco's Modified Eagle's medium (DMEM), DMEM/Ham's F12 (DMEM/F12) and RPMI-1640. Optimal growth for ECs under low serum (less than 1%) occurs in the presence of a high magnesium content, hydrocortisone, epidermal growth factor, cAMP, or isobutyl methyl xanthine *(12)*. Extracellular matrix (ECM) components are important for EC attachment and growth *(13)*. These include collagen, fibronectin, laminin, and gelatin, used when seeding cells onto plastic Petri dishes.

The limitations of EC culture include changes in ECs from a quiescent in vivo state (0.1% replications/d) to an activated state (1–10% replications/d). Specialized functions associated with different vascular beds may also be lost. A model does not exist, as yet, for generating resting ECs in vitro. Culture also involves the omission of shear forces and circulating proteins, plus the presence of activated ECs and exogenous growth factors. Additionally, extensive studies have been done on HUVEC, even though these cells are rarely affected by vascular disorders.

Emerging trends in endothelial cell biology include the concept of heterogeneity of cell function depending on source of vascular bed and even donors. Cells isolated from different vascular beds and species, large and small blood vessels display heterogeneity in antigenicity, biochemistry, morphology, and responses to stimulants *(6,14)*. Other future directions include the genetic manipulation of ECs with proteins such as tPA to overcome thrombosis and other disorders, coculture systems to mimic the natural environment, the clinical use of proangiogenic growth factors such as vascular endothelial cell growth factor (VEGF) to overcome coronary ischemia, and the therapeutic use of antiangiogenic factors to overcome tumor growth *(15)*. Commercially available sources of cells include Clonetics (MD, USA), Promocell (Heidelberg, Germany), and Technoclone (Vienna, Austria). Immortalized EC lines such as HMEC-1 are also available, although some EC characteristics may be lost *(16)*.

1.1. Isolation of Endothelial Cells from Umbilical Vein (Fig. 1A)

Human umbilical veins are traditionally used to isolate endothelial cells as large numbers of cells are obtained from readily available tissues *(2)*. Because their origin is fetal, HUVECs grow extremely well in culture. Isolation of large vessel ECs occurs by cannulation followed by perfusion of vessels with collagenase and flushing out of ECs. During isolation, veins undergo mild enzymatic digestion, with collagenase acting on the dominant component of the basement membrane, collagen IV. This strips endothelial cells off the vessel wall, as cell sheets, without disturbing the underlying smooth muscle cell layer. Cells are grown on ECM-coated Petri dishes in medium containing a high serum concentration and endothelial cell growth supplement (ECGS) or other growth factors such as basic fibroblast growth factor (bFGF) and VEGF. When cells reach confluency, they are transferred from one culture dish to another, i.e., subcultured, passaged, or split.

1.2. Isolation of Microvascular Cells from Foreskin (Fig. 1B)

Most studies on endothelial cell biology have focused on macrovascular cells isolated from the aorta or umbilical vein. With the recent development of simple, selective measures of isolating specific cell types, more studies involving microvascular ECs have begun. The first report of EC isolation from microvessels was by Wagner from fat in 1975 *(9)*. ECs from human newborn foreskin were first isolated 20 years ago *(7)*. Continuous density gradient centrifugation using Percoll was used to separate microvessels from nonendothelial cells in human skin *(17)*. However, microvascular cells are now isolated by enzymatic digestion of whole tissue followed by positive selection for ECs using magnetic beads coated with a lectin, *Ulex europaeus* (UEA-1), which binds with high affinity and specificity to α-fucosyl residues of glycoproteins associated with the EC surface *(4)*. Other investigators couple antibodies directed against PECAM-1/CD 31 to magnetic beads *(5)*. Beads are then collected with a magnet, plated out, and incubated in growth medium. The use of magnetic beads during cell isolation circumvents the use of expensive flow cytometry equipment.

1.3. Characterization of Endothelial Cells (Fig. 1C)

Isolated endothelial cells are characterized by light microscopy according to cell morphology and arrangement in culture. Both macrovascular and microvascular cells exhibit a cobblestone morphology. Furthermore, because cells stop growing when in contact with each other (contact inhibition), endothelial cells form monolayer cultures. On passaging, cells becoming elongated and display a less regular monolayer consisting of cells with overlapping

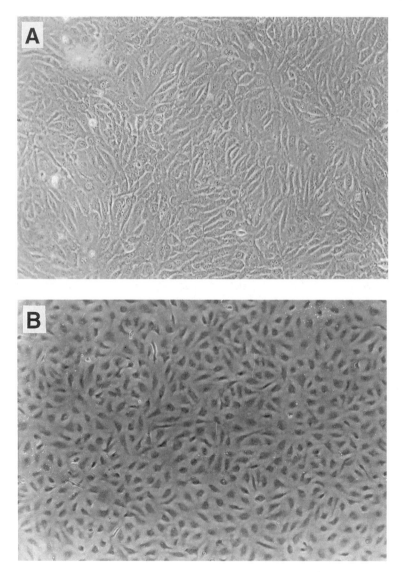

Fig. 1. Culture of human endothelial cells. (**A**) A monolayer of human umbilical vein endothelial cells showing typical cobblestone formation and contact inhibition, shown by phase microscopy (×100). (**B**) Human foreskin microvascular endothelial cells, by phase microscopy (×100). (Courtesy of Professors J. Wojta and B. Binder, University of Vienna.)

processes. At the end of their lifespan, monolayers may display multinucleated, senescent cells. A correlation exists between senescence and intracellular IL-1 accumulation *(18)*.

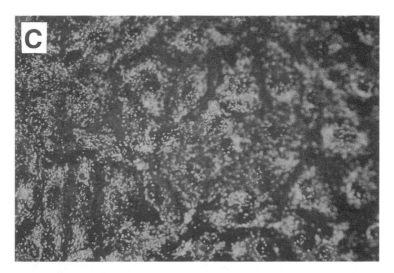

Fig. 1. (**C**) A monolayer of human umbilical vein endothelial cells showing granular fluorescent staining for von Willebrand factor (×250). (Courtesy of Professors J. Wojta and B. Binder, University of Vienna.)

Isolated ECs are also characterized by demonstrating the presence of granules of von Willebrand factor (vWF) in the cytoplasm of cells. vWF complexes with factor VIII and is stored in the ECs' Weibel-Palade (WP) bodies. Expression of vWF decreases with passaging *(8)*. WP bodies are present in large numbers in human ECs, although they may be expressed by all ECs *(2,8)*.

Live ECs also take up acetylated low-density lipoprotein (LDL) coupled to a fluorescent carbonic dye (1,1'-dioctadecyl-3,3,3'3'-tetramethyl-indo-carbocyanine perchlorate acetylated low-density lipoprotein; Dil-Ac-LDL) *(19)*. This is due to the presence of scavenger receptors on the EC membrane. Fibroblasts, smooth muscle cells, and pericytes do not have the scavenger receptor for LDL. LDL is taken up by lysosomes in which LDL is broken down and lipophilic carbocyanine dye (Dil) is incorporated into the lysosomal membrane, giving intense red punctate staining under fluorescence microscopy. LDL is also taken up by macrophages and monocytes. Negative staining by antibodies to α-actin and pan-cytokeratin rule out the presence of smooth muscle and ECs, respectively, in cultures. Since ECs demonstrate heterogeneity in expression of cell markers because of vascular source and passage number, a lack of EC markers does not preclude the EC origin of an isolate *(6)*. Other features of cells used to characterize ECs include tube formation in Matrigel, staining for PECAM-1, and thrombomodulin expression.

2. Materials

2.1. Isolation of Endothelial Cells from Umbilical Vein

1. Scalpel.
2. Straight artery forceps.
3. 50-mL sterile syringe.
4. 0.5-cm long blunt sterile needle.
5. Sterile tray.
6. Hank's Balanced Salt Solution (HBSS) may be bought as a solution (Sigma). To this is added 50 U/mL penicillin (Sigma), 50 µg/mL streptomycin (Sigma), 0.25 µg/mL amphotericin B (Sigma), 0.01M HEPES (Sigma; see **Note 1**) and 0.35 g/L sodium bicarbonate buffer (see **Note 2**). Penicillin, streptomycin, and amphotericin solutions may be aliquoted and stored at –20°C for up to 6 mo. Amphotericin is light sensitive and is thus stored in the dark. Avoid freeze thawing aliquots of antibiotics. HBSS containing antibiotics and buffers is stored at 4°C in the dark for up to 1 mo.
7. Calcium- and magnesium (Ca^{2+} and Mg^{2+})- free HBSS is also bought as a solution. It is prepared as for HBSS and stored in the dark at 4°C for up to 1 mo.
8. Medium 199 (M199) with Earle's salts may be bought as a solution without glutamine (Sigma; see **Note 3**). M199 working stock is made up by adding 50 U/mL penicillin, 50 µg/mL streptomycin, 0.25 µg/mL amphotericin B, 2 mM L-glutamine, and 2.2 g/L sodium bicarbonate to liquid M199 medium. L-glutamine may be aliquoted and stored at –20°C for up to 6 mo. Avoid freeze thawing aliquots of glutamine. M199 medium is stored at 4°C in the dark for up to 1 mo.
9. M199 growth medium is made up of 20%(v/v) bovine calf serum (BCS; see **Note 4**), 5 U/mL heparin (preservative free) and 200 µg/mL ECGS in M199 working stock (i.e., containing antibiotics, buffer and glutamine). M199 growth medium is stored at 4°C for up to 2 wk. Prewarm to 37°C before use. Do not leave at 37°C for longer than necessary as growth factors in serum and ECGS are heat labile. Avoid freeze thawing aliquots of ECGS.
10. Collagenase solution is made by adding 2 mg/mL collagenase IV or II (Worthington; see **Note 5**) in HBSS, filter sterilizing with a 0.22-µm filter and prewarming to 37°C. Make up fresh just before use.
11. Serum is heat inactivated at 56°C for 30 min to inactivate complement and destroy mycoplasma. Some sera are filtered through 0.1-µm filters to remove *Mycoplasma*. Serum is supplied frozen and should be thawed overnight at 4°C, then completely thawed at 37°C before heat inactivation. Heating serum at unnecessarily high temperature will destroy serum growth factors as will repeated freeze thawing.
12. 1%(w/v) gelatin (Sigma).
13. Serum starvation medium for experiments is made up of M199 working stock containing either 1–2% BCS or a compound solution containing 5 µg/mL insulin, 5 µg/mL transferrin, and 5 ng/mL sodium selenite.

2.2. Isolation of Microvascular Endothelial Cells from Foreskin

2.2.1. Coating Magnetic Beads with Lectin

1. 5 mg *Ulex europaeus* (Sigma).
2. Borate buffer: 0.618 g H_3BO_3 is dissolved in 100 mL H_2O and brought to a pH to 9.5.
3. Dynabeads (2 mL at 4×10^8 beads/mL; Dynal).
4. 10%(v/v)BCS/HBSS.
5. 0.1%(v/v)BCS/phosphate buffered saline (PBS).
6. Magnetic particle concentrator (MCP-1, Dynal).
7. 0.2-μm filter.

2.2.2. Isolating Endothelial Cells with Lectin Coated Beads

1. Sterile 100-μm nylon mesh covering a 6-cm diameter glass funnel.
2. Magnetic particle concentrator (MPC-1, Dynal).
3. 10-cm diameter Petri dish.
4. M199 growth medium.
5. 1%(w/v) gelatin.
6. HBSS.
7. 0.6%(w/v) trypsin/1%(w/v) EDTA/HBSS pH 7.4.
8. 5%(v/v)BCS/HBSS.
9. *Ulex europaeus* (UEA-1)-coated Dynabeads (4×10^8 beads/mL).

2.3. Endothelial Cell Characterization

2.3.1. Antibody Staining

1. Nunc culture chamber slides.
2. Fluorescence microscope with blue filter.
3. M199 growth medium.
4. 1%(w/v) gelatin.
5. HBSS.
6. 1%(w/v) bovine serum albumin (BSA)/PBS pH 7.4.
7. 3%(w/v) formalin/PBS pH 7.4.
8. Vectrashield (Vector Laboratories, Oakland, CA) or 5%(v/v) glycerol/PBS.
9. Acetone.
10. Calf serum.
11. Antihuman vWF (DAKOPatts).
12. Antihuman smooth muscle α-actin (Boehringer Mannheim).
13. Antihuman pan cytokeratin (Boehringer Mannheim).
14. Fluorescein isothiocyanate (FITC) conjugated secondary antibodies (fluorescein excitation/emission maxima 494/520 nm; Boehringer Mannheim).

2.3.2. Acetylated Low Density Lipoprotein Labeling

1. M199 growth medium.
2. 3%(w/v)formalin/PBS.
3. 1%(w/v) gelatin.
4. 1,1' Dioctadecyl-3,3,3'-tetramethyl-indocarbocyanine perchlorate acetylated LDL (Dil-Ac-LDL) (Biomedical Technologies, Stoughton, MA).
5. HBSS.
6. Vectrashield or 5%(v/v) glycerol/PBS.
7. Fluorescent microscope with green filter.

2.4. Passaging Endothelial Cells

1. 0.25%(w/v) trypsin/0.02%(w/v)EDTA in PBS.
2. Ca^{2+}- and Mg^{2+}-free HBSS.
3. 10%(v/v)BCS/M199.
4. M199 growth medium.
5. 1%(w/v) gelatin.

2.5. Freezing Endothelial Cells

1. 0.25%(w/v) trypsin/0.02%(w/v)EDTA in PBS.
2. Ca^{2+}- and Mg^{2+}-free HBBS.
3. 10%(v/v)BCS/M199.
4. M199 growth medium.
5. 2% gelatin.
6. 10% dimethyl sulfoxide (DMSO)/M199 growth medium.
7. Cryotubes.
8. Nalgene freezing container.

2.6. Thawing Endothelial Cells

1. 10%(v/v)BCS/M199.
2. M199 growth medium.
3. 2%(w/v) gelatin.
4. 10-cm diameter Petri dish.
5. Sterile 50-mL centrifuge tube.

3. Methods
3.1. Isolation of Endothelial Cells from Umbilical Vein

1. Collect blood vessel and place into a sterile bottle containing HBSS and antibiotics.
2. Fill 50-mL sterile syringe with HBSS.

3. Attach sterile blunt needle to syringe.
4. Clamp syringe to one end of blood vessel with artery forceps.
5. Wash clots out of blood vessel with HBSS-filled syringe.
6. Fill syringe with collagenase solution.
7. Perfuse blood vessel until collagenase exits.
8. Clamp free end of blood vessel with artery forceps.
9. Leave for 10 min.
10. Flush cells out of vessel with remaining collagenase solution into sterile 50-mL tube (*see* **Note 6**).
11. Refill syringe with HBSS and continue to flush cells.
12. Centrifuge at 1500 rpm for 5 min at 4°C.
13. Aspirate supernatant.
14. Resupend pellet in 7.5 mL M199 growth medium.
15. Incubate 2.5 mL of 1%(w/v) gelatin in a 10-cm diameter Petri dish for 5 min at 37°C.
16. Aspirate gelatin and add cell suspension.
17. Incubate cells in a 5% CO_2, 95% air humidified atmosphere.
18. Change medium next day and every second or third day thereafter.

3.2. Isolation of Microvascular Endothelial Cells from Foreskin

3.2.1. Coating Beads with Lectin

1. Dissolve 5 mg *Ulex europaeus* in 12.5 mL borate buffer.
2. Filter sterilize *Ulex europaeus*/borate solution with 0.2micron filter.
3. Add 2 mL *Ulex europaeus* solution to 2 mL of beads.
4. Mix overnight on a rotary shaker at room temperature.
5. Collect beads on magnet and wash two times with 2 mL of 10%(v/v)BCS/HBSS for 5 min on a rotary shaker.
6. Wash overnight in 2 mL of 10%(v/v) BCS/HBSS at 4°C on a rotary shaker.
7. Collect and resuspend 4×10^8 beads/mL in 2 mL 0.1%(v/v)BCS/PBS to 2 mL (*see* **Note 9**).

3.2.2. Isolating Endothelial Cells with Lectin-Coated Magnetic Beads

1. Cut foreskin into 5-mm^3 cubed pieces.
2. Place tissue in 3 mL of 0.6%(w/v)trypsin/1%(w/v)EDTA/HBSS in a Petri dish.
3. Incubate tissue for 20 min at 37°C in an incubator.
4. Tease tissue with back of scalpel blade in 5%(v/v)BCS/HBSS.
5. Filter through 100-μm nylon mesh.
6. Wash mesh with 5%(v/v)BCS/HBSS.
7. Centrifuge filtrate at 1500 rpm at 4°C for 5 min.
8. Resuspend cell pellet in 1 mL 5%(v/v)BCS/HBSS.
9. Add 20 μL of 4×10^8 Dynabeads/mL stock.
10. Incubate for 10 min at 4°C. Invert tube and shake after 5 min.

11. Wash cells with 1 mL of 5% BCS/HBSS for 1 min, five times.
12. Resuspend cells in 7.5 mL M199 growth medium (*see* **Note 12**).
13. Plate cells in gelatin-coated well of 6-well plate.
14. Incubate in a 5% CO_2, 95% air humidified atmosphere.
15. Change medium next day and every second or third day thereafter.

3.3. Characterization of Endothelial Cells
3.3.1. Antibody Staining

1. Coat Nunc chamber slides with gelatin by incubating at 37°C for 5 min.
2. Seed with endothelial cells and grow to confluence.
3. Aspirate medium and wash cells in HBSS.
4. Fix cells in acetone at –20°C for 8 min.
5. Wash cells in 1%(w/v)BSA/PBS.
6. Coat slides with calf serum and incubate for 10 min at 37°C.
7. Aspirate calf serum.
8. Incubate cells at room temperature for 1 h with primary antibody diluted according to manufacturers' recommendations in 1%(w/v)BSA/PBS.
9. Wash cells in 1%(w/v)BSA/PBS.
10. Incubate cells at room temperature for 2 hours with FITC labelled secondary antibody diluted in 1%(w/v)BSA/PBS according to manufacturers' recommendations.
11. Wash cells in 1%(w/v)BSA/PBS.
12. Fix cells in 3%(w/v)formalin/PBS for 10 min at room temperature.
13. Wash in water.
14. Mount in Vectashield.
15. View cells at 200× magnification under fluorescence.

3.3.2. Acetylated Low-Density Lipoprotein Labeling

1. Coat Nunc chamber slides with gelatin for 5 min at 37°C and aspirate.
2. Seed coverslips with endothelial cells and grow to confluence.
3. Wash cells in HBSS.
4. Add acetylated LDL (10 mg/mL in M199 growth medium).
5. Incubate cells for 4 h at 37°C.
6. Wash cells in 1%(w/v)BSA/PBS.
7. Fix cells in 3%(v/v) formalin/PBS.
8. Wash cells in water.
9. Mount in Vectashield.
10. View under fluorescent microscope at 200× magnification
11. Protect slides from light and store at 4°C.

3.4. Passaging Endothelial Cells

1. Rinse confluent endothelial cells with prewarmed (37°C) Ca^{2+}- and Mg^{2+}- free HBSS.
2. Add 1.5 mL prewarmed trypsin to each 10-cm diameter Petri dish.

3. Let sit for 5 min at 37°C.
4. Free cells by forcefully pipeting trypsin up and down.
5. Add cell suspension to 5 mL of 10%(v/v)BCS/M199.
6. Centrifuge 1500 rpm for 5 min.
7. Aspirate supernatant.
8. Resuspend pellet in 3 mL M199 growth medium.
9. Add 1 mL cell suspension to each of these three gelatin-coated Petri dishes each containing 7.5 mL M199 growth medium (*see* **Note 25**).

3.5. Freezing Endothelial Cells

1. Rinse confluent endothelial cells with prewarmed (37°C) Ca^{2+}- and Mg^{2+}- free HBSS.
2. Add 1.5 mL prewarmed trypsin to 10-cm diameter Petri dish.
3. Let sit for 5 min at 37°C.
4. Free cells by forcefully pipeting trypsin up and down.
5. Add cell suspension to 5 mL of 10%(v/v)BCS/M199.
6. Centrifuge at 1500 rpm for 5 min.
7. Aspirate supernatant.
8. Resuspend pellet in 1 mL cold (4°C) 10%(v/v)DMSO/M199 growth medium (*see* **Notes 26** and **27**).
9. Add to cryotube.
10. Store tube at –80°C overnight in Nalgene freezing container (*see* **Note 29**), then place into liquid nitrogen (–196°C).

3.6. Thawing Endothelial Cells

1. Take cryotube out of N_2 and quickly thaw in 37°C water bath.
2. Transfer cell suspension to a sterile tube.
3. Add 1 mL prewarmed 10%(v/v)BCS/M199 and wait 1 min (*see* **Note 32**).
4. Add 2 mL prewarmed 10%(v/v)BCS/M199 and wait 1 min.
5. Add 4 mL prewarmed 10%(v/v)BCS/M199 and wait 1 min.
6. Make up volume to 20 mL with prewarmed 10%(v/v)BCS/M199.
7. Centrifuge 1500 rpm, 5 min.
8. Aspirate supernatant.
9. Resuspend cells in M199 growth medium and dilute into three Petri dishes.
10. Change medium next day.

4. Notes
4.1. Isolation of Endothelial Cells from Umbilical Vein

1. HEPES buffer is known to be detrimental to some cell types and enhances the detrimental effect of fluorescent light on medium.
2. The amount of bicarbonate added to HBSS and M199 is for use in an incubator set for 5% CO_2, 95% air.

3. M199 medium without added L-glutamine and bicarbonate should be bought. L-glutamine is an essential amino acid that is unstable in solution so is best added just before use.
4. Various batches and sources of calf sera may be tried to ascertain the best growth promoter. Iron-supplemented bovine calf serum (Hyclone Labs, Logan, UT, USA) is a cheap alternative to many sera.
5. Collagenase types II or IV may be used with equal effect.
6. When flushing cells out of the blood vessel, exert some force on the syringe plunger to dislodge cells from the cell wall and therefore increase cell yield.
7. Umbilical cords and other human blood vessels may be stored for up to 24 h in physiological buffer at 4°C before cell isolation.
8. Because these cells grow faster than ECs, contaminating fibroblasts (less than 0.1% of population) can overgrow a culture. Some investigators substitute D-valine for L-valine in growth medium, which prevents fibroblast growth.

4.2. Isolation of Microvascular Endothelial Cells from Foreskin
4.2.1. Coating Magnetic Beads with UEA-1

9. UEA-1 coated beads are active for at least 1 yr.

4.2.2. Isolation of Endothelial Cells with Magnetic Beads

10. Foreskin may be stored in physiological buffer at 4°C for several hours. Overnight storage at 4°C is not recommended as cell yield markedly decreases. Cells grow without difficulty from neonatal foreskin. However, isolates from foreskin removed from infants more than 1 year old invariably show extensive fibroblast contamination.
11. Various groups report isolation of microvascular EC using anti-PECAM-1 antibodies (5). However, others report decreased growth of EC isolated in this manner, presumably because anti-PECAM-1 antibodies interfere with cell-to-cell contact.
12. It has been recommended that beads be taken off cells by incubation in fucose solution. However, this has not been successful in this author's hands. Instead, beads are yielded by cells into the culture medium after approximately 10 d in culture, i.e., by the first passage (4).
13. Coated magnetic beads have been used for the successful isolation of EC from tissues as diverse as synovium, fat, skin, and the uterine wall.
14. Contaminating cells may be removed by weeding with a pipet tip. Alternatively, the culture dish may be emptied of medium and contaminating cells killed by freezing with a scalpel handle exposed to liquid N_2.
15. Magnetic beads may also be used to remove contaminating cell types from cultures of ECs. Allow ECs to grow to confluence in a Petri dish and then expose trypsinized cells to lectin-coated Dynabeads. If cultures are heavily contaminated with another cell type, cells may not be completely dissociated into a single cell suspension. The nonspecific interaction of beads with aggregated cell clumps limits the purity of the final preparation.

16. Solutions used should be cold to prevent phagocytosis of Dynabeads by non-ECs.
17. Dynabeads are added at a bead-to-target cell ratio of 2:1, assuming ECs comprise 1–2% of the total cell count. High bead-to-cell ratios result in poor attachment of cells to the matrix.
18. UEA-1 also binds to α-fucosyl residues in the H blood group antigen as evidenced by the clumping of red blood cells. This does not present a problem during isolation.

4.3. Characterization of Endothelial Cells

4.3.1. Antibody Staining

19. Peroxidase-labeled secondary antibodies may be substituted for fluorescein-labeled antibodies and staining detected by light microscopy.
20. When viewing cells, note the morphology of cells, as well as the percentage of cells that actually label, to determine the purity of cultures.
21. Antibody specificity may be checked using the appropriate positive control cells, i.e., epithelial cells with pan cytokeratin antibodies and smooth muscle cells with anti-α-actin. Negative controls include ECs exposed to non-EC specific primary antibodies or smooth muscle cells and fibroblasts exposed to EC markers.
22. Sometimes ECs do not stick to gelatin-coated glass because of their origin or passage number. If this occurs, trypsinize cells, cytospin or air dry them onto a glass slide and proceed as for **step 4** onward.
23. Stained cells may be stored in the dark at 4°C for 2 wk.

4.3.2. Acetylated LDL

24. Acetylated LDL has a shelf life of approximately 2 mo from delivery.

4.4. Passaging Endothelial Cells

25. A split ratio of 1:3 is used. If the cell suspension is diluted too much, cellular growth factors are diluted and cells will die.

4.5. Freezing Endothelial Cells

26. Cells must be resuspended in DMSO solution as a single-cell suspension. If cells are in clumps the likelihood of these being viable on thawing decreases.
27. Gloves should be worn while handling DMSO as it is a skin penetrant.
28. Exposure to liquid nitrogen requires eye and hand protection. Preferably, face shields should be worn, together with protective gloves.
29. Vials should be placed in a Nalgene freezer container, which reduces the temperature slowly by 1 degree/minute when in the –80°C freezer.

4.6. Thawing Endothelial Cells

30. When thawing cryotubes, a face guard and protective gloves should be worn as tubes are liable to explode when submerged in liquid N_2 and not properly sealed.
31. Cryotubes may be labeled on the outside and color coded on top for quick identification of vials.
32. DMSO is harmful to cells and must be removed quickly.

References

1. Lewis, W. H. (1922) Endothelium in tissue culture. *Am. J. Anat.* **30,** 39–59.
2. Jaffe, E. A., Nachman, R. L., Becker, C. G., and Minick, C. R. (1973) Culture of human endothelial cells derived from umbilical veins. Identification by morphologic and immunologic criteria. *J. Clin. Invest.* **52,** 2745–2756.
3. Gimbrone, M. A., Jr, Cotran, R. S., and Folkman, J. (1974) Human vascular endothelial cells in culture. Growth and DNA synthesis. *J. Cell Biol.* **60,** 673–684.
4. Jackson, C. J., Garbett, P. K., Nissen, B., and Schrieber, L. (1990) Binding of human endothelium to *Ulex europaeus* 1-coated Dynabeads: Application to the isolation of microvascular endothelium. *J. Cell Sci.* **196,** 257–262.
5. Hewett, P. W. and Murray, J. C. (1993) Immunomagnetic purification of human microvessel endothelial cells using Dynabeads coated with monoclonal antibodies to PECAM-1. *Eur. J. Cell Biol.* **62,** 451–454.
6. Kumar, S., West, D. C., and Ager, A. (1987) Heterogeneity in endothelial cells from large vessels and microvessels. *Differentiation* **36,** 57–70.
7. Davison, P. M., Bensch, K., and Karasek, M. A. (1980) Isolation and growth of endothelial cells from the microvessels of the newborn foreskin and cell culture. *J. Invest. Dermatol.* **75,** 316–321.
8. Craig, L. E., Spelman, J. P., Strandberg, J. D., and Zink, M.C. (1998) Endothelial cells from diverse tissues exhibit differences in growth and morphology. *Microvasc. Res.* **55,** 65–76.
9. Wagner, R. C. and Matthews, M. A. (1975) The isolation and culture of capillary endothelium from epididymal fat. *Microvasc. Res.* **10,** 286–297.
10. van Hinsbergh, V. W., Kooistra, T., Scheffer, M. A., Hajo van Bockel, J., and van Muijen, G. N. (1990) Characterization and fibrinolytic properties of human omental tissue mesothelial cells. Comparison with endothelial cells. *Blood* **75,** 1490–1497.
11. Macphee, M. J., Wiltrour, R. H., McCormaick, K. L., Sayers, T. J., and Pilaro, A. M. (1994) A method for obtaining and culturing large numbers of purified organ-derived murine endothelial cells. *J. Leukoc. Biol.* **55,** 467–475.
12. Knedler, A. and Ham, R. G. (1987) Optimised medium for clonal growth of human microvascular endothelial cells with minimal serum. *In Vitro Cell Dev. Biol.* **23,** 481–491.
13. Madri, J. A. and Williams, S. K. (1983) Capillary endothelial cell cultures: Phenotypic modulation by matrix components. *J. Cell Biol.* **97,** 153–165.
14. Gerritsen, M. E. (1987) Functional heterogeneity of vascular endothelial cells. *Biochem. Pharmacol.* **36,** 2701–2711.

15. Gallicchio, M., Argyriou, S., Ianches, G., Filonzi, E. L., Zoellner, H., Hamilton, J. A., McGrath, K., and Wojta, J. (1994) Stimulation of PAI-1 expression in endothelial cells by cultured vascular smooth muscle cells. *Arterioscler. Thromb.* **14,** 815–823.

16. Ades, E. W., Candal, F. J., Swerlick, R. A., George, V. G., Summers, S., Bosse, D. C., and Lawley, T. J. (1992) HMEC-1: Establishment of an immortalized human microvascular endothelial cell line. *J. Invest. Dermatol.* **99,** 683–690.

17. Imcke, E., Ruszczak, Z., Mayer-da-Silva A., Detmar, M., and Orfanos, C. E. (1991) Cultivation of human dermal microvascular endothelial cells *in vitro*: immunocytochemical and ultrastructural characterization and effect of treatment with three synthetic retinoids. *Arch. Dermatol. Res.* **283,** 149–157.

18. Garfinkel, S., Brown, S., Wessendorf, J. H., and Maciag, T. (1994) Post-transcriptional regulation of interleukin 1 alpha in various strains of young and senescent human umbilical vein endothelial cells. *Proc. Natl. Acad. Sci. USA* **91,** 1559–1563.

19. Voyta, J. C., Via, D. P., Butterfield, C. E., and Zetter, B. R. (1984) Identification and isolation of endothelial cells based on their increased uptake of acetylated-low density lipoprotein. *J. Cell Biol.* **99,** 2034–2040.

14

Assay for Cell Migration and Invasion of Vascular Smooth Muscle Cells

George Karakiulakis, Eleni Papakonstantinou, and Michael Roth

1. Introduction

Chemotaxis is a critical event in the development of atherosclerotic lesions and in the restenosis that often occurs after surgical intervention and angioplasty *(1)*. Chemokines involved in atherogenesis include colony-stimulating factors *(2)*, oxidized low-density lipoproteins *(3)*, transforming growth factor-β *(4)* and fibroblast growth factor *(5)*, which induce chemotaxis of monocytes and endothelial cells. Other growth factors, such as platelet-derived growth factor (PDGF) *(6)* and insulin-like growth factor-1, induce chemotaxis of vascular smooth muscle cells (VSMCs) *(7)*, which play a major role in the formation of atherosclerotic lesions *(8,9)*. In normal human arteries, VSMC-reside mainly in the tunica media in a quiescent state and express a variety of differentiation-specific genes important to maintain the physiological regulation of vessel tone and blood pressure *(10)*. Under pathological conditions, such as vessel injury or atherosclerotic plaque development, VSMCs become exposed to certain growth factors and cytokines, such as PDGF, which induce a transformation from the contractile to a synthetic state *(7,11–13)*. Only in the latter state, VSMCs acquire the ability to migrate from the tunica media to the tunica intima. In vivo, VSMCs are surrounded by and embedded in a variety of extracellular matrices (ECMs) that must be traversed during migration. In the intact vessel, one of the main ECM barriers to cell movement is the basement membrane (BM) that surrounds each VSMC and separates the VSMC-containing medial cell layer from the endothelium *(14)*. Migrating VSMCs have been shown to digest BM *(14,15)*, an invasion process that is mediated by tightly regulated proteases *(16)*. Within this group of proteases, the family of matrix metalloproteinases (MMPs) are essential for the digestion of ECM components such as collagens, gelatins, or proteoglycans *(17,18)*.

From: *Methods in Molecular Medicine, vol. 52: Atherosclerosis: Experimental Methods and Protocols*
Edited by: A. F. Drew © Humana Press Inc., Totowa, NJ

In this chapter we describe the methodology for assessing VSMC migration and invasion.

2. Materials

2.1. Establishment of Primary Cultures of VSMC from Pulmonary Arteries

1. Hank's buffered salt solution (Seromed).
2. Cell culture flasks.
3. Dulbecco's minimal essential medium (DMEM) (Seromed).
4. HEPES buffer (Seromed).
5. Trypsin (Gibco AG).
6. Colostrum (Chemie Brunschwig).
7. Fetal bovine serum (FBS; Gibco AG).
8. L-glutamine (Seromed).

2.2. Characterization of VSMC

1. Monoclonal antibodies specific for smooth muscle cell actin and for von Willebrand factor (Boehringer Mannheim).
2. Lab Tek tissue culture chamber slides (Miles, Scientific Div.).
3. Phosphate-buffered saline (PBS).
4. 4% paraformaldehyde in PBS.
5. PBS supplemented with 0.5% (w/v) bovine serum albumin (Fluka).
6. Fluorescein isothiocyanate-coupled rabbit antimouse immunoglobulin (Boehringer Mannheim).
7. Fluorosave reagent (Calbiochem-Novabiochem).
8. Fluorescence microscope (e.g., Axiophot; Carl Zeiss).

2.3. Cell Migration and Invasion Assays

1. Boyden chamber systems equipped with cell-permeable filters (pore size 8 μm) (Becton Dickinson). For the invasion studies, the cell-permeable filters of the Boyden-chambers are precoated with a reconstituted BM (Matrigel, Collaborative Biolabs).
2. 4% paraformaldehyde in PBS.
3. Hoechst dye (33342).

3. Methods

3.1. Establishment of Primary Cultures of VSMC from Pulmonary Arteries

Primary cultures of VSMC can be established from pulmonary arteries obtained from patients undergoing lobectomy or pneumonectomy for peripheral lung cancer.

1. Keep arteries overnight in Hank's buffered salt solution at 4°C.
2. Strip off the intimal cell layer and residual adventitial tissue with forceps.
3. Cut the tunica media of the vessels into small pieces (3–5 mm^3) and transfer into prewetted cell culture flasks. Allow VSMC to grow out of the tissue by incubating the vessel tissue for 1 wk in Dulbecco's minimal essential medium (DMEM), supplemented with 5% fetal bovine serum (FBS) and 20 mM HEPES-buffer.
4. Wash away small pieces of vessel tissue with DMEM, treat cells with trypsin and subcultivate in DMEM, supplemented with 10% colostrum, 10% FBS, 20 mM HEPES, and 8 mM L-glutamine.
5. Primary VSMC can be used at passages 2–6.

3.2. Characterization of VSMC

Characterize VSMC by immunohistochemical staining using monoclonal antibodies specific for smooth muscle cell actin.

1. Allow cells to grow in Lab Tek tissue culture chamber slides until confluency and fix in 4% paraformaldehyde.
2. Block nonspecific protein binding by incubating the cells in PBS supplemented with 0.5% (w/v) bovine serum albumin, for 20 min.
3. Incubate slides with mouse anti–smooth muscle cell actin antibody for 60 min, wash with PBS (three times) and further incubate with fluorescein isothiocyanate-coupled rabbit antimouse immunoglobulin.
4. Wash slides with PBS (three times), mount with Fluorosave reagent, and examine, using a fluorescence microscope. Nonspecific binding of the fluorescein-linked antibody is detected using the second antibody alone. Possible contamination of cultures with endothelial cells is excluded by negative staining for von Willebrand factor.

3.3. Migration, Chemotaxis, and Invasion Assays

3.3.1. Assay for Spontaneous Migration

1. Seed VSMC (10^4 cells/mL) onto cell-permeable filters (pore size 8 mm) of Boyden chambers.
2. Bring cells to quiescence by incubating for 48 h in the presence of DMEM, supplemented with 0.1% FBS (quiescence medium), at 37°C, in a 5% CO_2 atmosphere.
3. Add the same medium to the lower compartment of the Boyden chamber.
4. Change the quiescence medium in both compartments every 12 h to avoid autostimulation of the cells.
5. Incubate for a further 24 h in the presence of quiescence medium, at 37°C, in a 5% CO_2 atmosphere.
6. At the end of the incubation period, remove filters and carefully scrape away VSMC remaining adherent to the upper side of the filters.
7. Fix VSMC on the lower side of the filters with 0.1 mL of 4% paraformaldehyde in PBS.

8. Stain with Hoechst dye for 2 min.
9. Assess spontaneous VSMC migration by counting the cells that appeared on the lower side of the filters using fluorescence microscopy ($\times 100$) by counting at least 4 randomly selected areas (1 mm^2) on the filter.

3.3.2. Assay for Agents Affecting Spontaneous Migration

1. Seed VSMC in Boyden chambers and bring to quiescence as described in **Subheading 3.3.1.**
2. Add agent to be tested as an inhibitor or inducer of spontaneous VSMC migration in the upper compartment of the Boyden-chamber.
3. Incubate cells for an additional 24 h in the presence of quiescence medium, at 37°C, in a 5% CO_2 atmosphere and assess VSMC migration, proceeding as described in **Subheading 3.3.1** (*see* **Note 1**).

3.3.3. Assay for Chemotaxis

1. Seed VSMC in Boyden chambers and bring to quiescence as described in **Subheading 3.3.1.**
2. Add agent to be tested as a chemoattractant in the lower compartment of the Boyden chamber.
3. Incubate cells for an additional 24 h in the presence of quiescence medium, at 37°C, in a 5% CO_2 atmosphere and assess VSMC chemotaxis, proceeding as described in **Subheading 3.3.1** (*see* **Note 2**).

3.3.4. Assay for Invasion

1. Precoat the cell-permeable filters of the Boyden chambers with a reconstituted BM (Matrigel).
2. Seed VSMC in Boyden invasion chambers and bring to quiescence as described in Subheading 3.3.1.
3. Add agent to be tested as an inhibitor or inducer of spontaneous VSMC invasion in either the upper or the lower compartment of the Boyden invasion-chamber.
4. Incubate cells for an additional 24 h in the presence of quiescence medium, at 37°C, in a 5% CO_2 atmosphere.
5. Assess VSMC invasion proceeding as described in **Subheading 3.3.1** (**Fig. 1A**; *see* **Note 3**).

4. Notes

1. If an agent induces spontaneous migration of VSMC when added in the upper compartment of the Boyden chamber, the effect may be referred to as chemokinesis.
2. The use of a known chemoattractant for VSMC, such as PDGF *(1)*, may be helpful as a positive control for VSMC chemotaxis. Addition of PDGF-BB (10

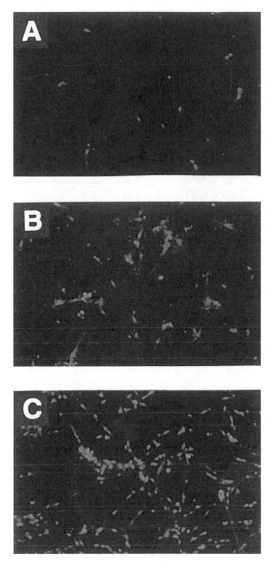

Fig. 1. Fluorescence microscopy (field ×100) of VSMC invasion. Invasion of VSMC was assessed using a Boyden invasion-chamber containing a cell-permeable filter membrane coated with reconstituted BM. Cells were seeded into the upper compartment of the Boyden chamber and brought to quiescence (0.1 % FBS, 48 h). Stimuli were then added to the upper or lower compartment and chambers were incubated for additional 24 h (37°C, 5% CO_2) before the filters were removed. Cells adherent to the upper side were removed, and cells on the lower side of the membranes were fixed with 0.1 mL of 4% paraformaldehyde in PBS and stained with Hoechst dye for 2 min. Invasion was assessed by counting the cells that appeared on the lower side of the filters by fluorescence microscopy. In all cases, four randomly selected areas (1 mm^2) were counted per filter. **(A)** control/control; **(B)** control/PDGF; **(C)** hyaluronic acid/PDGF. Compartments: upper/lower; Control: 0.1% FBS; PDGF-BB: 10 ng/mL; hyaluronic acid: 1 µg/mL.

ng/mL) in the lower compartment of the Boyden chamber will induce significant VSMC chemotaxis *(19)*.

3. The use of a known inducer of VSMC invasion, such as PDGF *(19)*, may be helpful as a positive control for VSMC invasion. Addition of PDGF-BB (10 ng/mL) in the lower compartment of the Boyden invasion-chamber will induce significant (×40–×50) VSMC invasion through BM (*19*; **Fig. 1B**). This phenomenon usually involves enzymatic breakdown of BM and is mediated by proteases *(16)*, the most common of which are MMPs *(17,18)*. An agent that enhances VSMC invasion may achieve this by inducing MMP activity when placed in the lower compartment of the Boyden invasion-chamber (e.g., PDGF-BB, 10 ng/mL, **Fig. 1B**). However, this may also be achieved if agents are placed in the upper compartment of the Boyden invasion-chamber together with the cells (e.g., hyaluronic acid, 1 µg/mL, **Fig. 1C**; *19*). VSMC invasion may also be enhanced via inhibition of tissue inhibitors of MMPs (TIMPs). MMP activity may be assayed employing gelatin zymography techniques *(19)*, and TIMPs may be measured by enzyme-linked immunosorbent assay *(20)*.

References

1. Ross, R. (1999) Atherosclerosis — An inflammatory disease. *N. Engl. J. Med.* **340,** 115–126.
2. Stanley, E. R. (1985) The macrophage colony-stimulating factor, CSF-1. *Methods Enzymol.* **116,** 564–587.
3. Rosenfeld, M. E., Palinski, W., Yla-Herttuala, S., and Carew, T. E. (1990) Macrophages, endothelial cells, and lipoprotein oxidation in the pathogenesis of atherosclerosis. *Toxicol. Pathol.* **18,** 560–571.
4. Sporn, M. B., Roberts, A. B., Wakefield, L. M., and de Crombrugghe, B. (1987) Some recent advances in the chemistry and biology of transforming growth factor-beta. *J. Cell Biol.* **105,** 1039–1045.
5. Folkman, J., Klagsbrun, M., Sasse, J., Wadzinski, M., Ingber, D., and Vlodavsky, I. (1988) A heparin-binding angiogenic protein—basic fibroblast growth factor—is stored within basement membrane. *Am. J. Pathol.* **130,** 393–400.
6. Ferns, G. A., Raines, E. W., Sprugel, K. H., Motani, A. S., Reidy, M. A., and Ross, R. (1991) Inhibition of neointimal smooth muscle accumulation after angioplasty by an antibody to PDGF. *Science* **253,** 1129–1132.
7. Ross, R. (1993) The pathogenesis of atherosclerosis: a perspective for the 1990s. *Nature* **362,** 801–809.
8. Ross, R., Masuda, A., and Raines, E. W. (1990) Cellular interactions, growth factors and smooth muscle proliferation in atherogenesis. *Ann. N.Y. Acad. Sci.* **598,** 102–112.
9. Stary, H. C. (1992) Composition and classification of human atherosclerotic lesions. *Virchows Arch.* **421,** 277–290.
10. Chamley-Campbell, J. H. and Campbell, G. R. (1981) What controls smooth muscle phenotype? *Atherosclerosis* **40,** 347–357.

11. Jawien, A., Bowen-Pope, D. F., Lindner, V., Schwartz, S. M., and Clowes, A. W. (1992) Platelet-derived growth factor promotes smooth muscle migration and intimal thickening in a rat model of balloon angioplasty. *J. Clin. Invest.* **89,** 507–511.

12. Ross, R. (1991) Polypeptide growth factors and atherosclerosis. *Trends Cardiovasc. Med.* **1,** 277–282.

13. Ross, R., Masuda, J., Raines, E. W., Gown, A. M., Katsuda, S., Sasahara, M., Malden, H., Masuko, L. T., and Sato, H. (1990) Localization of PDGF-B protein in all phases of atherogenesis. *Science* **248,** 1009–1012.

14. Pauly, R. R., Passaniti, A., Bilato, C., Monticone, R., Cheng, L., Papadopoulos, N., Gluzband, Y. A., Smith, L., Weinstein, C., Lakatta, E. G., and Crow, M. T. (1994) Migration of cultured vascular smooth muscle cells through a basement membrane barrier requires type IV collagenase activity and is inhibited by cellular differentiation. *Circ. Res.* **75,** 41–54.

15. Sperti, G., van Leeuven, R. T. J., Quax, P. H. A., Maseri, A., and Kluft, C. (1992) Cultured rat aortic vascular smooth muscle cells digest naturally produced extracellular matrix. *Circ. Res.* **71,** 385–392.

16. Quigley, J. P., Berkenpas, M. B., Aimes, R. T., and Chen, J. M. (1990) Serine protease and metalloprotease cascade systems involved in pericellular proteolysis. *Cell Differ. Dev.* **32,** 263–276.

17. Matrisian, L. M. (1990) Metalloproteinases and their inhibitors in matrix remodeling. *Trends Genet.* **6,** 121–125.

18. Woessner, J. F. (1991) Matrix metalloproteinases and their inhibitors in connective tissue remodeling. *FASEB J.* **5,** 2145–2154.

19. Papakonstantinou, E., Karakiulakis, G., Eickelberg, O., Perruchoud A. P., Block, L. H., and Roth, M. (1998) A 340 kDa hyaluronic acid secreted by human vascular smooth muscle cells regulates their proliferation and migration. *Glycobiology* **8,** 821–830.

20. Karakiulakis, G., Papanikolaou, C., Jankovic, S., Aletras, A., Papakonstantinou, E., Vretou, E., and Mirtsou-Fidani, V. (1997) Increased type IV collagen-degrading activity in metastases originating from primary tumors of the human colon. *Invas. Metast.* **17,** 158–168.

15

Collection and Processing of Arterial Specimens for Histological Analysis

Angela F. Drew

1. Introduction

After atherosclerotic development has proceeded for the allotted time, arteries can be harvested by several techniques to optimize both quantitative and qualitative histological analysis. A study design must include consideration of the parameters to be analyzed, to determine how tissue should be harvested. Often, studies increase the numbers of samples in each group to allow specimen collection by several techniques, and hence several different analyses can be performed.

It is often necessary to preserve the arterial shape or size, as much as possible, after the animal has been killed and the artery removed. Unlike solid tissue, which maintains much of its shape after fixation, hollow arteries require more effort to preserve after removal. In situ perfusion with a fixative solution is often performed to achieve structural integrity of the artery wall. While this is successful when performed on arteries from larger animals, smaller arteries from mice, such as the femoral aorta, can still become slightly squashed by gentle handling with forceps during embedding procedures, because of the difficulty in handling such small tissue. This reduces lumen size, which may be an important study parameter. Fortunately, these distortions are minor and rarely persist throughout the entire specimen. Generally, perfusion fixation results in preservation of much of the arterial structure of the specimen and is therefore the method of choice in quantitative procedures.

Perfusion fixation is best performed at physiological pressure, to prevent altering the size of the artery or dislodging arterial lesions. This can be achieved either with a perfusion fixation apparatus or with the setup described in the text.

From: *Methods in Molecular Medicine, vol. 52: Atherosclerosis: Experimental Methods and Protocols*
Edited by: A. F. Drew © Humana Press Inc., Totowa, NJ

The main disadvantage of perfusion fixing and processing arteries is that fixatives can destroy some antigens required for immunohistological staining of cell surface molecules. Unfixed, snap-frozen tissue is optimal for such immunohistology procedures. The advantage of using processed, paraffin-embedded tissue is greatly enhanced morphology, including shape and tissue structure. Most routine histological procedures can be performed successfully on processed tissue. Depending on the parameters of the study, both frozen and processed tissue may be required.

Many popular staining procedures are restricted by constraints during tissue collection. Several examples are provided for consideration. Oil red O or other lipid stains are often used in the quantitation of lesion area of arteries. Since lipid is removed during processing, this technique can be performed only on frozen tissue, either fixed in formalin or unfixed. Immunohistochemical procedures for the detection of cell surface antigens, including T-cell markers such as CD3, 4, and 8, are optimally performed on frozen tissue.

Most routine histological or immunohistological procedures can be performed on frozen tissue, but morphology will always be compromised. The following stains work well on processed, paraffin-embedded tissue: hematoxylin and eosin (H&E), trichrome procedures (collagen/muscle), Verhoef's (elastin), and many immunohistological stains, depending on the stability of the antigenic epitope.

Quantitative analyses can be performed on H&E-stained tissue sections. Best results, however, are obtained with an elastin stain. The enhanced delineation of arterial layers, achieved with an elastin stain, is especially beneficial when creating digitized images for computer-assisted planimetry. A highly suitable method for elastin staining is provided elsewhere *(1)*.

2. Materials
2.1. Perfusion-Fixed Tissue

1. Dissection board and equipment.
2. Gauze.
3. Disposable pressure infusor (Infusable, Vital Signs Inc., Totowa, NJ).
4. Blunted needle (*see* **Note 1**).
5. Catheter (optional).
6. Clamp.
7. Normal saline bags (0.9% sodium chloride irrigation).
8. Perfusion fixative solution (*see* **Note 2**), e.g., 10% neutral buffered formalin (Sigma Diagnostics, St. Louis, MO).
9. Tissue marking dyes (optional) (Triangle Biomedial Sciences, Durham, NC).
10. Disposable embedding cassettes (Omnisette, Fisher Scientific, Pittsburgh, PA).
11. Tissue processor.

2.2. Frozen Tissue

1. OCT (Tissue–Tek, Sakura Finetek USA Inc., Torrance, CA).
2. Plastic cryomolds, (Tissue-Tek, Miles Inc., Elkhart, IN).
3. Liquid nitrogen or dry ice.
4. Isopentane (optional), (2-methylbutane 99+%, Aldrich Chemical Co., Milwaukee, WI).

3. Methods

3.1. Perfusion Fixation at Physiological Pressure

Setup: Perfusion fixation can be achieved with a perfusion apparatus. If unavailable, the following setups can achieve the same result. Perfusion solutions, typically saline and formalin, must be elevated. Physiological pressure can be achieved by elevating perfusion solutions 100–120 cm above the animal and the outlet for the solution. This results in a physiological pressure of 100–120 mm Hg. This pressure can also be obtained by attaching solutions to a pressure infusion device. Inflation of this device to the desired pressure (shown by the gage) provides a simple method for maintaining the correct pressure. Empty saline bags can be filled with fixative to fit into the infusion device. A three-way tap attached to tubing will allow switching between perfusion solutions without removing the needle/catheter from the vasculature.

1. Anesthetize animals and pin to a dissection board.
2. Depending on the arterial segment required, entry inside the vasculature may be gained through the left ventricle (collection of the aortic arch, carotid artery, or thoracic aorta) or directly through the descending aorta for more distal arteries (femoral artery). Commonly, a small incision is made in the left ventricular wall, or arterial wall, and a blunted needle (attached to the perfusion solution) is inserted and clamped in place with a hemostat. Alternatively, insertion of a catheter provides a simple method for infusing solutions into the artery wall.
3. Make an incision in the left atrium to allow an outlet for perfusion solutions.
4. Perfuse saline or PBS through the vasculature for 5 min to eliminate blood cells and plasma proteins.
5. Perfuse fixative solution, such as 10% neutral buffered formalin, for 15 min.
6. Blot dry before marking small arteries with dye, if desired (*see* **Note 3**).
7. Remove arteries and place in fixative for 24 h, prior to processing (*see* **Notes 4** and **5**).

3.2. Collection of Unfixed, Frozen Tissue

1. Remove arteries from anesthetized animals.
2. Rinse arteries in saline or PBS to remove blood cells.
3. Gently blot tissue dry on gauze.

4. Immerse arteries in freezing embedding medium (OCT), in plastic embedding molds, and take care to prevent bubbles from forming.
5. Snap-freeze molds in liquid nitrogen (*see* **Notes 10** and **11**) or freeze on dry ice.
6. Store blocks at –20°C or –80°C until required for sectioning (*see* **Note 12**).

4. Notes

1. A blunted needle can be made by cutting the tip from a needle with scissors and filing any sharp edges.
2. Perfusion fixing can be performed with various fixatives, depending on the tissue *(2)*. For light microscopy, fixation in 10% neutral buffered formalin results in suitable quality morphology for arteries and is stable and available ready made. For best results, tissue should be placed in formalin for 24 h, then transferred to 70% alcohol and processed as soon as possible. Prolonged storage in formalin may cause the tissue to be brittle when sectioning and may cause excessive masking of antigenic epitopes.
3. Small arteries can be marked with insoluble dyes to identify sham-operated arteries from contralateral control arteries then embedded in the same mold; this halves the cutting time.
4. Non-perfusion-fixed tissue should be no larger than 5 mm to allow uniform penetration of fixative.
5. Immerse tissue in at least 20 times the volume of fixative.
6. Small vessels such as mouse arteries can be difficult to find in cassettes after processing into wax. Marking periadventitial tissue with a dye will help to find small tissue and will not interfere with cross-sectional intimal/medial analyses. Biopsy bags or biopsy cassettes should be used with such small tissue.
7. Shorter processing cycles can be used with arterial tissue since it is thin and hollow.
8. The tissue processing cycle can be altered for optimal processing of atherosclerotic arteries, because of their high fat content. After dehydrating the blocks and placing in the first clearing agent reservoir (xylene or xylene substitute), blocks are placed in a further absolute alcohol reservoir before placing in two further clearing agent reservoirs.
9. Sections should be collected onto treated slides, which optimize adhesion of the section and do not contribute to background staining. Such slides are commercially available from Fisher (Superfrost Plus Disposable Microscope Slides; Pittsburgh, PA) and other suppliers. Alternatively, silane-coated slides can be prepared in the laboratory by assembling cleaned slides in a rack, and rinsing slides in acetone, before coating in 2% 3-aminopropyltriethoxysilane for 15 min, followed by a further rinse in acetone, then leaving slides to dry in a dust-free environment.
10. When snap-freezing tissue, examine specimens after removal from liquid nitrogen to ensure complete coverage of tissue sample. Areas of exposure will result in dehydration of the tissue, over time, which will prevent successful cryosectioning.
11. Isopentane can be used when snap-freezing tissue to slow the freezing process down. This may be an advantage if freezing is violent enough that some

embedding medium is forced from the cryomold, exposing tissue. Isopentane is placed in a thermoplastic beaker that can be lowered into the liquid nitrogen container. The isopentane is precooled in the liquid nitrogen prior to placing the specimens on the surface of the isopentane. The beaker is then lowered into the isopentane to allow complete freezing of the tissue.

12. Immunostaining with frozen tissue is best performed on the same day as the sections are cut. This allows for optimal preservation of the antigens.

References

1. Sheehan, D. C. and Hrapchak, B. B. (1980) Connective tissue and muscle fiber stains, in *Theory and Practice of Histotechnology*. Batelle Press, Columbus, OH, pp. 180–201.
2. Luna, L. G. (1992) Histopathologic methods and color atlas of special stains and tissue artifacts. American Histolabs, Inc., Gaitheresburg, MD.

16

Intravascular Ultrasound Imaging in the Quantitation of Atherosclerosis in Vivo

Hannu I. Manninen

1. Introduction

A number of imaging modalities have been used for evaluating the severity of atherosclerotic lesions in vivo. X-ray angiography, using iodine contrast agent, has been the standard imaging technique so far, in spite of its limitations. The severity of lumen-narrowing lesions is generally underestimated in X-ray angiography when compared to operative and histological findings, especially in cases of diffuse atherosclerosis or concentric stenosis. Because of compensatory enlargement of the vessel, human atherosclerotic plaques do not encroach on the lumen until the lesion occupies up to 40% of the combined arterial wall and lumen volume *(1)*. Contrast angiography provides only indirect signs of atherosclerosis on the basis of analysis of the longitudinal silhouette of the vessel lumen, but does not give information about the structure of the vessel wall or morphology of the atherosclerotic lesions, with the exception of heavy calcifications. Magnetic resonance angiography (MRA) is already competing with X-ray angiography in many clinical applications *(2)*. Preliminary data have suggested that magnetic resonance imaging (MRI) is able to provide information about the vessel wall and plaque characteristics ex vivo *(3,4)* and in vivo *(5)*, but poor spatial and temporal resolution impairs thus far the utility of MR techniques in quantitation of atherosclerosis in animal models *(6,7)*.

Intravascular ultrasound (IVUS) imaging is widely used in human peripheral and coronary arteries for the diagnosis, quantitation, and characterization of atherosclerotic lesions. IVUS is currently recognized as the "gold standard" for imaging of atherosclerosis *(8)*. In IVUS imaging, a high-frequency ultrasound transducer attached to the tip of a catheter is inserted into the artery and

From: *Methods in Molecular Medicine, vol. 52: Atherosclerosis: Experimental Methods and Protocols*
Edited by: A. F. Drew © Humana Press Inc., Totowa, NJ

advanced selectively to the site of interest. Since US beam is transmitted and received in a perpendicular orientation to the catheter, IVUS does not provide any data about the longitudinal location of the probe in the vessel; thus, fluoroscopic and angiographic controls are to be used. IVUS offers valuable and unique information about the structure and pathology of the vessel wall. Current catheter technology facilitates IVUS examination in vessels 2 to 3 mm in diameter and makes the method potentially feasible also for imaging vessels in small animals, for example, the aorta of rabbits. Theoretically, this method might become beneficial also in the assessment of effectiveness of experimental therapeutic interventions such as gene therapy.

This chapter describes the principle of IVUS study, technical performance IVUS imaging on an animal model (abdominal aorta of a hyperlipidemic rabbit; *9*), and principles of interpretation and quantitation of atherosclerotic changes on IVUS.

2. Materials

2.1. Angiographic Equipment

A digital fluoroscope, preferably with road mapping and subtraction facilities, should be available. Modern movable surgical C-arm image intensifiers with a 6-in. image field and an electronic zooming function and a minimum of 2 frames/s exposure rates are very well suited. The equipment should include a video printer or a laser film printer. Pressure- and volume-controlled automated injectors of the X-ray contrast media are very useful, but not absolutely mandatory.

2.2. IVUS Equipment

IVUS equipment is basically composed of the US unit, the imaging catheter, and SuperVHS video for the long-term image storage. Some new equipment utilizes digital image data registration and storage. Several types of IVUS catheters are available in sizes 3–8 French (1–2.7 mm external diameter) used at 10–40 MHz. Typically, catheters with smaller diameter and higher frequency are intended for smaller arteries, since they provide better spatial resolution and are more flexible facilitating navigation in small and tortuous vessels, such as coronary arteries. Catheters with lower imaging frequency offer a wider imaging field, necessary in large-caliber arteries. Catheters 3–3.5 French in diameter used at 30–40 MHz are mandatory for imaging arteries of small animals, e.g., rabbit aorta. Both mechanical and phased-array transducers are available. In the former type, the ceramic US probe or a mirror rotates inside the catheter. Thus, the catheter is to be connected to a motor-driven unit. A fluid-filled tip is also necessary to produce an acoustic pathway from the transducer to the exterior of the catheter. In phased-array catheters the direction of the US beam is controlled electronically. IVUS catheters contain a channel for a guide wire, either for the whole length of the catheter (over-the-wire type) or at a short distance near the tip of the catheter (monorail or rapid-exchange type). The former type provides better pushability and trackability characteristics, while the latter type has an advantage for easier change of the catheter, a valuable feature especially in complex interventions with several types of catheters used.

2.3. Experimental Animals

The animals used for the following protocol for IVUS imaging are Watanabe heritable hyperlipidemic (WHHL) rabbits. Hyperchlolesterolemic (1% cholesterol diet for 5 wk) New Zealand White (NZW) rabbits, usually after balloon denudation, can also be used. The imaging procedures are performed under general anesthesia with intravenous injection of phentanyl-fluonisone (0.2 ml/ kg, Hypnorm, Janssen Pharmaceutica, Belgium), and midazolam (1.5 mg/kg, Dormicum, Roche, France; **9**).

3. Methods
3.1. Arterial Access

The right or left carotid artery is prepared, preferably under an operation microscope, and surgically ligated immediately beneath the carotid bifurcation. Another loose, temporary ligation is performed about 2 cm more proximally, and a small incision is made into the closed arterial segment. A 0.035-in. hydrophilic (Terumo Inc) or Teflon-coated guide wire (for practical reasons, preferably not more than 40 cm long) is advanced under visual control into the artery after partial loosening of the proximal ligature, followed by a size 4 French introducer sheath (e.g., Cordis). The ligation around the sheath is tightened to avoid bleeding. To avoid thrombosis, 300–500 U heparin is administrated into the side arm of the introducer sheath.

3.2. Catheterization of the Descending Aorta

After cannulation the animal is tranferred into the angiographic laboratory. A 0.014–0.018-in. guide wire (e.g., Control wire, Boston Scientific), with a 3–5-cm floppy distal end, is advanced into the aortic arch under fluoroscopic control (*see* **Note 1**). The distal end of the guide wire should be slightly angled (degree of the angle can usually be increased by gentle manual compression). A no. 4 French pigtail or Judkins right coronary catheter is advanced over the guide wire into the aortic arch and navigated into the descending aorta (**Fig. 1**). In case of difficulty, contrast agent injection into the thoracic arch can be done through the side arm of the sheath to obtain a "road map." When the catheter is in the descending thoracic aorta, contrast angiography is performed. About 5 mL of preferably nonionic contrast agent (e.g., Omnipaque 240 mgI/mL,

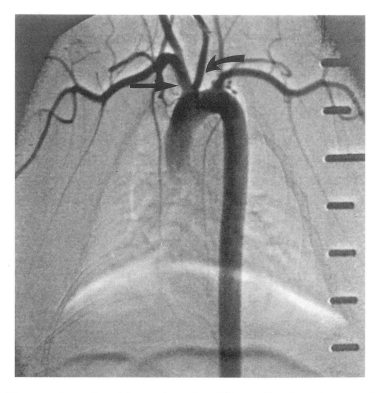

Fig. 1. X-ray angiography of the aortic arch and descending thoracic aorta of a rabbit. Note that both the brachiocephalic trunk *(straight arrow)* and left *(curved arrow)* carotid artery originate from the ascending aorta, an anatomical condition that necessitates some guide wire manipulation to get a catheter into the descending aorta.

Nycomed Inc., Oslo, Norway) is injected at a flow of 5 mL/s and image registration is done at 2–6 frames/s. If manual injections are performed, 5-mL syringes are preferable.

3.3. Performance of IVUS Imaging

After removal of the diagnostic catheter, the IVUS catheter is advanced over the guide wire to the distal abdominal aorta. IVUS imaging can be performed by a standard pull-back technique and recorded on super VHS video. Use of a motorized pull-back device, if available, facilitates more versatile postprocessing and analyzing protocols (*see* **Note 2**). Numerous spot images are taken during the IVUS imaging to register the longitudinal location of the imaging probe in relation to various bony landmarks, external X-ray positive ruler, and angiographic side branches (**Fig. 2A**). Time point or number of each X-ray spot image is to be marked by annotations into the IVUS video. Alternatively, digital road mapping control can be applied to exactly locate the imaging probe (*see* **Note 3**) if also recorded on another super VHS video.

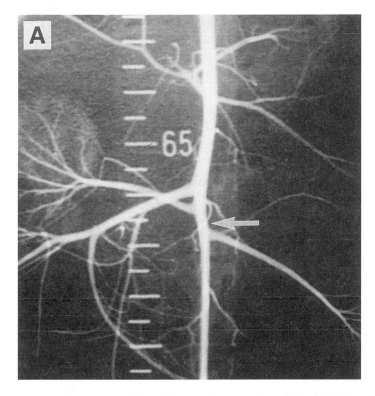

Fig. 2. X-ray angiography of the abdominal aorta of a rabbit. (**A**) Note the radio-paque ruler. An arrow between the right and left renal artery indicates the level of the IVUS image in (**B**).

After the IVUS examination, the introducer sheath is removed and the prepared common carotid artery is ligated. Rabbits generally tolerate closure of one carotid artery well, without neurological sequelae, and the IVUS study can be repeated through the other carotid artery or by femoral artery access later. The animal can be sacrificed with an overdose of phentanyl-fluonisone.

3.4. Analysis of the IVUS Images

By using the renal, superior mesenteric, and celiac arteries, located from the X-ray angiography as anatomical landmarks, the longitudinal location of each IVUS frame can be verified with sufficient accuracy. If performing a comparison of two different IVUS studies on the same animal, or correlating IVUS results with histological findings, identification of exact longitudinal location is needed. Slices that are close to identified side branches, of considerable size, are the most suitable.

The most simple and straightforward quantitative technique is to select the anatomical slice with the most severe lesion in each predetermined arterial segment and measure the maximum thickness and the area of the plaque with the software provided with the IVUS equipments (**Fig. 2B**). Alternatively, the area of the plaque can be measured (**Fig. 2C**). The equipment also provides determination of diameter stenosis by measuring the smallest diameter of the free lumen at the site of the lesion. Especially in cases with concentric lesions, the plaque burden is best characterized by the difference of the area delineated by the intima-media interface (known as the media-bounded area) and the free lumen (**Fig. 3** *see* **Notes 6** and **7**). If a motor-driven pull-back device and sophisticated postprocessing equipment, facilitating three-dimensional reconstruction, are available, the three-dimensional and longitudinal reconstructions are demonstrative and facilitate determination of plaque volumes.

4. Notes
4.1. Technical Considerations of IVUS

1. The IVUS catheter should be strictly prepared according to the instructions of the manufacturer, and pretesting for correct function, e.g., in a water-filled 1-mL syringe, is mandatory. The exact location of the imaging probe inside the catheter should be checked by fluoroscopy, beforehand, to correlate each IVUS frame with the longitudinal position inside the artery.
2. IVUS imaging suffers often from various artifacts, identification and prevention of which, if possible, is crucial for successful application of the technique. In particular, the catheters with a mechanical transducer can easily jam during the examination if pushed when the motor is active or if there is a sharp angle at the catheter shaft. Another problem is the bright halo artifact, 1 to several millimeters around the catheter echo ("ring-down" artifact) that deteriorates the visibility of any structures falling within this zone (*see* **Figs. 2** and **3**). It is important to identify this artifact and try to change the location of the imaging probe inside the arterial lumen by rotating the imaging catheter so that all sectors of the arterial wall can get enough distance from the transducer to be reliably visualized.
3. IVUS does not provide any information about the axial directions (right, left, anterior, or posterior) unless anatomical landmarks such as visceral and renal arteries, or, e.g., vena cava or renal veins, are utilized. This direction orientation is lost immediately when the catheter is rotated within the artery, however.

4.2. Performance of IVUS Study

4. We prefer arterial access from the carotid artery, since difficulties can be encountered in advancement of the guide wire and imaging catheter through the diseased femoral artery of WHHL rabbits. Preferably, the right common carotid artery should be used, since it offers a more straightforward route to the descending

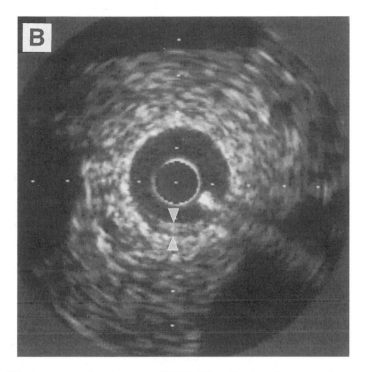

Fig. 2. **(B)** An eccentric plaque at IVUS. The distance between the arrowheads denotes the maximum thickness of the plaque. Note the bright artifact of the guide wire at 4 o'clock.

thoracic aorta (*see* **Fig. 1**). Great care is to be taken not to advance the guide wire, and especially the introducer sheath, more than 5 cm into the carotid artery to avoid damage of the aortic arch or unintended catheterization of the left ventricle. Instead of frontal fluoroscopy, 45-degree left anterior oblique projection may be better when navigating the guide wire and catheter into the descending aorta.

5. During imaging, care should be taken to get the imaging catheter as coaxially as possible with the artery. Marked errors in plaque quantitation are unavoidable in angled arteries, since the US beam is transmitted and perceived perpendicular to the catheter.

4.3. Analysis of IVUS Images

6. The normal wall of a rabbit aorta is too thin (<200 µm) to facilitate visualization of vessel wall layers in IVUS at 30 MHz. In an atherosclerotic vessel, the intralesional structure can, however, be evaluated. In human arteries, IVUS has been proven to be useful in distinguishing fibrotic, "lipid-rich," and calcified components of the plaques (*10,11*). Several factors, such as gain settings and

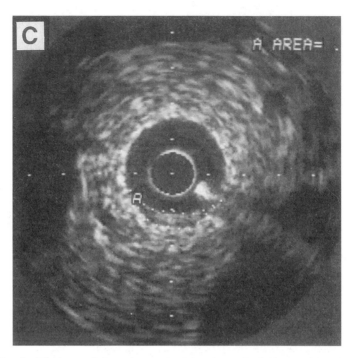

Fig. 2. (C) Area of the atherosclerotic plaque is delineated by dots.

eccentric situation of the imaging catheter within the vessel lumen, can interfere with the accuracy of the method *(12)*. Moreover, elastic arteries such as the abdominal aorta, exhibit a nonlayered structure in IVUS *(13)*, a fact that further complicates visual assessment of plaque echogenicity. We have found some correlation between the echogenicity and histopathological findings in thick atherosclerotic plaques of WHHL rabbits *(9)*. In less severe lesions, evaluation of intraplaque structure is beyond the resolution of IVUS equipment (axial resolution of approximately 150 μm and lateral resolution of 250 μm according to the manufacturer).

7. The maximum thickness and the cross-sectional area of the plaque are the most reproducible measures, according to our experience (*see* **Fig. 2**). We found the determination of the media-bounded area often troublesome because of the difficulty in identifying arterial layers (borderline between media and adventitia) and sometimes even the adventitial-periadventitial border in a rabbit aorta. Sophisticated postprocessing programs, providing semiautomatic edge detection and volume determination of three-dimensional reconstructions, have been successfully applied in human arteries. This technique is theoretically ideal to measure plaque burden, but there are scant publications about its utility in animal models.

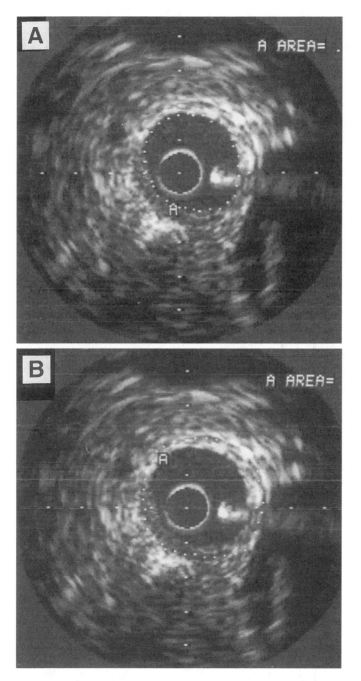

Fig. 3. A concentric plaque of a rabbit aorta. (**A**) The area of the free lumen is delineated by dots. (**B**) The dots delineate media-adventitia interface and give the media-bounded area. The media-bounded area minus the area of the free lumen represents the plaque burden.

References

1. Glagov, S., Weisenberg, E., Zarins, C. K., Stankunavicins, R., and Kolettis, G. D. (1987) Compensatory enlargement of human atherosclerotic coronary arteries. *N. Engl. J. Med.* **316,** 1371–1355.
2. Anderson, C. M., Lee, R. E., Levin, D. L., de la Torre, A. S., and Saloner, D. (1994) Measurement of internal carotid artery stenosis from source MR angiograms. *Radiology* **193,** 219–226.
3. Halliburton, S. S. and Paschal, C. B. (1996) Atherosclerotic plaque components in human aortas contrasted by ex vivo imaging using fast spin-echo magnetic resonance imaging and spiral computed tomography. *Invest. Radiol.* **31,** 724–728.
4. Toussaint, J.-F., Southern, J. F., Fuster, V., and Kantor, H. L. (1995) T2-weighted contrast for NMR characterization of human atherosclerosis. Arterioscler. *Thromb. Vasc. Biol.* **15,** 1533–1542.
5. Toussaint, J.-F., LaMuraglia, G. M., Southern, J. F., Fuster, V., and Kantor, H. L. (1996) Magnetic resonance images lipid, fibrous, calcified, hemorrhagic, and thrombotic components of human atherosclerosis in vivo. *Circulation* **94,** 932–938.
6. Yuan, C., Skinner, M. P., Kaneko, E., Mitsumori, L. M., Hayes, C. E., Raines, E. W., Nelson, J. A., and Ross, R. (1996) Magnetic resonance imaging to study lesions of atherosclerosis in the hyperlipidemic rabbit aorta. *Magn. Reson. Imaging.* **14,** 93–102.
7. Skinner, M. P., Yuan, C., Mitsumori, L., Hayes, C. E., Raines, E. W., Nelson, J. A., and Ross, R. (1995) Serial magnetic resonance imaging of experimental atherosclerosis detects lesion fine structure, progression and complications in vivo. *Nature Med.* **1,** 69–73.
8. Waller, B., Pinkerton, C., and Slack, J. (1992) Intravascular ultrasound: A histological study of vessels during life. The new "gold standard" for vascular imaging. *Circulation* **85,** 2305–2310.
9. Manninen, H. I., Vanninen, R. L., Laitinen, M., Räsänen, H., Vainio, P., Luoma, J. S., Pakkanen, T., Tulla, H., and Ylä-Herttuala, S. (1998) Intravascualr ultrasound and magentic resonance imaging in the assessment of atherosclerotic lessions in rabbit aorta. *Invest. Radiol.* **33,** 464–471.
10. Potkin, B. N., Bartorelli, A. L., Gessert, J. M., Neville, R. F., Almengor, Y., Roberts, W. S., and Leon, M. B. (1990) Coronary artery imaging with intravascular high-frequency ultrasound. *Circulation* **81,** 1575–1585.
11. Manninen, H. I., Räsänen, H., Vanninen, R. L., Berg, M., Hippeläinen, M., Saari, T., Yang, X., Karkola, K., and Kosma, V.-M. (1998) Human carotid arteries: Correlation of intravascular US with angiographic and histopathologic findings. *Radiology* **206,** 65–74.
12. Kimura, B. J., Bhargava, V., and DeMaria, A. N. (1995) Value and limitations of intravascular ultrasound imaging in characterizating coronary atherosclerotic plaque. *Am. Heart J.* **130,** 386–396
13. Nishimura, R. A., Edwards, W. D., Warnes, C. A., Reeder, G. S., Holmes, D. R. Jr., Tajik, A. J., and Yock, P. G. (1990) Intravascular ultrasound imaging.; In vitro validation and pathological correlation. *J. Am. Coll. Cardiol.* **16,** 145–154.

17

Identification of Cell Types and Quantification of Lesion Composition

Rodney J. Dilley

1. Introduction

Many different cell types have been identified in atherosclerotic plaques, including endothelial cells, smooth muscle cells, monocytes, monocyte-derived macrophages, lymphocytes, and mast cells. Examining the role each cell type plays in the formation and pathophysiology of atherosclerotic plaques relies upon the identification of these cells within plaques and early plaque-like structures, which in turn depends on their expression of recognizable and stable morphological characteristics. Cell-type characterization was limited in early studies to light microscopy, and then electron microscopy increased the number of different cell types identified. There is still substantial information to be gained by the use of these methods alone, but more recently the increasing use of immunohistochemistry with a panel of cell-type–specific antibodies has simplified and expanded these earlier methods *(1)*. There are now examples of commercially available antibodies for most cell types thought to be involved in the atherosclerotic process. The protocol for utilizing these antibodies for cell identification requires three steps: tissue collection, sectioning, and staining; this chapter will deal in detail with the last only.

Quantitation of lesion composition depends on adequate staining for specific tissue components, and on the establishment of reliable quantitative methods to measure their abundance. The predominant quantitative methods used are based on the now widely available image analysis tools, usually in conjunction with videomicroscopy *(2,3)*. These methods are ideal for measuring areas on sections or area fractions (e.g., percentage area) to give estimates of the changes in proportions of tissues or cell types in atherosclerotic lesions. While it is

From: *Methods in Molecular Medicine, vol. 52: Atherosclerosis: Experimental Methods and Protocols*
Edited by: A. F. Drew © Humana Press Inc., Totowa, NJ

tempting to count the number of stained cells in sections, counting three-dimensional structures in two-dimensional sections produces a bias, so that apparent changes in number may simply reflect changes in cell size or orientation *(4)*. Over the last 10–15 yr there have been remarkable advances in stereological methods for unbiased estimation of cell number *(5,6)*, but these have not found their way into the atherosclerosis literature to date. Percentage area measurements are generally not affected by size or orientation and may give useful information regarding the composition of tissues and their role in atherogenesis *(2,7)*.

The rapidly developing field of systematic genomics will likely identify many new cell characteristics *(8)* and provide new tools for examining cell populations and their roles in atherogenesis. As a result, cell-type identification and quantification methodology will become more widely applied to study cell-type distribution in sections of atherosclerotic plaque. This chapter presents a simple method for identification of cell types in paraffin-embedded tissues by immunohistochemistry and quantification by image analysis of the area of stained material, as an estimator of the amount of tissue affected.

2. Materials

2.1. Immunohistochemistry

1. Tissues: postmortem, endarterectomy, transplant, or vascular graft material is suitable. Tissues should be fresh-frozen or fixed in a suitable fixative and sectioned onto adhesive-coated slides (e.g., gelatin, polylysine, silane).
2. Phosphate-buffered saline (PBS) (0.01 M sodium phosphate, 0.9% saline, pH 7.4).
3. Primary antibodies: A panel of antibodies specific to cellular characteristics is in the table.

Antigen	Cell type
Von Willebrand factor	Endothelium
Smooth muscle cell α-actin	Smooth muscle
CD68	Macrophage/monocyte
CD3	T-lymphocytes
Tryptase	Mast cells

All antibodies are available from DAKO Corporation (Carpinteria, CA) as antihuman monoclonal antibodies raised in mouse. Similar reagents are available from other suppliers.

4. Negative control antibodies: an unrelated antibody with similar isotype (e.g., antihuman cytokeratin mouse IgG_1, DAKO Corp, Carpinteria CA).
5. Secondary antibodies: labeled (biotinylated) antibody raised against mouse IgG (Vector Laboratories, Burlingame CA).
6. Detection system: Vector Elite ABC kit (Mouse IgG/peroxidase) (Vector Laboratories, Burlingame CA).

7. Chromogen: 3'3'-diaminobenzidine (DAB) tablets (Sigma Chemical Company, St Louis MO).
8. Histology reagents: Slides, staining racks, ethanol dehydration/rehydration series, mounting media and counterstain.
9. PAP pen: hydrophobic marker for restricting volume of solutions applied to sections (DAKO Corp, Carpinteria CA).
10. Humid chamber for incubations: Purpose-built chambers are available, but a resealable household food storage container or a dampened paper pad with an upturned tray for a cover can be used.

2.2. Image-Analysis Equipment

1. Microscope, with monochrome or color video camera (e.g., Olympus BX 50 microscope, JVC KYF-55B 3 CCD color camera).
2. Computer with color video framegrabber card (Intel Pentium III 600 MHz system, Imaging Technology IC PCI framegrabber).
3. Image analysis software (Optimas, Media Cybernetics, Silver Spring MD).

Current system used in this laboratory is shown in parentheses. Other systems are available from various suppliers.

3. Methods
3.1 Immunohistochemistry
3.1.1. Collection of Material

When necessary, tissues may be collected fresh and snap-frozen for cryostat sections or, as appropriate to the antibody/antigen combination, fixed in a suitable fixative solution (generally an aldehyde-based solution; *see* **Note 1**) and embedded in paraffin or resin (epoxy/methacrylate; *see* **Notes 2** and **3**). Sections are cut and placed onto slides with adhesive coating.

3.1.2. Immunohistochemical Staining of Paraffin-Embedded Sections

1. Deparaffinize sections in xylene or xylene substitute (2 changes, 5 min each;all treatments are at room temperature).
2. Rehydrate sections in ethanol series 100% ethanol, 95%, 90%, 70%, and water — 2 changes, 5 min each.
3. Wash in PBS, 5 min.
4. Incubate 5 min with fresh 3% H_2O_2 solution in PBS to quench endogenous peroxidase activity.
5. Wash in PBS, 5 min
6. Wipe dry around sections with tissue or filter paper and mark a ring around sections with PAP pen to restrict spread of solutions and minimize solution volume required.

7. Incubate 30 min in normal serum to block nonspecific antibody binding (10% nonimmune serum from same species that the secondary antibody was raised in, e.g. normal horse serum).

8. Tap slides on their sides to remove serum-blocking solution.

9. Incubate with primary antibody, or appropriate controls (*see* **Note 6**) at recommended dilution for 1 h, or test dilution by titration (range of 0.2–20 µg/mL is a good starting point).

10. Wash in PBS 2 changes, 5 min each on rotary platform.

11. Incubate in secondary biotinylated antibody (diluted to 1 µg/mL in PBS) for 1 h.

12. Wash in PBS 2 changes, 5 min each.

13. Incubate in avidin/biotin/HRP complex (ABC reagent diluted 1:100 in PBS, made 30 min prior to use) for 1 h.

14. Wash in PBS 2 changes, 5 min each.

15. Incubate in fresh chromogen solution (DAB, 0.5 mg/mL in PBS with 0.015% H_2O_2), monitoring stain intensity under low-magnification objective on the microscope; 5–10 min is a convenient time. Antibody dilutions may be altered to adjust time.

16. Wash in water to stop reaction.

17. Counterstain with a contrasting nuclear dye (e.g., Harris' hematoxylin) for up to 5 min.

18. Wash in water.

19. Dehydrate in ethanol series and clear in xylene or similar clearing agent.

20. Mount in permanent mounting medium (Depex).

3.2. Quantification of Lesion Composition

The aim of this protocol is to identify and quantitate stained material in sections of atherosclerotic lesions based on the intensity of tissue staining. The protocol can be divided into four major steps.

1. Image capture and enhancement.
2. Feature of interest (region of interest) identification.
3. Measurement.
4. Analysis of data.

The measurement method of choice depends on the distribution of stain. For example, to measure a large or diffusely stained structure such as the plaque fibrous cap or lipid core, the method is to draw an outline around the structure and measure the area within the outline. Several discrete areas may be measured, e.g., total plaque area, fibrous cap, lipid core, and then a percentage area calculated for each component. For more numerous and/or smaller objects distributed throughout the tissue, such as specifically stained cells in an area of tissue, a range (threshold) of stain intensity or color can be selected to distinguish the objects from their surrounding tissue background intensity. The intensity values for all picture elements (pixels) in the image can be displayed as an intensity histogram. The image analysis program will count the number of pixels in the image that fall within this defined range, as well as the total number of pixels, and then calculate the percentage of the total area that is comprised of the selected structure.

1. The light microscope, video camera, and computer are turned on and allowed to warm up before use.
2. A slide is placed on the microscope, and an appropriate magnification objective lens is selected to allow imaging of the area to be measured within the field of view given on the video monitor. The light microscope is set up for bright-field imaging, ensuring an even field of illumination throughout the image (e.g., Koehler illumination). The analysis is simpler if the image on the computer display appears similar to the image viewed through the microscope. Brightness and contrast should be adjusted to allow the range of pixel intensities from the image to fall within the range of the intensity histogram. A broad range will allow more precise selection of threshold.
3. The area measurements taken may be calibrated by selecting a calibration factor appropriate to the objective lens being used (*see* **Notes 10** and **11**). This allows each pixel of the image to have a defined size, and therefore measurements will represent actual area units (square millimeters or square microns), not just pixel counts.
4. A focused image of the region of interest is gathered (acquired) and stored.
5. The structure to be measured (e.g., atherosclerotic plaque) is defined by drawing around the edge of the structure with a drawing tool (mouse or drawing tablet). The data (pixel counts) are then acquired from the image.
6. When numerous small objects (e.g., cells) are to be measured, it is necessary to set a threshold. This is done by using either an intensity histogram to observe peaks or by selecting a range of representative pixels from the image directly. The threshold data can be presented as a colored image overlay to show the position of the pixels that lie within the range selected. When the area of interest is defined, and a threshold set to represent stained material, the percentage area of stained material can be calculated directly by dividing the area of thresholded pixels by that of the total and multiplying by 100.
7. Data can be exported directly to a spreadsheet program for further analysis.

4. Notes

4.1. Immunohistochemistry

1. Fixation is critical for some antibodies, the chemical crosslinking caused by aldehyde fixatives, such as routine formalin fixation, can destroy tissue antigenicity. In this case it may be possible to treat tissues so as to retrieve sufficient antigenicity (*see* **Note 4**). Alternatively, it may be necessary to prepare more tissue with a different fixative, such as those that coagulate protein (ethanol, acetone) rather than crosslinking, or prepare fresh-frozen samples. In this labora-

tory, the order of fixative potency in degrading tissue binding of commonly used antibodies is glutaraldehyde > formaldehyde > Zamboni's fixative (formaldehyde/picric acid) > Carnoy's fixative (ethanol/acetic acid/chloroform) > cold ethanol, or acetone. For screening fixative effects on an unknown antibody it is possible to bind antigen to nitrocellulose membranes and test different fixatives on those samples before immunostaining, or to use frozen sections postfixed in a panel of fixatives.

2. The level of resolution required may determine the method of tissue embedding. Highest resolution may be available in resin-embedded tissues *(9)*, even allowing electron microscopic examination *(10)*. Frozen sections give lower resolution but higher levels of antigen preservation and greater volumes of tissue available for analysis.

3. Epoxy resin sections may be immunostained after removal of resin by brief incubation in saturated sodium ethoxide (sodium hydroxide in absolute ethanol) *(9)*.

4. A high level of staining (background) with negative control tissue or negative control antibody can be due to a number of factors.

   Endogenous peroxidase activity may produce background signal, particularly from erythrocytes and macrophages, and should be blocked with incubation in 3% H_2O_2, 5–10 min.

   Nonspecific tissue binding of antibodies may occur and can be blocked by preincubation with 2–20% bovine serum albumin or addition of normal serum to the antibody mixture (2%).

   Endogenous tissue biotin may be blocked with avidin/biotin blocking solutions added sequentially. These are available from major suppliers in kit form (e.g., DAKO Corp., Vector Laboratories).

5. Low-intensity (none) or uneven staining may be due to epitope loss by overfixation of tissues. The epitope may be retrieved by microwave or enzyme-digestion protocols.

   a. Microwave antigen retrieval: Place slides in plastic 60-mL coplin jars, fill with citrate buffer, pH 6. Microwave 3 coplin jars, each filled with buffer and blank or test slides for 5 min at 650–700 W power, change solutions and microwave again at 650–700 W for 5 min. Allow to stand for 20 min.

   b. Enzyme treatment: 0.1% trypsin in PBS or 0.1% protease in PBS for 15–30 min at 37°C.

6. Control antibodies are essential components of an immunohistochemistry experiment. A positive control antibody tests suitability of the tissue preparation and antibody detection systems. It typically is an antibody against a protein constitutively expressed in the tissue of interest (such as smooth muscle α-actin or endothelial von Willebrand factor for vascular tissues). A negative control antibody does not specifically recognize components of the tissue, but is the same antibody isotype as the test antibody, and applied at the same concentration. Any staining observed in these samples is regarded as background to be compared against positive staining in the test sample.

4.2. Image Analysis

7. Image capture can be performed a number of ways, traditionally via film-based photography, but increasingly with video- or digital- camera–based methods. We routinely use videomicroscopy, but have also used either a digital camera or a 35-mm slide scanner adapted for microscope slides to gather images of large samples and en face preparations. We have also scanned 35-mm film to gather images (for example, for fluorescence microscopy) from the microscope at high resolution.

8. The raw image may be analyzed when the illumination is even across the field. When illumination is not even, it may introduce a shift in the stain intensity and affect the setting of a threshold. A correction to uneven images can be made by a simple arithmetic operation. Two images are collected, a bright field from a blank area of slide, and a dark field (e.g., light source covered). The image is then corrected by applying the following formula:

$$I = (I_o - I_d)/ (I_b - I_d)$$

where corrected image (I) is derived by subtracting the dark field image (I_d) from both the original image (I_o) and the bright field image (I_b) and dividing the corrected original image by the corrected bright field image.

4. The principal issue in feature-of-interest identification is contrast. This is generally provided by staining methods, such as immunohistochemical or specific histochemical (e.g., oil red O method for lipids, Verhoeff's elastic stain, trichrome methods for collagen) staining procedures on tissue sections. There must be sufficient contrast generated by the stain to separate the feature of interest from the surrounding tissue background. When the contrast is low and positive staining is difficult to distinguish from the background, or inconsistent from slide to slide within the experiment, the use of quantitative image analysis is not appropriate.

5. For the total area method of measurement, most systems can be calibrated spatially to provide data in mm^2 or μm^2. Calibration factors can be established by forming an image of a stage micrometer with the same magnification objective lens on the microscope and calibrating pixel dimensions against a user-defined length. Calibrations may be saved and used in subsequent sessions with the same optical magnification. Percentage area is largely independent of magnification and can be used on an uncalibrated system where the microscopy parameters of magnification and illumination intensity are held constant.

6. For spatial calibration it may also be necessary to determine the aspect ratio of the system by calibrating in both vertical and horizontal orientation.

References

1. Katsuda, S., Boyd, H. C., Fligner, C., Ross, R., and Gown, A. M. (1992) Human atherosclerosis. III. Immunocytochemical analysis of the cell composition of lesions of young adults. *Am. J. Pathol.* **140,** 907–914.

 2. Sukhova, G. K., Schonbeck, U., Rabkin, E., Schoen, F. J., Poole, A. R., Billinghurst, R. C., and Libby, P. (1999) Evidence for increased collagenolysis by interstitial collagenases-1 and -3 in vulnerable human atheromatous plaques. *Circulation* **99,** 2503–2509.

 3. Chen, Y. X., Nakashima, Y., Tanaka, K., Shiraishi, S., Nakagawa, K., and Sueishi, K. (1999) Immunohistochemical expression of vascular endothelial growth factor/ vascular permeability factor in atherosclerotic intimas of human coronary arteries. *Arterioscler. Thromb. Vasc. Biol.* **19,** 131–139.

 4. Sterio, D. C. (1984) The unbiased estimation of number and sizes of arbitrary particles using the disector. *J. Microsc.* **134,** 127–136.

 5. Gundersen, H. J., Bagger, P., Bendtsen, T. F., Evans, S. M., Korbo, L., Marcussen, N., Moller, A., Nielsen, K., Nyengaard, J. R., and Pakkenberg, B. (1988) The new stereological tools: Disector, fractionator, nucleator and point sampled intercepts and their use in pathological research and diagnosis. *APMIS* **96,** 857–881.

 6. Mayhew, T. M. and Gundersen, H. J. (1996) If you assume, you can make an ass out of u and me: A decade of the disector for stereological counting of particles in 3D space. *J. Anat.* **188,** 1–15.

 7. Falkenberg, M., Giglio, D., Bjornheden, T., Nygren, H., and Risberg, B. (1998) Urokinase plasminogen activator colocalizes with CD25+ cells in atherosclerotic vessels. *J. Vasc. Res.* **35,** 318–324.

 8. Schwartz, S. M. (1999) The definition of cell type. *Circulation* **84,** 1234–1235.

 9. Bobik, A., Agrotis, A., Kanellakis, P., Dilley R., Krushinsky, A., Smirnov, V., Tararak, E., Condron, M., and Kostolias, G. (1999) Distinct patterns of transforming growth factor B isoform and receptor expression in human atherosclerotic lesions. *Circulation* **99,** 2883–2891.

10. Taatjes, D. J., Wadsworth, M., Absher, P. M., Sobel, B. E., and Schneider, D. J. (1997) Immunoelectron microscopic localization of plasminogen activator inhibitor type 1 (PAI-1) in smooth muscle cells from morphologically normal and atherosclerotic human arteries. *Ultrastruct. Pathol.* **21,** 527–536.

18

Nonradioactive *In Situ* Hybridization in Atherosclerotic Tissue

Jim Apostolopoulos

1. Introduction

In situ hybridization (ISH) is a powerful and important technique that allows the detection and microscopic localization of nucleic acids within the specific cell, tissue, or chromosome of interest. In addition, it offers increased sensitivity over traditional filter hybridization, since low-copy mRNA molecules in individual cells can be detected. At the time the ISH technique was developed by Pardue and Gall *(1)*, there were restrictions in it since radioisotopes were the only labels for nucleic acids available and autoradiographic film was the only detection system. Current molecular biological cloning techniques have now enabled most researchers to prepare almost any specific probe of choice and, more importantly, modern nonradioactive labels with colorimetric detection have removed all the limitations and restrictions of radioactive labels. The principal advantages of nonradioactive hybridization compared with isotopic hybridization are increased speed, greater resolution, lower costs, and reduced radioactive exposure. Furthermore, it allows the opportunity for combining different labels in one ISH experiment. The procedures behind ISH localization of DNA or RNA are very similar and may be summarized in five areas: (1) sample and glass slide preparation, including fixation, mounting, and ISH pretreatment, (2) probe preparation/labeling, (3) hybridization, (4) probe removal/washing, and (5) detection. Nonradioactive probe labeling itself can be divided into two methods, i.e., direct and indirect. This chapter describes the preparation of atherosclerotic tissue for ISH, indirect labeling of probes with digoxigenin (DIG), and the detection protocols suitable for this type of

From: *Methods in Molecular Medicine, vol. 52: Atherosclerosis: Experimental Methods and Protocols*
Edited by: A. F. Drew © Humana Press Inc., Totowa, NJ

tissue. The DIG labeling method was developed by Kessler *(2)* and is based on the steroid digoxigenin, which is isolated from *Digitalis purpurea and D. lanata*. The DIG molecule is linked to the C-5 position of uridine (UTP, dUTP, or ddUTP) via a spacer arm. The DIG-labeled nucleotides can be incorporated easily into nucleic acid probes by DNA polymerases such as DNA polymerase I, Taq DNA polymerase, T7 DNA polymerase, RNA polymerases, and terminal transferase. These various enzymes therefore allow DIG labeling by random priming, nick translation, PCR, 3'-end labeling/tailing, and in vitro transcription. Following hybridization, DIG-probes may be detected with high-affinity specific anti-DIG antibodies *(3)*. These antibodies are conjugated with alkaline phosphatase, peroxidase, fluoroscein, rhodamine, AMCA (amino-methylcoumarin-acetic acid), or colloidal gold (for electron microscopy) enabling a very versatile detection system. This system can be made even more versatile and sensitive by using unconjugated anti-DIG followed by conjugated secondary antibodies. A detection sensitivity of about 0.1 pg (as determined by Southern blot) can be achieved with combinations of anti-DIG-alkaline phospatase and NBT or BCIP. In this chapter, I describe a protocol that we developed for nonradioactive in situ hybridization of atherosclerotic tissue for the detection of interleukin 8, tissue factor, and tissue factor pathway inhibitor in both frozen and paraffin-embedded tissue *(4–7)*.

2. Materials
2.1. Slide Subbing Solution

1. Slowly add 9.25 g porcine gelatin to 1.8 L heated, distilled water (40–50°C) while stirring. (Do not add the gelatin to water that exceeds 50°C as it will denature the gelatin).
2. Once the gelatin is thoroughly dissolved, add 900 mg chromium potassium sulfate.
3. Filter while still warm through Whatman no. 1 filter paper.

2.2. In vitro Transcription of DIG-Labeled RNA

1. NTP labeling mixture (10X): 10 mM ATP, 10 mM CTP, 10 mM GTP, 6.5 mM UTP, 3.5 mM DIG-ll-UTP; in Tris-HCI, pH 7.5.
2. 10X transcription buffer: 400 mM Tris-HCl, pH 8.0, 60 mM MgCl$_2$, 100 mM DTT, 100 mM NaCI, 20 mM spermidine, RNase inhibitor 1 U/µL.
3. Dnase I, RNase-free, 10 U/mL.
4. RNase inhibitor, 20 U/µL.
5. SP6 RNA Polymerase, 20 U/mL.
6. T7 or T3 RNA Polymerase, 20 U/mL.
7. 200 mM EDTA, pH 8.0

2.3. 3'-Tailing of Oligonucleotides

1. dATP: 10mM dATP in Tris buffer, pH 7.5.
2. Terminal transferase: 50 U/µL in 200 mM potassium cacodylate, 1mM EDTA, 200 mM KCl, 0.2 mg/mL BSA, 50% (v/v) glycerol, pH 6.5.
3. 25 mM CoCl$_2$.
4. 5X reaction buffer: 1 M potassium cacodylate, 125 mM Tris-HCl, 1.25 mg/mL BSA, pH 6.6.
5. Glycogen solution: 20 mg/mL glycogen in redistilled water.

2.4. Proteinase K Digestion

1. Proteinase K 1–2µg/mL.
2. Glycine: 0.2% glycine in PBS (pH 7.4).
3. 0.25% acetic anhydride/0. 1 M TEA.
4. 2X standard saline citrate (SSC).

2.5. Prehybridization and Hybridization

1. Buffer 1: 100 mM maleic acid, 150 mM NaCl; pH 7.5.
2. Buffer 2: 1% blocking reagent (final concentration).
3. Buffer 3: 100 mM Tris-HCl, pH 9.5, 100 mM NaCl, 50 mM MgCl$_2$ (add Tris to H$_2$O, then add NaCl and MgCl$_2$ to avoid precipitating to Mg(OH)$_2$.
4. 20X SSC: 3 M NaCl, 0.3 M trisodium citrate, pH 7.0.
5. DEPC-treated H$_2$O: Distilled water treated with 0.1% diethylpyrocarbonate (DEPC) and autoclaved.
6. Tissue fixing solution: 3% paraformaldehyde dissolved in 0.1 M phosphate buffered saline (PBS), pH 7.4 containing 0.02% diethylpyrocarbonate.

2.6. Color Detection of mRNA

1. NBT: 50 mg 4-nitroblue tetrazolium chloride in 70% (v/v) dimethyl formamide (50 mg/mL).
2. X-phosphate: 50 mg 5-bromo-4-chloro-3-indolyl phosphate toluidinium salt in 100% dimethyl formamide (50 mg/mL).
3. Anti-DIG-AP monoclonal antibody: Fab fragments (Boehringer Mannheim Cat. no. 1093274).
4. DIG-11-UTP (Boehringer Mannheim Cat. no. 1093274).
5. Prehybridization buffer: 50% (v/v) formamide, 0.075 M trisodium citrate, 0.75 M NaCl, 0.1% (w/v) PVP, 0.1% (w/v) BSA, 0.1% (w/v) Ficoll, 50 mM NaH$_2$PO$_4$ (pH 6.5), denatured herring sperm DNA 250 µg/mL.
6. Hybridization buffer: 50% (v/v) formamide, 0.075 M trisodium citrate, 0.75 M NaCl, 0.02% (w/v) PVP, 0.02% (w/v) BSA, 0.02% (w/v) Ficoll, 50 mM NaH$_2$PO$_4$ (pH 6.5), denatured herring sperm DNA 100 µg/mL.

3. Methods

3.1. Subbed Slide Preparation

Tissue sections or cells will undergo various treatments during in situ hybridization and washing which are relatively harsh. The tissue sections must therefore be mounted in a manner that will allow the tissue to resist the worst possible outcome during these procedures, namely, detachment from the slide! A suitable coating agent is required, and although various agents have been used for this process (subbing), one such method is described below (*see* **Note 1**).

1. Load required number of slides into a metal rack (a rack available from Thomas Scientific holds 50 slides), and soak in 0.1 M HCl for 30 min (4.3 mL conc. HCl, [11.65 M], in 500 mL dH$_2$0).
2. Rinse in dH$_2$0 3 times.
3. Soak in 95% ethanol for 1 h.
4. Allow slides to dry completely (in dust-free container).
5. Soak slides in subbing solution (*see* **Materials**) for 2 min, then dry at 4°C (at least 30 min).
6. Dip slides in subbing solution again (once or twice) and allow to dry at 4°C between each coating.
7. Allow slides to dry in dust-free container overnight at room temperature (RT).

3.2. Preparation of the Tissue on the Slide

Fixation is a very important procedure and needs to be optimized (empirically) for different tissues, as each type of tissue may require a specific fixative to meet in situ requirements (no shortcuts here!). Fixation affects target retention, hybridization efficiency, and, most importantly, preservation of morphology (*see* **Note 2**). This in situ–hybridization procedure has been optimized for frozen sections, paraffin-embedded sections, and cytocentrifuge preparations. Following are the procedures (listed separately) for preparing each type of sample.

3.2.1. Frozen Sections

1. Remove required tissue from animal and immediately place it in optimal cutting temperature (OCT) medium. Dip section in and out of liquid nitrogen quickly until OCT has frozen (white). Store tissue at –70°C.
2. Cut sections (5 μm) on a cryostat and thaw-mount onto subbed slides at –20°C; store these at –70°C until ready for prehybridization.
3. Immediately before prehybridization, quickly bring tissue sections to RT and allow to dry (approx 15 min).
4. Fix tissue in ice-cold fixative (3% paraformaldehyde) for 5 min with *gentle* rocking on rocking platform.
5. Wash slides in 1X PBS, 3 times, 5 min per wash, with *gentle* shaking.
6. Wash slides in 2X SSC, 10 min with *gentle* shaking.
7. Proceed to prehybridization step (or proteinase K digestion) *immediately*.

3.2.2. Paraffin-Embedded Sections

1. Submerge paraffin-embedded sections in xylene for 10 min to remove paraffin.
2. Rinse twice for 10 min in 100% ethanol.
3. Air dry for 10 min.
4. Rehydrate the tissue sections through a series of graded ethanol dilutions: 95%, 80%, and 70%, 1 min for each wash.
5. Wash in PBS three times, 5 min for each wash.
6. Incubate in 2X SSC for 10 min.
7. Proceed to prehybridization step (or proteinase K digestion) *immediately*.

3.2.3. Cytocentrifuge Preparations

Cells fixed in 4% paraformaldehyde, and deposited on subbed slides with a cytocentrifuge, should be treated according to the procedure below to minimize nonspecific background (binding):

1. Wash in PBS containing 5 mM MgCl$_2$ 3 times, 5 min for each wash.
2. Wash in 0.1 M triethanolamine containing 0.25% (v/v) acetic anhydride for 10 min.
3. Wash in 0.2 M Tris-HCl containing 0.1 M glycine, pH 7.4 for 10 min.
4. Incubate in 2X SSC for 10 min.
5. Proceed to prehybridization step (or proteinase K digestion) *immediately*.

3.3. Probe Preparation

Either DNA or RNA probes can be used to localize DNA or RNA in in situ hybridization. However, the quality of the final result will vary depending on the type of probe used. Generally, I use RNA probes for the following reasons: (a) RNA: RNA hybrids are highly stable; (b) no probe denaturation is required; (c) no reannealing occurs during hybridization; (d) probes are strand specific (may be sense or antisense); (e) probe is free of vector sequence; (f) the template is removed easily and (g) posthybridization RNase treatment removes nonhybridized probe. RNA probes are most effient when used as smaller fragments of 50–200 nucleotides. Labeling such probes is described in **Subheading 3.3.1.**

3.3.1. In vitro Transcription of DIG-Labeled RNA

Before starting the transcription reaction, the DNA template must be linearized at a restriction enzyme site downstream of the cloned insert. To avoid transcription of undesirable sequences, use a restriction enzyme that leaves 5' overhangs or blunt ends. After the restriction digest, purify the DNA by phenol/chloroform extraction and subsequent ethanol precipitation.

1. Add the following reagents to a sterile, RNase-free microfuge tube (on ice) in the following order:

Reagent	Volume	Final concentration
Purified DNA template	(variable) 1pg	0.05 µg/µL
NTP labeling mixture (10X)	2 µL	1X
10X transcription buffer	2 µL	1X
DEPC-treated H_2O	to 18 µL	
RNA polymerase (SP6, T7, or T3)	2 µL	2 U/µL
Total volume	20 µL	

2. Mix gently and centrifuge briefly. Incubate for 2 h at 37°C.
3. If desired, add 2 µL DNase I, RNase-free, and incubate for 15 min at 37°C to remove the DNA template. Because the amount of DIG-labeled RNA transcript greatly exceeds the amount of DNA template, removal of the DNA template is usually unnecessary.
4. With or without prior DNase treatment, add 2 µL EDTA solution to stop the transcription reaction.
5. Precipitate the labeled RNA with 0.1 vol 4 M LiCl and 2.5–3.0 vol chilled absolute ethanol. Mix well and incubate at –70°C for 30 min or at –20°C overnight.
6. Remove from the –70°C incubation, and centrifuge the reaction at 13,000g for 15 min in a microcentrifuge at 4°C.
7. Decant the ethanol and wash the pellet with 100 µL cold 70% ethanol. Centrifuge at 13,000g for 5 min in a microcentrifuge at 4°C then decant the 70% ethanol.
8. Dry the pellet and resuspend in 100 µL DEPC-treated H_2O. If not used immediately, store the labeled probe at –20°C.

The amount of newly synthesized DIG-labeled RNA depends on the amount, size (site of linearization), and purity of the template DNA. When 1 µg of template DNA, which has been linearized to give "run-off" transcripts of 760 bases, is labeled according to the standard reaction, approximately 37% of the nucleotides are incorporated into about 10 µg of transcribed DIG-labeled RNA. The RNA can be analyzed by agarose gel electrophoresis and ethidium bromide staining under RNase-free conditions. RNA yield can be estimated from the ratio of DNA to RNA bands. Labeling efficiency can be more accurately checked by direct detection of the labeled RNA probe with an anti-digoxigenin-alkaline phosphatase.

3.3.2. 3'-Tailing of Oligonucleotides (see **Note 3**)

The oligonucleotide to be labeled should be purified by high-pressure liquid chromatography (HPLC) or gel electrophoresis after synthesis.

1. Add the following reagents to a sterile microfuge tube (on ice) in the following order shown in the table (*see* **Note 4**).

Reagent	Volume	Final concentration
5X reaction buffer	4 µL	1X
$CoCl_2$ solution	4 µL	5 mM
DIG-11-dUTP	1 µL	0.05 mM
Oligonucleotide	(Variable) 100 pmol	5 µM
dATP	1 µL	0.5 mM
Terminal transferase	1 µL	2.5 units/µL
H_2O	to 20 µL	Variable
Total volume	20 µL	

(When upscaling the labeling reaction, all components have to be increased proportionally. Increasing only the oligonucleotide concentration results in insufficient labeling).

2. Incubate the reaction at 37°C for 15 min and then place on ice.
3. Add 1 µL glycogen solution and 1 µL EDTA to the reaction tube.
4. Precipitate the labeled oligonucleotide with 0.1 vol (2.5 µL) 4 M LiCl and 2.5–3.0 vol (75 µL) prechilled ethanol. Mix well and incubate at –70°C for at least 30 min or 2 h at –20°C.
5. Remove from the –70°C incubation and centrifuge the reaction at 13,000g for 15 min in a microcentrifuge at 4°C.
6. Decant the ethanol and wash the pellet with 50 µL cold 70% ethanol. Centrifuge at 13,000g for 5 min in the microcentrifuge at 4°C, then remove the 70% ethanol.
7. Dry the pellet and resuspend in 20 µL sterile distilled water. If not used immediately, store the labeled probe at –20°C. *See* **Note 5** for estimating the DIG-labeled DNA or RNA yield.

3.4. In Situ Hybridization

3.4.1. Proteinase K Digestion

Proteinase K digestion enables the permeabilization of the tissue to allow entry of the probe. This is a critical step.

1. Determine best concentration and incubation time for tissue of choice empirically.
2. Circle tissues with wax pen.
3. Incubate tissues in humid chamber (e.g., plastic household food storage container with wet paper towels on bottom and airtight lid) with appropriate concentration of proteinase K (1–2 µg/mL, 15 min at 37°C (*see* **Notes 6** and **7**).
4. Wash slides in dH_2O for 5 min with *gentle* shaking.
5. Wash slides in 0.2% glycine in PBS (pH 7.4) for 10 min with *gentle* shaking.
6. Wash slides in 0.25% acetic anhydride/0. 1 M TEA for 10 min with *gentle* shaking.
7. Rinse in 2X SSC briefly.

3.4.2. Prehybridization and Hybridization

1. Place slides in humid chamber and circle sections with wax pen.
2. Apply approx. 50 μL (depending on tissue section size) of *prehybridization* solution (with 500 μg/mL denatured herring sperm DNA).
3. Incubate sections at 42°C for 1.5 h.
4. Wash slides briefly in 2X SSC.
5. Apply approx. 25 μL *hybridization* solution (with 500 μg/mL denatured herring sperm DNA) *avoiding bubbles*. Typical probe concentrations are: cDNA, 0.25–5 ng/μL; cRNA, 5–10 ng/μL; oligonucleotides, 0.34–6 ng/μL (1–10 fmol/μL; 21 mer=700 ng=100pmol; 30 mer=1 μg=100 pmol). cDNA probes require denaturation as usual. No cover slips are required if solution in humid chamber has a vapor pressure similar to the hybridization solution (e.g., 4X SSC/50% formamide).
6. Incubate in humid chamber at 50°C overnight.
7. Rinse slides *very carefully* by dipping slide in 2X SSC, 1 min.
8. When using cRNA probes, digest unbound or nonspecific cRNA with RNase A (100 μg/mL in 2X SSC), for 30 min at 37°C (or can use RNase cocktail: 200 μg/mL RNase A, 5000 U/mL RNase T1 in 50 m*M* NaCI, pH 7.0).
9. Wash slides, with *gentle* shaking, in the following order:
   15 min, 2X SSC, RT
   15 min, 1X SSC, RT
   15 min, 0.5X SSC, 50°C (prewarm buffer to 50°C *before* use)
   15 min, 0.5X SSC, RT

3.5. Color Detection of mRNA

1. Briefly wash slides for 1 min in buffer 1 (*see* **Subheading 2.5.**) with *gentle* shaking.
2. Put blocking solution on slides in humid chamber for 1 h at RT.
3. Repeat **step 1**.
4. Incubate tissue with anti-DIG-AP antibodies (1:5000) for 1.5 h at RT in humid chamber (approx. 40 μL per section).
5. Wash slides 2 times, 10 min each wash, in buffer 1 with *gentle* shaking.
6. Equilibrate tissue 2 min in buffer 3 (*see* **Subheading 2.5.**) to "activate" alkaline phosphatase.
7. Add approx. 40 μL color solution (e.g., NBT or any other color substrate for alkaline phosphatase), previously filtered with a 0.22 μm in filter to remove crystals, and incubate slides in humid chamber in the dark at RT for a variable time (unpredictable, therefore must be determined empirically; *see* **Note 8**).
8. Stop reaction by dipping slides in TE (pH 8.0) for 5 min.
9. Optional: Dehydrate sections if color substrate is alcohol insoluble.
70% alcohol	30 s
Absolute ethanol	30 s
Absolute ethanol	30 s
Allow to dry thoroughly	

10. The color of mRNA detected with NBT is dark purple, so choose a counterstain for the tissue that provides best contrast. I found hematoxylin to be a bad choice. I stain with 1% methyl green for approx. 3 min , then rinse in dH_20 and mount coverslip with 90% glycerol (in PBS) for temporary mounting. Mount with DPX for *permanent* fixing. Color reaction seems to fade with time in DPX, so photograph as soon as possible.

4. Notes

1. Esco Superfrost/Plus microscope slides (Erle Scientific, USA) are presubbed and ideal for in situ work. Alternatively, prepare own slides by the following method, as described above. To prepare subbed slides, microscope slides are cleaned, submerged into a subbing solution (gelatin/chromium), and dried. Wear gloves throughout the procedure (subbed slides are stable 6–8 wk if stored at RT). Fresh subbing solution should be prepared for each use.
2. Best results are obtained when all tissues are removed and prepared as close as possible to time of hybridization.
3. Important notes for labeling: (a) make sure linearization leaves no 3' overhangs; (b) make sure DNA is very pure/clean and that concentration is accurate; (c) use 5X scaled-up reaction with 1 µg linearized plasmid DNA; and (d) cDNA labeling by "random priming" or by "nick translation" can also be performed. The in vitro transcription labeling reaction may be scaled up to increase the yield of RNA. This is especially recommended if SP6 RNA polymerase is used. This is done by keeping the amount of template DNA constant while increasing the amount of the other components in the labeling reaction. For example, in a 5X scaled-up reaction with 1 µg linear control DNA (e.g., pSPT1 8-Neo DNA) as template, more than 40 µg RNA is synthesized after 2 h of incubation at 37°C.
4. When target sequence is DNA, add 100 µg/mL poly (A) and 5 µg/mL poly (dA) in the prehybridization and hybridization buffer when using 3'-tailed oligonucleotides. This prevents nonspecific hybridization of the tail to complementary sequences in the target DNA. Hybridization buffers containing SSC are preferable when "longtailed" probes are used. Both the optimal concentration of labeled probe in the hybridization buffer and the time required for hybridization depend on the amount of DNA or RNA. Heat-denature the oligonucleotide prior to hybridization if secondary structures are expected from the oligonucleotide sequence.
5. To estimate the DIG-labeled DNA or RNA yield, use the following method: All incubations are performed at RT and, except for the color reaction, with shaking or mixing.
   a. Make 10-fold serial dilutions of the labeled control DNA or RNA in DNA or RNA dilution buffer (*see* table). The concentration of the labeled control RNA is 100 µg/mL. Dilute 1:5 to a concentration of 20 µg/mL.

Serial Dilutions of Labeled Control DNA or RNA

Labeled control DNA or labeled control RNA, starting concentration 20 µg/mL		Dilution	Final concentration	Total dilution
(1)	20 ng/µL	2 µL/38 µL	1 ng/µL	1:20
(2)	1 ng/µL	5 µL/45 µL	100 pg/µL	1:200
(3)	100 pg/µL	5 µL/45 µL	10 pg/µL	1:2,000
(4)	10 pg/µL	5 µL/45 µL	1 pg/µL	1:20,000
(5)	1 pg/µL	5 µL/45 µL	0.1 pg/µL	1:200,000
(6)	0.1 pg/µL	5 µL/45 µL	0.01 pg/µL	1:2,000,000

Make fivefold serial dilutions of the DIG-ll-ddUTP–labeled control oligonucleotide or of the DIG-11-dUTP/dATP–tailed control oligonucleotide in TE-buffer (*see* table).

Dilution Series for Oligonucleotide Labeling Reactions

DIG-11-dUTP/dATP, DIG-11-dUTP concentration		Dilution	Final concentration	Total dilution
(1)	2.5 pmol/µL	2 µL/98 µL	50 fmol/µL	1:50
(2)	50 fmol/µL	10 µL/40 µL	10 fmol/µL	1:250
(3)	10 fmol/µL	10 µL/40 µL	2 fmol/µL	1:1,250
(4)	2 fmol/µL	10 µL/40 µL	0.4 fmol/µL	1:6,250
(5)	0.4 fmol/µL	10 µL/40 µL	0.08 fmol/µL	1:31,250

  b. Mark the membrane lightly with a pencil to identify each dilution. Spot 1 µL of the control dilutions onto a positively charged nylon membrane. For DNA/RNA probes, use dilutions 2–6. For oligonucleotides, use dilutions 1–5.

  c. Make serial dilutions of the labeled experimental DNA, RNA, or oligonucleotide in DNA/RNA dilution buffer or TE buffer according to **Step 1**.

  d. Mark the membrane lightly with a pencil to identify each dilution and spot 1 µL of each of the labeling reaction dilutions onto the nylon membrane.

  e. Fix DNA/RNA or oligonucleotide to the membrane by crosslinking with a UV transilluminator for 3 min or by baking for 30 min at 120°C (Boehringer Mannheim Nylon Membrane).

  f. Wash the membrane in buffer 1.

  g. Incubate the membrane in buffer 2 for 30 min.

  h. Dilute anti-DIG-alkaline phosphatase 1:5000 in buffer 2.

  i. Incubate the membrane in the diluted antibody for 30 min. The diluted antibody solution must cover the entire membrane.

  j. Wash the membrane twice, 15 min per wash, in buffer 1.

  k. Incubate the membrane in buffer 3 for 2 min. Application of this buffer "activates" the alkaline phosphatase that is conjugated to the antibody.

l. Mix 67.5 µL (50 mg/µL) NBT solution and 35 µL X-phosphate (50 mg/mL) solution in 10 mL buffer 3. This freshly prepared color substrate solution will be used immediately in the next step.

m. Decant the buffer and add the color substrate solution. Allow color development to proceed in the dark. The color precipitate starts to form within a few minutes, and the reaction is usually complete within 16 h. Do not shake or mix while the color is developing.

n. When the desired intensity spots or bands have developed, stop the reaction by washing the membrane for 5 min with 50 mL TE.

o. Compare spot intensities of the control and experimental dilutions to estimate the concentration of the experimental probe.

6. A negative control slide for in situ (RNase treatment) should be included in in situ experiments by the following method: (a) digestion by treatment with Rnase A (100 µg/mL in 2X SSC) for 30 min at 37°C. (or can use Rnase cocktail: 200 µg/mL Rnase A, 5000 U/mL Rnase T1 in 50 mM NaCI, pH 7. 0). (b) rinse in 2X SSC briefly, and (c) proceed to prehybridization step.

7. The proteinase K digestion step is crucial. Too-high a concentration or too-long an incubation with proteinase K can destroy tissue morphology.
Therefore, this procedure must be determined empirically and optimized for each different tissue and probe. A guide for proteinase K concentrations in paraformaldehyde-fixed, paraffin-embedded tissues, for example, is: brain 0.25 mg/mL, lung 0.25 mg/mL, liver 0.5 mg/mL, kidney 0.5 mg/mL, stomach 0.75 mg/mL, lymph node 0.75 mg/mL, muscle 1 mg/mL , placenta 1 mg/mL, and heart 1 mg/mL.

8. The NBT color reaction is time and temperature dependent (as well as light sensitive). The reaction can be at RT at 37°C (very fast, possible high background) or overnight at 4°C (slow). The time required for the color reaction also depends on the staining intensity required and amount of RNA or DNA present. *Suggestion*: Check reaction regularly under microscope whenever possible.

Acknowledgements

This work was performed at the Monash University Department of Medicine, Monash Medical Centre in the laboratories of Dr. Peter Tipping and Professor Stephen Holdsworth. My thanks, gratitude, and appropriate acknowledgment go to them. In addition, I also acknowledge the help of Angela Drew and Piers Davenport with some of the in situ work. The methods described within this protocol were developed and improved in our laboratory over several years. Some parts (labeling, estimation of yield, and color detection) were based on protocols derived from the Boehringer Mannheim *Nonradioactive in Situ Hybridization Application Manual*, since we used their reagents extensively.

References

1. Pardue, M. L. and Gall, J. G. (1969). Molecular hybridization of radioactive DNA to the DNA of cytological preparations. *Proc. Natl. Acad. Sci. USA* **64,** 600–604.

2. Martin, R., Hoover, C., Grimme, S., Grogan, C., Holtke, J., and Kessler, C. (1990) A highly sensitive, nonradioactive DNA labeling and detection system. *Biotechniques* **9,** 762–768.
3. Nonradiactive In situ Hybridization Application Manual, 2nd ed., 1996. Boehringer Mannheim.
4. Tipping, P. G., Erlich, J., Apostolopoulos, J., Mackman, N., Loskutoff, D., and Holdsworth, S. R. (1995) Glomerular tissue factor expression: Correlations between antigen, activity and mRNA in crescentic glomerulonephritis in rabbits. *Am. J. Pathol.* **147,** 1736–1748.
5. Apostolopoulos, J., Davenport, P., and Tipping, P. G. (1996) Interleukin-8 production by macrophages from atheromatous plaques. *Arterioscler. Thromb. Vasc. Biol.* **16,** 1007–1012.
6. Erlich, J., Apostolopoulos, J., and Tipping , P. (1996) Characterisation of Tissue Pathway Inhibitor in a Rabbit Model of Anti-Glomerular Basement Membrane Glomerulonephritis. *J. Clin. Invest.* **98,** 325–335.
7. Drew, A. F., Davenport, P., Apostolopoulos, J., and Tipping, P. G. (1997) Tissue pathway inhibitor expression in atherosclerosis. *Lab. Invest.* **77,** 1–8.

19

Evaluation of Angiogenesis

Marcy Silver and Jeffrey M. Isner

1. Introduction

Every year, thousands of individuals around the world suffer from severe lower extremity vascular disorders that are amenable to neither medical nor surgical treatment, and thus amputation is required. A substantial portion of these amputations might be avoided by stimulating blood vessel growth to the affected lower extremity. In a new therapeutic approach, certain recombinant growth factors, administered as genes or recombinant proteins, have been used successfully to promote neovascularization *(1,2)*. However, prior to the investigation of such therapy in human patients, it is necessary to obtain specific information in animal studies regarding the basic mechanisms involved in lower-extremity collateral vessel development. In particular, the use of genetically engineered mice (e.g., mice that have specific genes deleted or overexpressed) allows one to investigate relevant key factors for neovascularization that can be related to human subjects *(3–6)*. Accordingly, we developed a murine model of angiogenesis *(7)*. In this model, the left femoral artery, including all major side branches of one hind limb, is excised, rendering the limb ischemic. The subsequent development of collateral blood vessels in the ischemic limb can then be monitored in vivo at arbitrarily selected time-points by laser Doppler perfusion imaging, and measured ex vivo by immunohistochemistry to determine capillary density.

Laser Doppler perfusion imaging (LDPI) is used to record serial blood flow measurements over the course of 5 wk postoperatively **(Fig. 1.)**. The LDPI system uses collimated laser radiation generated by a visible red helium neon laser operating at a wavelength of 632.8 nm and a maximum accessible power of 2 mW. This generates a beam that sequentially scans a 12-×12-cm tissue surface to a depth of 800 μm. Low-power laser light is directed via a moving mirror to execute a raster pattern across the tissue surface. The incident light is

From: *Methods in Molecular Medicine, vol. 52: Atherosclerosis: Experimental Methods and Protocols*
Edited by: A. F. Drew © Humana Press Inc., Totowa, NJ

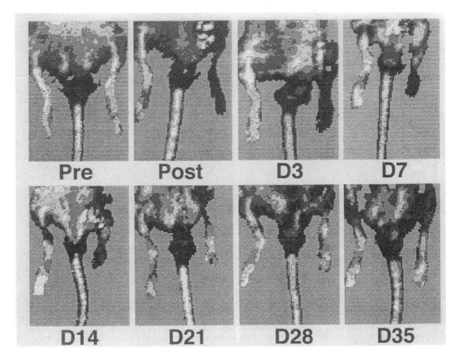

Fig. 1. Hindlimb blood flow monitored serially in vivo by laser Doppler perfusion imaging (LDPI). In color-coded images, normal baseline (pre) perfusion in both hindlimbs is depicted in white. Immediately after operative excision of one femoral artery (post), marked reduction in blood flow of one hindlimb is depicted in black. Perfusion remained severely impaired for 7 d, increased by d 14, and ultimately returned to near-normal levels by d 28.

scattered by static tissue and by moving blood. The perfusion signal is split into six different intervals, and each is displayed as a separate color.

The information generated in this model should yield insight and understanding to the basic processes involved in limb neovascularization due to occlusive artery disease and provide implications for novel strategies for the treatment of ischemia (**Fig. 2.**). Particularly, the application of the laser-Doppler perfusion-imager will provide valuable information regarding the vascular changes that occur in response to acute limb ischemia and how they can be modified by angiogenic growth factors. The user of this model and LDI system will find it very straightforward and reproducible.

2. Materials
2.1. Equipment

1. Laser Doppler Imager System (Moor Instruments Inc, Wilmington, DE). This system consists of an LDI scanhead (633 nm red and 780 nm infrared laser), LDI

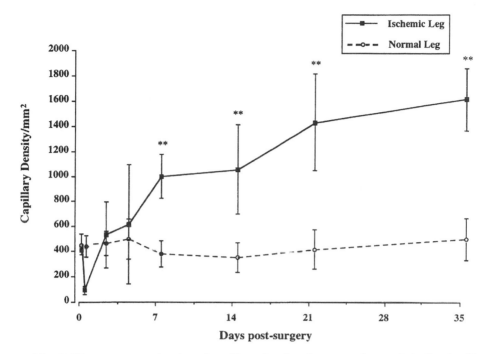

Fig. 2. Time-course evaluation of capillary density, demonstrating statistically significant increase in capillary density in the ischemic limb as early as d 7; this was sustained at d 14, and further increased at d 21 and 35. In contrast, histological examinations of the contralateral normal hindlimb disclosed no significant alteration in capillary density between 0 and 35 d.

control box, two LDI interconnecting leads, one main lead, one RS232 interface lead, LDI software, LDI user manual, one desktop stand (including bolts), one large desktop mirror, one pentium desktop computer and accessories, one SVGA color monitor, one pair of protective glasses.

2. Surgical instruments, which include: one small scissors, two small rat-tooth forceps, one curved forceps, one spring scissors (Fine Science Tools, Foster City, CA). Surgical autoclipper with 9-mm wound clips (Baxter Corp, McGaw Park , IL) .

3. Suture 3-0 Vicryl (Ethicon, Inc., Somerville, NJ).

4. Depilatory cream (local drug store).

5. Slide warmer or heating pad (Baxter Corp., McGaw Park, IL).

6. 1-mL 25-gage syringe (Baxter Corp., McGaw Park, IL).

7. 4×4 gauze sponges (nonsterile) (Kendall Co., Mansfield, MA).

2.2. Anesthestic and Analgesic

1. Nembutal sodium, 50 mg/mL (Abbott Laboratories, North Chicago, IL).

2. Levodromoran, 2 mg/mL (Hoffmann-La Roche Inc., Nutley, NJ).

3. Methods

1. Turn on LDI system and make sure temperature in room is at 70°F.
2. Anesthetize mouse by individual body weight (Nembutal, 45 mg/kg; *see* **Note 1**).
3. Administer analgesia (Levodromoran, 60 mg/kg).
4. Apply depilatory cream to lower abdomen and both hindlimbs.
5. After several minutes, gently remove hair from lower abdomen and hindlimbs (*see* **Note 2**).
6. Place mouse for 5 min between several gauze squares or on slide warmer to minimize temperature variation (*see* **Notes 3** and **4**).
7. Take control scan picture of mouse with LDI System.
8. Make small incision in the skin overlying the middle portion of the left hindlimb of each mouse. Remove small amount of fat around immediate incision. This fat will contain a small branch of the femoral artery that leads to the skin. It is important to excise this branch. Ligate the proximal end of the femoral artery and the distal portion of the saphenous artery. The femoral artery and all side branches are dissected free, then excised. Close overlying skin using the surgical stapler.
9. Take postsurgical scan picture of mouse with LDI System (*see* **Notes 5** and **6**).
10. Place mouse on slide warmer or heating pad until fully awake (*see* **Note 8**).
11. Post surgical follow-up scans should be taken at d 3, 7, 14, 21, 28, 35.

4. Notes

1. The most critical element to the success of imaging is achieving and maintaining proper anesthetic levels in the mice. If the mouse is not at the proper anesthetic level (either too light or too deep), the LDI will give inappropriate scan values. If the mouse is moving or light, the image will appear to show more red. In contrast, if the mouse is too deep, the image will appear more blue. Weighing each mouse and giving the appropriate dose of anesthesia is of the utmost importance.
2. Depilatory cream should be removed very gently. It can be abrasive to the skin and cause irritation. This can lead to false imaging values.
3. It is very important to keep the mice warm at all times when they are anesthetized. Scans should be taken in a room with a set temperature of 70°F. Mice should be kept between gauze squares before scan to minimize temperature variation. If limbs appear blue on scan, most likely the animal is cold. If limbs appear too red while scanning, the mouse may be too warm.
4. Be careful not to touch or squeeze limbs (especially feet) when arranging the mice for scan. This can bring flow into the limbs, which will also lead to false imaging values.
5. Low or no perfusion is displayed on the monitor as dark blue, whereas maximum perfusion is displayed as red.
6. LDPI is used to record perfusion of both right and left limbs, preoperatively and at predetermined time-points postoperatively. Consecutive measurements are obtained over the same region of interest (leg and foot). Color-coded images are

recorded, and analysis is performed by calculating the average perfusion for each (ischemic and nonischemic) foot. To account for variables including ambient light and temperature, calculated perfusion is expressed as a ratio of left (ischemic) to right (normal) limb.

7. Occasionally, one might experience unexplained high values (red) of the ischemic limb early during the time-course. This mouse most likely has an infection. Sterile technique should be used to reduce the incidence of infection.

8. Most mice recover without difficulty from the surgery. Most do not use their ischemic hindlimb during the first postoperative week; then progressively they begin to use the limb again. By the fifth week it is difficult to detect a difference between the ischemic and nonischemic limbs. Toe and/or limb necrosis is common in this model, depending on the strain of mouse.

References

1. Isner, J. M., Pieczek, A., Schainfeld, R., et al. (1996) Clinical evidence of angiogenesis following arterial gene transfer of phVEGF$_{165}$. *Lancet* **348,** 370–374.
2. Baumgartner, I., Pieczek, A., Manor, O., Blair, R., and Isner, J. M. (1997) Evidence of therapeutic angiogenesis in patients with arterial limb ischemia after intramuscular phVEGF$_{165}$ gene transfer (Abstract). *Circulation* **96,** I-32 (Abstract).
3. Murohara, T., Asahara, T., Silver, M., et al. (1998) Nitric oxide synthase modulates angiogenesis in response to tissue ischemia. *J.Clin.Invest.* **101,** 2567–2578.
4. Rivard, A., Fabre, J.-E., Silver, M., et al. (1999) Age-dependent impairment of angiogenesis. *Circulation* **99,** 111–120.
5. Rivard, A., Silver, M., Chen, D., et al. (1999).Rescue of diabetes related impairment of angiogenesis by intramuscular gene therapy with adeno-VEGF. *Am. J. Pathol.* **154,** 355–364.
6. Couffinhal, T., Silver, M., Kearney, M., et al. (1999).Impaired collateral vessel development associated with reduced expression of vascular endothelial growth factor in ApoE^{-1-} mice. *Circulation,* **99,** 3188–3198.
7. Couffinhal, T., Silver, M., Zheng, L.P., Kearney, M., Witzenbichler, B., and Isner, J.M. (1998).A mouse model of angiogenesis. *Am. J. Pathol.* **152,** 1667–1679.

20

Evaluation of Cell Proliferation in Human Atherosclerotic Lesions

Elena R. Andreeva and Alexander N. Orekhov

1. Introduction

Local accumulation of cells (hypercellularity) in the intima of the arterial wall is recognized as one of the major manifestations of human atherosclerosis, which may result from local cell proliferation (1–3). This assumption was raised both on the comparative analysis of cell number in nondiseased and atherosclerotic areas of human arteries (3–5) and on the basis of the analysis of cell replication in experimental atherosclerosis (for review see **ref. 1**). In experimental atherosclerosis, cell replication was identified in several models, including mechanical injury of the arteries and experimental hypercholesterolemia. The experimental approach permits the direct determination of DNA replication using radiolabeled precursor—[^{3}H]-thymidine, but it is impossible to demonstrate proliferation in human vessels directly, using standard procedures with labeling of replicating DNA. Villaschi and coworkers (6) labeled human arteries with [^{3}H]-thymidine-ex vivo. They found a low level of replication in both grossly normal tissues and atherosclerotic plaques. In the case of ex vivo labeling, the questions of diffusion and of thymidine incorporation into ex vivo incubated tissue (6) make it difficult to be sure that this procedure reflects replication rates in vivo. Use of proliferation-specific antibodies is advantageous, since proliferating cells are detected directly. Antibodies to the cell-cycle related protein, PCNA (cyclin), are now commonly used in the study of human tissues (7–12). PCNA is an auxiliary protein of mammalian DNA polymerase-δ and is a stable cell-cycle–regulated nuclear protein (synthesized mainly in the S-phase but also present in G1 and G2 phases of the cell cycle), the presence of which correlates directly with a proliferative state of normal cells (7–9).

From: *Methods in Molecular Medicine, vol. 52: Atherosclerosis: Experimental Methods and Protocols*
Edited by: A. F. Drew © Humana Press Inc., Totowa, NJ

A good correlation between PCNA immunostaining and thymidine labeling of rat intestine, as well as with a different proliferation-specific antibody to Ki-67 antigen *(11,13,14)* on both human atherosclerotic plaques and tonsil tissue, has been demonstrated *(10,11)*.

In this chapter we describe the immunocytochemical evaluation of proliferative activity of cells in the human aorta using anti-PCNA antibody and cell-typing of proliferating cells.

2. Materials

2.1. Tissue Sample Preparation

1. Samples of human arteries (surgical or autopsy; **see Note 1**).
2. Samples of rat small intestine.
3. Set of scissors and forceps.
4. Phosphate buffered saline (PBS) (pH 7.4).
5. 10-cm diameter Petri dish.
6. Fixatives:
   a. Methanol-Carnoy's (Methacarn) (methanol:chloroform:glacial acetic acid in 60:30:10 volume ratio) for paraffin embedding.
   b. 4% formaldehyde in PBS + 95% ethyl alcohol for postfixation of frozen sections.
7. Ethyl alcohol: 100%, 95%, 70%.
8. Xylenes.
9. Microscope slides and cover glasses.
10. Histomount or any other synthetic mounting medium.

2.2. PCNA Immunostaining

1. PBS–0.05% Tween-20.
2. 3% hydrogen peroxide.
3. 1% bovine serum albumin (BSA) in PBS.
4. Antiproliferating cell nuclear antigen (PCNA) antibody (PC10, Dako Corp., Carpenteria, CA).
5. Cell-type–specific antibodies against smooth muscle α-actin to identify smooth muscle cells, CDLC to identify common leukocyte antigens, CD14 to identify monocyte-macrophages.
6. Normal (nonimmune) mouse serum.
7. Biotinylated horse antimouse IgG antibody (Vector Laboratories, Burlingame, CA).
8. Avidin-biotin-peroxidase complex (ABC) standard or Elite Kit (Vector).
9. Streptavidin-alkaline phosphatase Substrate Kit I (red) (Vector).
10. 0.05 M Tris-HCl (pH 7.6–7.7) as substrate buffer for peroxidase reaction.
11. 0.1 M Tris-HCl (pH 8.2) as substrate buffer for alkaline phosphatase reaction.
12. 3-3'-Diaminobenzidine (DAB) tetrahydrochloride: 5 mg/mL stock solution in 0.05 M Tris-HCl (pH 7.6-7.7; toxic). Store at –20°C in aliquots.

13. Nickel chloride: 8% in H_2O.
14. Methyl green: 2% in 0.1 M acetate buffer (pH 4.2).
15. Levamisol.
16. Streptavidin-alkaline phosphatase (Vector).
17. OCT compound (Miles Inc., Elkhart, IN).
18. 0.2 M glycine buffer (pH 2.4).

3. Methods

3.1. Tissue Sample Preparation

1. Wash samples of human arteries or rat intestine in PBS, thoroughly, to remove blood and other foreign particles.
2. Remove excess PBS with filter paper
3. Either paraffin-embedded or snap-frozen tissue can be used.
   Paraffin-embedded:
   a. Fix in Methacarn overnight, process, and embed in paraffin
   b. Prepare 5-μm sections on microscope slides.
   c. Deparaffinize sections in three changes of xylenes—5 min. in each.
   d. Rehydrate by passing slides through 100% ethyl alcohol: 3 changes, 5 min total; 95% ethyl alcohol: 2 changes, 5 min total; 70% ethyl alcohol: 1 change, 1 min. Wash with distilled H_2O and leave in PBS–Tween-20.
   Snap-frozen:
   a. Freeze unfixed tissue in OCT compound.
   b. Prepare 5-μm cryostat sections.
   c. Air-dry sections and fix for 2 min at room temperature with 4% formaldehyde/PBS and then for 10 min at room temperature with 95% ethyl alcohol.
   d. Rehydrate in 70% ethyl alcohol: 1 change, 1 min. Wash with distilled H_2O and leave in PBS–Tween-20.
4. Dilute all antibodies in 1% BSA-PBS.
5. Block endogenous peroxidase by placing slides in 3% hydrogen peroxide for 5 min.
6. Wash in one change of PBS–Tween-20 for 5 min.

3.2. PCNA Immunostaining

3.2.1. Single PCNA Labeling

1. Apply enough of the appropriately diluted anti-PCNA antibody (1:1000 for DAKO PC10) to cover tissue and incubate overnight at 4°C in a moist chamber. Use sections of rat small intestine as positive control (*see* **Note 2**). Use non-immune mouse serum or irrelevant monoclonal antibody, with matched IgG isotype and concentration, as negative control.
2. Wash in 3 changes of PBS–Tween-20 (2 min each).
3. Apply biotinylated antimouse IgG antibody (1:200) and incubate for 30 min at room temperature in a moist chamber.

4. Wash in 3 changes of PBS–Tween-20 (2 min each).
5. Apply avidin-biotin peroxidase complex and incubate 30 min at room temperature in a moist chamber. (This complex needs to be made per kit instructions at least 30 min in advance).
6. Wash in one change of PBS–Tween-20 and 0.05 M Tris-HCl buffer (kept at 37°C) for 5 min total.
7. Prepare developing solution in warm (37°C) 0.05 M Tris-HCl buffer: 0.5 mg/mL DAB·4HCL (dilute aliquot of DAB 5 mg/mL thawed stock solution 1:10), 0.03% H_2O_2, and 0.08% $NiCL_2$. Mix prior to using, and keep at 37°C. Solution should be used within 1 h.
8. Incubate slides in DAB solution for 5–10 min (*see* **Note 3**).
9. Wash in distilled water—one change.
10. For single labeling, counterstain in methyl green.
11. Dehydrate sections and coverslip with Histomount.
    Results: PCNA-positive nuclei—black; PCNA-negative nuclei—green.

3.2.2. Cell Typing of PCNA-Positive cells (Double Labeling)

12. After step 8, incubate slides in glycine buffer 1 h at room temperature to remove unbound antibody (*see* **Note 4**).
13. Neutralize with 3.5 M Tris-HCl 20 min at room temperature.
14. Wash in several changes of PBS–Tween-20 at 4°C overnight.
15. Apply cell-type–specific antibody in appropriate dilution for 1 h at room temperature in a moist chamber. Use nonimmune serum or irrelevant antibody, raised in the same species as the cell-type–specific antibody, with matched IgG concentration, as negative control.
16. Wash in 3 changes of PBS–Tween-20 (2 min each).
17. Apply appropriate biotinylated anti- (host of the cell-type–specific antibody) IgG antibody and incubate for 30 min at room temperature in a moist chamber.
18. Wash in 3 changes of PBS–Tween-20 (2 min each).
19. Apply streptavidin-alkaline phosphatase (dilute according to manufacturer's instructions) and incubate for 30 min at room temperature in a moist chamber.
20. Prepare ABC-AP substrate I (red) as described in the Substrate Kit instructions.
21. Incubate sections with alkaline phosphatase substrate up to 30 min in a dark chamber. Appropriate time should be determined individually by microscopic examination.
22. Wash in PBS–Tween-20.
23. Wash in distilled H_2O.
24. Counterstain in methyl green.
25. Dehydrate sections and cover slip with Histomount (*see* **Note 5**).
Results: PCNA-positive nuclei: black; red cytoplasmic staining in cells expressing cell-type–specific antigens. PCNA-negative nuclei: green, with red cytoplasmic staining in cells, expressing cell-type–specific antigens.

4. Notes
4.1. Tissue Sample Preparation

1. Autopsy samples of human arteries with postmortem intervals up to 24 h may be used, but shorter postmortem intervals are preferable (up to 6 h).

4.2. PCNA Immunostaining

2. Single PCNA staining. It is very important to use a positive control in every run when revealing PCNA. Any tissue with particular localization of proliferating cells may be used. Rat small intestine is very good control tissue, because one can always find specific nuclear staining localized to the crypt epithelium of intestinal mucosa.
3. The time required for developing the peroxidase reaction should be monitored carefully, under the microscope, using sections of the rat intestine. The reaction should be stopped when nuclei in the crypts are black but nuclei of the smooth muscle cells in the tunica muscularis are unstained.
4. It is very important to remove all unbound antibodies after PCNA staining. This can be done with glycine buffer or by dehydration of tissue sections and subsequent rehydration.
5. Do not dehydrate sections in xylenes after use of alkaline-phosphatase Substrate Kit I, because the red reaction product dissolves in xylenes. Aqueous mounting medium can be used instead.

References

1. Ross, R. (1993) The pathogenesis of atherosclerosis: A perspective for the 1990s. *Nature* **362,** 801–809.
2. Benditt, E. P. and Benditt, J. M. (1993) Evidence for monoclonal origin of human atherosclerotic plaques. *Proc. Natl. Acad. Sci. USA* **70,** 1753–1756.
3. Geer, J. S. and Haust, M. D. (1972) Smooth muscle cell in atherosclerosis, in *Monographs on Atherosclerosis.* Karger, Basel.
4. Orekhov, A. N., Karpova, I. I., Tertov, V. V., Rudchenko, S. A., Andreeva, E. R., Krushinsky, A. V., and Smirnov, V. N. (1984b) Cellular composition of atherosclerotic and uninvolved human aortic subendothelial intima. Light-microscopic study of dissociated aortic cells. *Am. J. Pathol.* **115,** 17–24.
5. Orekhov, A. N., Andreeva, E. R., Krushinsky, A. V., Novikov, I. D., Tertov, V. V., Nestaiko, G. V., Khashimov, K. A., Repin, V. S., and Smirnov, V. N. (1986) Intimal cells and atherosclerosis. Relationship between the number of intimal cells and major manifestations of atherosclerosis in the human aorta. *Am. J. Pathol.* **125,** 402–415.
6. Villaschi, S. and Spagnoli, L. G. (1983) Autoradiographic and ultrastructural studies on the human fibro-atheromatous plaque. *Atherosclerosis* **48,** 95–100.

7. Gerdes, J., Schwab, U., Lemke, H., and Stein, H. (1983) Production of a mouse monoclonal antibody reactive with a human nuclear antigen associated with cell proliferation. *Int. J. Cancer* **31**, 1–20.

8. Kurki, P., Vanderlaan, M., Dolbeare, F., Gray, J., and Tan, E. M. (1986) Expression of proliferating cell nuclear antigen (PCNA)/cyclin during cell cycle. *Exp. Cell Res.* **166**, 209–219.

9. Bravo, R., Frank, R., Blundell, P. A., and Macdonald-Bravo, H. (1987) Cyclin/PCNA is the auxiliary protein of DNA-polymerase-δ. *Nature* **326**, 515–517.

10. Rekhter, M. D. and Gordon, D. (1995) Active proliferation of different cell types, including lymphocytes, in human atherosclerotic plaques. *Am. J. Pathol.* **147**, 668–677.

11. Gordon, D., Reidy, M. A., Benditt, E. P., and Schwartz, S. M. (1990) Cell proliferation in human coronary arteries. *Proc. Natl. Acad. Sci. USA* **87**, 4600–4604.

12. Andreeva, E. R., Mikhailova, I. A., Orekhov, A. N., and Gordon, D. (1998) Cell proliferation in normal and atherosclerotic human aorta: Proliferative splash in lipid-rich lesions. *Atherosclerosis* **139**, 41–48.

13. Kamel, O. W., Franklin, W. A., Ringus, J. C., and Meyer, J. S. (1989) Thymidine labeling index and Ki-67 growth fraction in lesions of the breast. *Am. J. Pathol.* **134**, 107–113.

14. Catoletti, G., Becker, M. H., Key, G., Duchrow, M., Schluter, C., Galle, J., and Gerdes, J. (1992) Monoclonal antibodies against recombinant parts of the Ki-67 antigen (MIB 1 and MIB 3) detect proliferating cells in microwave-processed formalin-fixed paraffin sections. *J. Pathol.* **168**, 357–363.

21

Gene Transfer to the Vasculature

Historical Perspective and Implications for Future Research Objectives

Sarah J. George and Andrew H. Baker

1. Introduction

Since the first demonstration of gene transfer to vascular tissue in 1990 *(1)*, the field of gene therapy has grown at an astonishing pace. This is due to the lack of an effective and safe pharmacological treatment for certain vascular diseases and the availability of different gene transfer vehicles to the researcher. Gene transfer offers the opportunity to study the effects of gene replacement, gene overexpression, or gene knockout on the phenotype of vascular cells in culture and in vivo. In terms of gene therapy, while much research has focused on identification of candidate therapeutic genes and optimization of delivery techniques, many obstacles remain before routine gene therapy will be available in clinical situations for treatment of diverse vascular pathologies. These situations include:

1. Identification of therapeutic gene(s) for individual applications.
2. Analysis of gene overexpression in vitro and in vivo in suitable animal models.
3. Generation and optimization of the most effective and least toxic gene delivery vehicle.

Gene delivery to vascular tissue, including endothelium and smooth muscle, is relatively inefficient using existing delivery systems, especially in vivo. For in vitro investigations of gene function, genes can be delivered to both endothelial cells (ECs) and smooth muscle cells (SMCs) with relative ease, thus allowing initial experimentation designed to determine the applicability of novel gene therapeutic strategies. However, transversing from in vitro to in vivo applications in vascular disease requires careful consideration of both the

From: *Methods in Molecular Medicine, vol. 52: Atherosclerosis: Experimental Methods and Protocols*
Edited by: A. F. Drew © Humana Press Inc., Totowa, NJ

method of gene transfer and the vascular disease model. In this brief review we discuss the applicability of currently available gene transfer vehicles for the assessment of gene transfer in different animal models.

2. Methods for Gene Transfer to Vascular Cells

Gene transfer initially relied on crude and simple methods, including calcium phosphate–mediated gene transfer and the use of naked plasmid DNA. Plasmid DNA alone has been shown to transduce vascular cells both in vitro and in vivo *(1)*, and a number of clinical trials using naked DNA are in progress aimed at promoting angiogenesis in vascular and myocardial tissue. However, the use of such simple technologies is undermined by the lack of efficiency of gene delivery both to the vascular cell itself and, once in the cell, to the nucleus where gene expression occurs. This results in the requirement for a relatively high concentration of DNA to achieve a therapeutic window for gene transfer and often results in diverse side effects in vivo. Much attention has therefore focused on development and optimization of more efficient and selective delivery vehicles. The advantages and disadvantages of the different vectors are summarized in **Table 1**.

2.1. Non-Viral Vectors

2.1.1. Naked DNA

Plasmid DNA, engineered to express the gene of interest, can be manipulated and produced in the laboratory quickly, efficiently, and without the requirement for specialized equipment. Modification of plasmid DNA for more successful gene delivery would therefore allow many laboratories to enter gene transfer experiments with relative ease. A number of different options are available to achieve this, as outlined below.

2.1.2. Liposome–Mediated Gene Transfer

Plasmid DNA can be complexed with liposomes, resulting in a more efficient delivery vehicle. Both cationic and anionic liposomes exist, and many are commercially available. In brief, to deliver genes to cells using this system, the plasmid DNA and liposomes are premixed to form a complex, and the mixture is then added to the cells. The liposomes fuse with the cell membrane and become internalized. Much of the plasmid DNA is released into the cytosol, prior to degradation, and is thus available for translocation to the nucleus. A small percentage of the DNA enters the nucleus, and gene expression then occurs. This method is suitable for analysis of gene expression in isolated SMCs, where results can be obtained with a small percentage of transduced genes (e.g., for analysis of promoter function and analysis of secreted proteins).

Table 1
Advantages and Disadvantages of Gene Delivery Systems for the Vasculature

Delivery vehicle	Advantages	Disadvantages
	Nonviral	
Naked plasmid DNA	Suited for intramuscular injection Applicable for DNA vaccination Simple to generate and use Relatively nonimmunogenic	Very low transduction rate No specific cell-entry mechanism Rapid clearance in vivo
Cationic lipids	Relatively simple to make Good safety profile	Poor efficiency in vivo Inactivated by serum None specific
	Viral	
Retroviruses	Relatively safe Well characterized Easy to produce	Integrates randomly Infects dividing cells only
Adenoviruses	Infects dividing and nondividing cells High efficiency transduction with high titers Well characterized	Endothelial and smooth muscle Low CAR levels Highly immunogenic Expression low for first 2 wk
Adeno-associated viruses	Long-term expression Stable integration on chromosome 19 Excellent safety profile Infects dividing and non-dividing cells Well characterized	4.5–5 kb cloning capacity Difficult to produce

However, endothelial cells are highly resistant to liposome–mediated gene transfer and exert significant levels of toxicity. Furthermore, the efficiency of liposome–mediated gene transfer to vascular tissue in vivo is low, which makes it less suitable for analysis of gene therapeutics.

2.2. Viral Gene Transfer

A number of different viral gene delivery vehicles have been developed over the last few years, and a number are now in routine use in many laboratories. These include retroviruses, adenoviruses, and adeno-associated viruses.

2.2.1. Retroviruses

This system of gene delivery has been used for many years; most of the systems are based on the Molony murine leukemia virus (MMLV). Retroviral–mediated gene transfer involves replacement of one of the gag, pol, or env genes with an expression cassette containing the gene of interest and a suitable promoter. Because of lack of one or more of the gag, pol, or env genes, the retrovirus is rendered replication defective, and production is required in a helper cell line engineered to express the required function *in trans*. However, this system has three main drawbacks for use in vascular gene therapy in vivo:

1. Retroviruses cannot be grown to very high titers.
2. The retrovirus will infect and express only the transgene in proliferative cells because of the requirement for proviral integration into the host genome prior to the onset of gene expression. As the majority of vascular cells have a low proliferative index at the required time of gene transfer, the system is inefficient for high-level gene transfer.
3. The provirus integrates randomly, and thus insertional mutagenesis is a possibility.

Despite these disadvantages, retroviruses are still extremely useful for a number of applications: for example, targeting proliferating vascular cells, and generation of stable cell lines overexpressing the gene of interest for research purposes.

2.2.2. Adenoviruses

Adenoviruses are icosahedral particles of approximately 70 nm in diameter and have been the preferred gene delivery vehicle for many research groups. Adenoviruses are highly suited for gene delivery to vascular tissue for the following reasons:

1. They are nonpathogenic and well characterized.
2. Over 50 serotypes of adenoviruses exist with the absence of any relationship between significant human disease and adenoviral infection.
3. They can be genetically modified with relative ease.

4. The generation of the 293 helper cell line and the availability of shuttle and gene vectors greatly enhance the use of adenovirus–mediated gene transfer within the laboratory *(2,3)*, which has strongly, and positively, influenced the field of vascular gene transfer.
5. They are engineered to be replication defective by removal of the E1 gene region.
6. They can be grown to high titer.
7. They infect both dividing and nondividing vascular cells with high efficiency, both in vitro and in vivo. Adenoviruses, because of the episomal existence in the nucleus of infected cells, results in high–level gene expression in both dividing and nondividing cells. This is particularly important for vascular cells, as they have a low proliferative index, and at the time of gene transfer in vivo, for angioplasty and vein grafting, the majority of cells are quiescent.

However, adenoviruses have inherent problems that preclude their use for human gene therapy in their present form: (1) Standard first-generation adenoviruses evoke a significant immune response in vivo because of viral load and excessive viral gene synthesis following infection of cells. (2) First-generation adenoviruses lack the capacity for cloning of large transgenes. (3) A number of strategies for generation of adenoviruses also have the inherent ability to generate significant levels of replication-competent adenovirus.

2.2.3. Adeno-associated Adenoviruses (AAVs)

AAVs are parvoviruses that have not been linked with any human illness and are remarkably prevalent in society. As a result of their good safety profile, AAVs are becoming more and more interesting as a gene therapeutic vector. AAVs are small viruses and have a packaging capacity for foreign DNA of approximately 4.7 kb following removal of the viral rep and cap genes. Only the AAV inverted terminal repeats are required in the delivery vehicle, and hence no viral genes are expressed following delivery of AAV to cells. Wild-type AAV integrates into the host chromosome at a specific and non-oncogenic site on chromosome 19, resulting in long-term viral integration. Thus vectors based on AAV have the capability of delivering therapeutic genes long term, and thus are particularly suited to applications in which this is required, e.g., hemophilia and other genetic diseases *(4)*. However, for site-specific integration, the rep protein is required, and caution is required in the design and implementation of studies using rep–deleted AAV vectors, as nonspecific integration may occur.

3. Gene Transfer Models

Two different approaches have been used to introduce recombinant genes into the vessel wall: cell-mediated and direct transfer into the vessel wall (ex vivo and in vivo).

3.1. Cell-Mediated Gene Transfer

Cell–mediated gene transfer involves harvesting vascular wall cells, transducing them in vitro, and then seeding them onto the vascular wall. This strategy is potentially useful for site-specific gene transfer at regions of vascular injury, coating vascular devices such as grafts and stents, and as a vehicle for systemic gene delivery. The disadvantages of this approach include: the requirement for syngeneic cell lines, technology intensive transfection of cells in culture, and a time delay between cell harvest and implantation. Both SMCs and ECs can be modified for vascular gene transfer. Cell–mediated gene transfer using SMCs and ECs has been demonstrated in several animal models, including seeding of genetically modified ECs on canine prosthetic grafts *(5)* and denuded porcine iliofemoral arteries *(6)*; seeding of genetically modified SMCs on denuded rat arteries *(7)* and denuded pig arteries *(8)*; seeding of stents with genetically modified sheep ECs *(9)*; and seeding of autologous transduced ECs onto rat skeletal muscle capillaries *(10)*.

Although most of these studies have used reporter genes, this technique has also been used to obtain biological effects. For example, SMCs transduced with tissue inhibitor of metalloproteinase-1 (TIMP-1), using a retroviral vector, were seeded into injured rat carotid arteries and caused decreased intimal thickening *(11)*. Using the same model and strategy, overexpression of endothelial nitric oxide synthase (eNOS) resulted in reduced intimal thickening and marked vessel dilatation *(12)*. In addition, SMC-based gene transfer may be used as a means of systemic gene delivery. For example, seeding rat arteries with SMCs transduced with erythropoietin by a retroviral vector caused an increase in red blood cell mass for up to 11 wk *(13)*. Genetically modified ECs have also been used to investigate biological effects. For example, sheep ECs expressing human tissue plasminogen activator (tPA) seeded onto balloon-expandable stents possessed prolonged survival when exposed to pulsatile flow *(14)*. Furthermore, decreased platelet deposition and fibrin formation were observed when ECs transduced with tPA and urokinase-type plasminogen activator (uPA) were seeded in a baboon model of arteriovenous shunt thrombosis *(15)*.

3.2. Direct Gene Transfer to the Vessel Wall

Direct gene transfer is simpler than cell-mediated transfer because it eliminates modification of cell lines in culture. However, current disadvantages of this strategy include the inability to target either SMCs or ECs, the possibility of systemic release of the vector, and an immune response to the vector. Direct gene transfer has been performed in several canine, rabbit, rat, and porcine models of vascular disease in normal, injured, and atherosclerotic arteries and bypass grafts.

3.2.1. Ex vivo Gene Transfer to the Vessel Wall

Ex vivo gene transfer is clinically well suited for genetic modification of venous or arterial bypass grafts since the vessel is removed from the individual prior to graft implantation. Grafts are easily genetically engineered ex vivo with optimized transfection efficiency and minimization of toxicity. The harvested vein or artery intended to be used as a bypass graft can by transduced ex vivo by either placing it in or filling the lumen with a vector solution before implantation. This strategy is applicable to liposome-mediated or viral-mediated gene transfer. The feasibility of ex vivo gene transfer of grafts was demonstrated using reporter genes in porcine and rabbit models *(16–18)*. This led to the investigation of potential therapeutic strategies employing the most commonly used conduit for coronary artery bypass grafting, human saphenous vein. Infection of human saphenous veins with eNOS using an adenovirus vector increased nitric oxide release and affected vessel reactivity *(19)*. Furthermore, exposure to adenoviral vectors expressing TIMP-1 or TIMP-2 reduced intimal thickening *(20,21)*.These studies suggest that gene transfer may be clinically useful for reducing early and late vein graft failure.

3.2.2. In vivo Gene Transfer to the Vascular Wall

The first in vivo gene transfer to the vascular wall was carried out in 1990 in porcine iliofemoral arteries using a double-balloon catheter and retroviral and plasmid vectors *(1)*. Since this initial study, many studies have been performed with different transgenes in several animal models, using various delivery techniques and vectors. The elastic laminae act as barriers to the vectors, and therefore expression of the transgene can be limited to the endothelium, media, or adventitia.

The endothelium is an accessible and large target for gene transfer. Since the endothelium plays a major role in the pathogenesis of hypertension and atherosclerosis, expression of recombinant proteins may be potentially useful. Intraluminal delivery of vectors leads to relatively specific gene transfer to the endothelium because the internal elastic lamina restricts deeper penetration. Exposure of the rat carotid artery to an adenoviral vector caused infection of 35% of ECs with little affect on intimal formation *(22)*. Although there have been very few studies that have assessed biological effects using this strategy, one study has demonstrated that endothelium-specific expression of eNOS caused alterations in vascular reactivity *(23)*.

The media contains the SMCs that are the major cell type in arteries and veins. The SMCs play a key role in vascular diseases such as atherosclerosis, restenosis, vein graft disease, and transplant vasculopathy, since SMC migration, proliferation, and extracellular matrix production lead to intimal thickening *(24)*. Consequently, SMCs have become a major target of various systemic and local therapies to limit intimal thickening. Luminal gene delivery can result in transduction of medial SMCs if the internal elastic lamina is previously disrupted by balloon injury or if the vector is injected into the vessel wall using high pressure. Many studies have investigated the effect of various transgenes on intimal thickening. The involvement of growth factors, including platelet-derived growth factor B (PDGFB) *(25)*, acidic fibroblast growth factor (FGF-1) *(26)*, and transforming growth factor β1 (TGFβ1) *(27)*, in intimal thickening has been demonstrated using transfection of porcine iliofemoral arteries using cationic liposomes. Furthermore, recombinant hirudin *(28)* and TIMP-2 *(29)* expression using adenoviral vectors reduced intimal thickening after balloon injury in rat carotid arteries, demonstrating the involvement of proteases in intimal thickening.

The adventitia is an attractive target since it is involved in remodeling and intimal thickening after arterial injury *(30,31)*, and it may influence atherogenesis *(32)* and hypertrophy caused by hypertension *(33)*. The advantages of adventitial gene transfer are that blood flow and the endothelium are not disrupted, and systemic distribution of the vector is avoided. Adventitial gene delivery has been achieved using a periadventital sheath in several animal models, including rabbits and normal and atherosclerotic cynomolgus monkeys *(34–36)*. Adventitial delivery of vectors has also been easily achieved in large peripheral arteries by direct application during surgery and in cerebral arteries by instillation into cerebrospinal fluid *(37)*. Novel strategies, such as delivery to the pericardial space *(38)* and percutaneous intervention using special catheters *(39)*, may also make adventitial delivery to the coronary arteries possible. Adventitial gene transfer has also been utilized to study biological effects in several models. Expression of eNOS in the adventitia of rabbit carotid arteries caused an alteration in vascular reactivity *(34)*, as did delivery of eNOS to the cerebral vessels via the cerebrospinal fluid in dogs *(40)*. Several studies have examined whether stimulating the formation of new blood vessels by transducing vascular wall cells with angiogenic factors affects vascular disease. Overexpression of vascular endothelial growth factor (VEGF) increased angiogenesis and reduced intimal thickening in rabbit carotid arteries *(41)* and reduced ischemia in rabbits *(42)*, and gene transfer of FGF-1 reduced ischemia in rabbits *(43)*. These studies indicated that direct gene transfer may be clinically useful. In fact, a phase-I study of VEGF gene transfer via intramuscular injection of plasmid DNA in patients with inoperable lower extremity ischemia has reported encouraging results *(44)*.

4. Summary

In the last decade, major advances have been made in the use of gene transfer to the vasculature (as summarized in Table 2). With the employment of various animal models, vascular gene transfer has been utilized to alter intimal thickening (restenosis and late vein graft failure) and vasomotor reactivity (endothelial

Table 2
The Use of Animal Models for Gene Transfer to the Vasculature

Delivery vehicle	Ref.	Delivery method	Transgene	Model	Effect	Potential clinical use
Naked DNA	42	In vivo	VEGF	Rabbit hindlimb ischemia	Reduced ischemia	Peripheral vascular disease
	43	In vivo	FGF-1	Rabbit hindlimb ischemia	Reduced ischemia	
Liposomes	25	In vivo	PDGFB	Pig iliofemoral injury model	Increased intimal thickening	Restenosis
	26		FGF-1			
	27		TGFβ1			
Retroviruses	11	Cell-based	TIMP-1	Rat carotid injury	Reduced intimal thickening	Restenosis
	12	Cell-based	eNOS	Rat carotid injury	Reduced intimal thickening	Restenosis
	14	Cell-based	tPA	Balloon extendable stent in sheep	Increased EC survival	Stent improvement
	15	Cell-based	tPA uPA	Baboon arteriovenous shunt thrombosis	Reduced platelet deposition and fibrin formation	Early graft failure
	41	In vivo	VEGF	Rabbit carotid artery adventitia	Increased angiogenesis and reduced intimal thickening	Restenosis
Adenoviruses	19	Ex vivo	eNOS	Human saphenous vein	Altered vessel reactivity and increased NO	Early graft failure
	20	Ex vivo	TIMP-1	Human saphenous vein	Reduced intimal thickening	Late vein graft failure
	21		TIMP-2			
	23	In vivo	eNOS	Rat carotid injury	Altered vascular reactivity	Endothelial dysfunction
	28	In vivo	Hirudin	Rat carotid injury	Reduced intimal thickening	Restenosis
	29		TIMP-2			
	40	In vivo	eNOS	Dog cerebral artery adventitia	Altered vascular reactivity	Endothelial dysfunction
	34	In vivo	eNOS	Rabbit carotid artery adventitia	Altered vascular reactivity	Endothelial dysfunction

dysfunction) and to stimulate angiogenesis. However, transfer of this technology to humans is still a major step, since the animal models are not a true reflection of the human situation and the current vectors have many deficiencies. Furthermore, safety and cost-effectiveness issues also need to be considered.

References

1. Nabel, E. G., Plautz, G., and Nabel, G. J. (1990) Site-specific gene expression in vivo by direct gene transfer into the arterial wall. *Science* **249,** 1285–1288.
2. Graham, F. L. and Prevec, L. (1992) Adenovirus-based expression vectors and recombinant vaccine, in *Vaccines: New Approaches to Immunological Problems* (Ellis, R.W., ed.), Butterworth-Heinemann, Boston, pp. 363–390.
3. Bett, A. J., Haddara, W., Prevec, L., and Graham, F. L. (1994) An efficient and flexible system for construction of adenovirus vectors with insertions or deletions in early regions 1 and 3. *Proc. Natl. Acad. Sci. USA* **91,** 8802–8806.
4. Synder, R. O., Miao, C. H., Patijn, G. A., Spratt, S. K., Danos, O., Nagy, D., Gown, A. M., Winther, B., Meuse, L., Cohen, L. K., Thompson, A. R., and Kay, M. A. (1997) Persistent and therapeutic concentrations of human factor IX in mice after hepatic gene transfer of recombinant AAV vectors. *Nat. Gene. 16,* 270–276.
5. Wilson, J. M., Birinyi, L. K., Salomon, R. N., Libby, P., Callow, A. D., and Mulligan, R. C. (1989) Implantation of vascular grafts lined with genetically modified endothelial cells. *Science* **244,** 1344–1346.
6. Nabel, E. G., Plautz, G., Boyce, F. M., Stanley, J. C., and Nabel, G. J. (1989) Recombinant gene expression in vivo within endothelial cells of the arterial wall. *Science* **244,** 1342–1344.
7. Lynch, C. M., Clowes, M. M., Osborne, W. R. A., Clowes, A. W., and Miller, A. D. (1992) Long-term expression of human adenosine deaminase in vascular smooth muscle cells of rats: A model for gene therapy. *Proc. Natl. Acad. Sci. USA* **89,** 1138–1142.
8. Plautz, G., Nabel, E. G., and Nabel, G. J. (1991) Introduction of vascular smooth muscle cells expressing recombinant genes in vivo. *Circulation* **83,** 578–583.
9. Dichek, D. A., Neville, R. F., Zwiebel, J. A., Freeman, S. M., Leon, M. B., and Anderson, W. F. (1989) Seeding of intravascular stents with genetically engineered endothelial cells. *Circulation* **80,** 1347–1353.
10. Messina, L. M., Podrazik, R. M., Whitehill, T. A., Ekhterae, D., Brothers, T. E., Eilson, J. M., Burkel, W. E., and Stanley, J. C. (1992) Adhesion and incorporation of lacZ-transduced endothelial cells into the intact capillary wall in the rat. *Proc. Natl. Acad. Sci. USA* **89,** 12018–12022.
11. Forough, R., Koyama, N., Hasenstab, D., Lea, H., Clowes, M., Nikkari, S. T., and Clowes, A. W. (1996) Overexpression of tissue inhibitor of matrix metalloproteinase-1 inhibits vascular smooth muscle cell functions in vitro and in vivo. *Circ. Res.* **79,** 812–820.
12. Chen, L., Daum, G., Forough, R., Clowes, M., Walter, U., and Clowes A. W. (1998) Overexpression of human endothelial nitric oxide synthase in rat vascular smooth muscle cells and in balloon-injured carotid artery. *Circ. Res.* **82,** 862–870.

13. Osborne, W. R. A., Ramesh, N., Lau, S., Clowes, M. M., Dale, D. C., and Clowes, A. W. (1995) Gene therapy for long-term expression of erythropoietin in rats. *Proc. Natl. Acad. Sci. USA* **92**, 8055–8058.

14. Flugelman, M. Y., Virmani, R., Leon, M. B., Bowman, R. L., and Dichek, D. A. (1992) Genetically engineered endothelial cells remain adherent and viable after stent deployment and exposure to flow in vitro. *Circ. Res.* **70**, 348–354.

15. Dichek, D. A., Anderson, J., Kelly, A. B., Hanson, S. R., and Harker, L. A. (1996) Enhanced in vivo antithrombic effects of endothelial cells expressing recombinant plasminogen activators transduced with retroviral vectors. *Circulation* **93**, 301–309.

16. Chen, S.-J., Wilson, J. M., and Muller, D. W. M. (1994) Adenovirus-mediated gene transfer of soluble vascular cell adhesion molecule to porcine interposition vein grafts. *Circulation* **89**, 1922–1928.

17. Takeshita, S., Losordo, D. W., Kearney, M., Rossow, S. T., and Isner, J. M. (1994) Time course of recombinant protein secretion after liposome-mediated gene transfer in a rabbit arterial organ culture model. *Lab. Invest.* **71**, 387–391.

18. Kupfer, J. M., Ruan, X. M., Liu, G., Matloff, J., Forrester, J., and Chaux, A. (1994) High-efficiency gene transfer to autologous rabbit jugular vein grafts using adenovirus-transferrin/polylysine-DNA complexes. *Hum. Gene Ther.* **5**, 1437–1443.

19. Cable, D. G., O'Brien, T., Schaff, H. V., and Pompili, V. J. (1997) Recombinant endothelial nitric oxide synthase-transduced human saphenous veins: gene therapy to augment nitric oxide production in bypass conduits. *Circulation* **96**(suppl. 9), II-173–II-178.

20. George, S. J., Johnson, J. L., Angelini, G. D., Newby, A. C., and Baker, A. H. (1998) Adenovirus-mediated gene transfer of the human TIMP-1 gene inhibits smooth muscle cell migration and neointima formation in human saphenous vein. *Hum. Gene Ther.* **9**, 867–877.

21. George, S. J., Baker, A. H., Angelini, G. D., and Newby, A. C. (1998) Gene transfer of tissue inhibitor of metalloproteinase-2 inhibits metalloproteinase activity and neointima formation in human saphenous veins. *Gene Ther.* **5**, 1552–1560.

22. Schulick, A. H., Dong, G., Newman, K. D., Virmani, R., and Dichek, D. A. (1995) Endothelium-specific in vivo gene transfer. *Circ. Res.* **77**, 475–485.

23. Kullo, I. J., Mozes, G., Schwartz, R. S., Gloviczki, P., Tsutsui, M., Katusic, Z. S., and O'Brien, T. (1997) Enhanced endothelium-dependent relaxations after gene transfer of recombinant endothelial nitric oxide synthase to rabbit carotid arteries. *Hypertension* **30**, 314–320.

24. Ross, R. (1993) The pathogenesis of atherosclerosis: A perspective for the 1990s. *Nature* **362**, 801–809.

25. Nabel, E. G., Yang, Z., Liptay, S., San, H., Gordon, D., Haudenschild, C. C., and Nabel, G. J. (1993) Recombinant platelet-derived growth factor B gene expression in porcine arteries induces intimal hyperplasia in vivo. *J. Clin. Invest.* **91**, 1822–1829.

26. Nabel, E. G., Yang, Z., Plautz, G., Forough, R., Zhan, X., Haudenschild, C. C., Maciag, T., and Nabel, G. J. (1993) Recombinant fibroblast growth factor-1 promotes intimal hyperplasia and angiogenesis in arteries in vivo. *Nature* **362**, 844–846.

27. Nabel, E. G., Shum, L., Pompili, V. J., Yang, Z.-Y., San, H., Hong, B.-S., Liptay, S., Gold, L., Gordon, D., Derynck, R., and Nabel, G. J. (1993) Direct transfer of transforming growth factor beta 1 gene into arteries stimulates fibrocellular hyperplasia. *Proc. Natl. Acad. Sci. USA* **90,** 10759–10763.
28. Rade, J. J., Schulick, A. H., Virmani, R., and Dichek, D. A. (1996) Local adenoviral-mediated expression of recombinant hirudin reduces neointima formation after arterial injury. *Nat. Med.* **2,** 293–298.
29. Cheng, L., Mantile, G., Pauly, R., Nater, C., Felici, A., Monticone, R., Bilato, C., Gluzband, Y. A., Crow, M. T., Stetler-Stevenson, W., and Capogrossi, M. C. (1998) Adenovirus-mediated gene transfer of the human tissue inhibitor of metalloproteinase-2 blocks vascular smooth muscle cell invasiveness in vitro and modulates neointimal development in vivo. *Circulation* **98,** 2195–2201.
30. Shi, Y., Pieniek, M., Fard, A., O'Brien, J., Mannion, J. D., and Zalewski, A. (1996) Adventitial remodelling after coronary arterial injury. *Circulation* **93,** 340–348.
31. Scott, N. A., Cipolla, G. D., Ross, C. E., Dunn, B., Martin, F. H., Simonet, L., and Wilcox, J. N. (1996) Identification of a potential role for the adventitia in vascular lesion formation after balloon overstretch injury of porcine coronary arteries. *Circulation* **93,** 2178–2187.
32. Barker, S. G. E., Tilling, L. C., Miller, G. C., Beesley, J. E., Fleetwood, G., Stavri, G. T., Baskerville, P. A., and Martin, J. F. (1994) The adventitia and atherogenesis: Removal initiates intimal proliferation in the rabbit which regresses on generation of a 'neoadventitia.' *Atherosclerosis* **105,** 131–144.
33. Chatelain, R. E. and Dardik, B. N. (1988) Increased DNA replication in the arterial adventitia after aortic ligation. *Hypertension* **11**(suppl. I), I130–I134.
34. Kullo, I. J., Mozes, G., Schwartz, R. S., Gloviczki, P., Crotty, T. B., Barber, D. A., Katusic, Z. S., and O'Brien, T. (1997) Adventitial gene transfer of recombinant endothelial nitric oxide synthase to rabbit carotid arteries alters vascular reactivity. *Circulation* **96,** 2254–2261.
35. Laitnen, M., Pakkanen, T., Donetti, E., Baetta, R., Luoma, J., Lehtolainen, P., Viita, H., Agrawal, R., Miyanohara, A., Friedmann, T., Risau, W., Martin, J. F., Soma, M., and Ylä-Herttuala, S. (1997) Gene transfer into the carotid artery using an adventitial collar: Comparison of the effectiveness of the plasmid-liposome complexes, retroviruses, pseudotypes retroviruses, and adenoviruses. *Hum. Gene Ther.* **8,** 1645–1650.
36. Rios, C. D., Ooboshi, H., Piegors, D., Davidson, B. L., and Heistad, D. D. (1995) Adenovirus-mediated gene transfer to normal and atherosclerotic arteries. A novel approach. *Arterioscler. Thromb. Vasc. Biol.* **15,** 2241–2245.
37. Ooboshi, H., Welsh, M. J., Rios, C. D., Davidson, B. L., and Heistad, D. D. (1995) Adenovirus-mediated gene transfer in vivo to cerebral blood vessels and perivascular tissues. *Circ. Res.* **77,** 7–13.
38. March, K. L., Woody, M., Mehdi, K., Zipes, D. P., Brantly, M., and Trapnell, B. L. (1999) Efficient in vivo catheter-based pericardial gene transfer mediated by adenoviral vectors. *Clin. Cardiol.* **22**(suppl. 1), 123–129.

39. Mehdi, K., Wilensky, R. L., Baek, S. H., Trapnell, B. C., and March, K. L. (1996) Efficient adenovirus-mediated perivascular gene transfer and protein delivery by a transvascular injection catheter. *J. Am. Coll. Cardiol.* **27**(suppl. A), 164A.

40. Chen, A. F. Y., Jiang, S.-W., Crotty, T. B., Tsutsui, M., Smith, L. A., O'Brien, T., and Katusic, Z. S. (1997) Effects of in vivo adventitial expression of recombinant endothelial nitric oxide synthase gene in cerebral arteries. *Proc, Natl. Acad. Sci. USA* **94**, 12568–12573.

41. Laitnen, M., Zachary, I., Breier, G., Pakkanen, T., Häkkinen, T., Luoma, J., Abedi, H., Risau, W., Soma, M., Laakso, M., Martin, J. F., and Ylä-Herttuala, S. (1997) VEGF gene transfer reduces intimal thickening via increased production of nitric oxide in carotid arteries. *Hum. Gene Ther.* **8**, 1737–1744.

42. Takeshita, S., Zheng, L. P., Ashara, T., Riessen, R., Brogi, E., Ferrara, N., Symes, J. F., and Isner, J. M. (1993) In vivo evidence of enhanced angiogenesis following direct arterial gene transfer of the plasmid encoding vascular endothelial growth factor. *Circulation* **88**, I–476.

43. Tabata, H., Silver, M., and Isner, J. M. (1997) Arterial gene transfer of acidic fibroblast growth factor for therapeutic angiogenesis in vivo: Critical role of secretion signal in use of naked DNA. *Cardiovasc. Res.* **35**, 470–479.

44. Baumgartner, I., Pieczek, A., Manor, O., Blair, R., Kearney, M., Walsh, K., and Isner, J. M. (1998) Constitutive expression of phVEGF165 after intramuscular gene transfer promotes collateral vessel development in patients with critical limb ischemia. *Circulation* **97**, 1114–1123.

22

A Pig Model of Vein Graft Disease

Applications for Potential Gene Therapies

Clinton T. Lloyd, Sarah J. George, Gianni D. Angelini, Andrew C. Newby, and Andrew H. Baker

1. Introduction

The development of an effective and safe gene therapy for prevention of vein graft failure, either acute or chronic, relies on the use of applicable and reproducible models of vein graft failure. Evaluation of potential new therapies usually involves assessment of beneficial phenotypic changes to vascular cells in isolated cells, in more complex organ cultures, and in in vivo models. We have extensively utilized gene transfer in isolated human vein vascular smooth muscle cells (SMCs) and endothelial cells (ECs) *(1)*. Furthermore, we have extended our initial studies and evaluated potential gene therapies in a human saphenous vein organ culture model *(2,3)*. The use of human saphenous vein, in this context, is advantageous as it is the most commonly used conduit for bypass grafting in the clinic. However, the organ culture model is static, and additionally studies need to be carried out in an in vivo model. In this chapter we describe a porcine model of vein graft neointima formation. Pig arteriovenous bypass grafting provides a reproducible model of intimal thickening, which is associated with late vein graft failure, and the effect of potential gene therapies can be assessed over long periods (up to 6 mo) *(4; see* **Fig. 1**). Furthermore, the saphenous vein is removed prior to grafting, and ex vivo genetic manipulation can be performed, providing a simple, controllable and safe method of gene transfer prior to grafting in vivo.

From: *Methods in Molecular Medicine, vol. 52: Atherosclerosis: Experimental Methods and Protocols*
Edited by: A. F. Drew © Humana Press Inc., Totowa, NJ

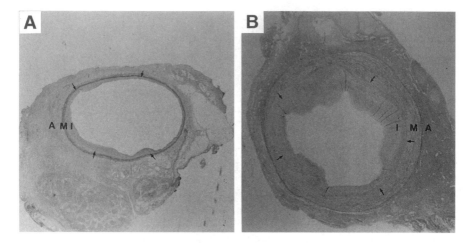

Fig. 1. Neointima formation in porcine saphenous vein grafts. Removal of grafts at 7 d (**A**) and 28 d (**B**) reveals extensive and progressive neointima formation. The intimal/medial border is indicated with arrows in each case. A, adventitia; M, media; I, intima.

1.1. Pathophysiology of Vein Graft Disease

Unlike their arterial counterparts, vein grafts undergo a series of adaptive changes when exposed to the arterial circulation, which leads to chronic occlusion. In human disease this attrition rate is 1–2% /yr with over 40% occluded at 10 yr (*5*). The underlying process of vein-wall thickening comprises three integrated processes of intimal damage with subsequent thrombosis, intimal hyperplasia, and the development of an accelerated atherosclerotic process within the neointima.

The surgical preparation of vein grafts inevitably leads to endothelial damage, which stimulates adherence and activation of platelets and neutrophils (*4*) and sets up a cascade of prothrombotic events mediated by decreased levels of prostacyclin, nitric oxide, and tissue plasminogen activator among others. The regeneration of a neoendothelium coincides with the release of a number of growth factors, among them platelet–derived growth factor (PDGF), basic fibroblast growth factor (bFGF), insulin-like growth factor (IGF-1), and transforming growth factor (TGF) α and β (*6*). These growth factors are produced also as a result of increased wall tension and reduced shear stress, and act in concert to alter the phenotypic expression of the vasoactive smooth muscle cells (VSMCs) in the vein media. They change from a contractile to a proliferative phenotype and they migrate across the internal elastic lamina, where, along with the production of extracellular matrix, they cause the formation of the thickened neointima. This migration of

VSMCs within the extracellular matrix is regulated by the balance of matrix metalloproteinases (MMPs) *(7)*, a series of proteases that digest components of the extracellular matrix, and their endogenous tissue inhibitors (TIMPs). These enzymes and inhibitors are themselves under the regulatory control of activators and inhibitors, particularly the products of the thrombus re-organization such as thrombin, plasminogen activator, and plasmin. Finally, subsequent to this is the rapid development of a diffuse concentric atherosclerosis caused by increased lipid uptake and synthesis and slower lipolysis in the neointima.

Strategies to reduce this process are numerous and include pharmacological intervention, physical external support *(8)*, and more recently molecular biological approaches, including antisense oligonucleotide inhibition and gene therapy *(2,3,9)*. The complexity of the processes involved and our limited understanding, however, require a great deal more work to be done.

2. Materials
2.1. Animals

1. Pigs. We use the *Large white* breed of pigs, although *Landrace* pigs have been used previously with success. Animals between 30 and 40 kg are of optimal weight for ease of handling and adequate vessel size.

2.2. Gene Transfer

All materials should be sterile.

1. Vein bathing solution: Dulbecco's modified Eagle's medium (DMEM) containing 20 mM HEPES, 2 mM L-glutamine, 8 µg/mL gentamicin, 100 IU/mL penicillin, and 100 µg/mL streptomycin. Store at 4°C. Prewarm to 37°C before use.
2. Infection dishes: Any presterilized plastic dish can be used, but it must be large enough (minimum 15 cm × 15 cm).
3. Crocodile clips.
4. 18 gage × 32-mm catheter needle (Abbocath®-T, Venisystems™, Abbott Ireland, Sligo, Republic of Ireland).
5. Lockable 3-way stopcock (Vygon, Ecouen, France).
6. Recombinant adenovirus. We use adenoviruses that have been cesium chloride banded and extensively dialyzed. Minimum titer is 2.5 × 10^{10} plaque forming units (pfu)/mL *(see* **Note 1***)*.

2.3. Surgery
2.3.1. General Equipment

1. Operating suite with table.
2. Autoclave.

3. Transport crate.
4. Diathermy unit and handle.
5. 2.5 magnifying operating spectacles.

2.3.2. Anesthetic

1. Boyle's anesthetics machine with circle circuit and O_2 and N_2O supply.
2. Laryngoscope with a straight blade.
3. Ketamine (Ketaset; Fort Dodge, Southampton, UK).
4. Halothane (Rhone Merieux Ltd. Harlow, UK).
5. Endotracheal tube 5.0–7.O mm cuffed (Centaur Services, Castle Cary, UK).
6. Endotracheal connector (Intersurgical Ltd, Wokingham, UK, ref: 3509).

2.3.3. Instruments

1. One no. 10 scalpel blade (Paragon, Sheffield, UK).
2. One scalpel blade holder.
3. Two Adson self retaining retractors.
4. One Mayo scissors.
5. One Lanes toothed tissue forcep.
6. One Potts fine scissors.
7. One Potts fine-needle holder.
8. Two Spencer Wells artery forceps.
9. Two Debakey angled vascular clamps.
10. One Castroviejo needle holder.
11. One Ryder needle holder.
12. Eight Shardle towel clips.

All the above instruments are available from South Western Surgical, Bristol, UK.

2.3.4. Disposables

1 One 1-mL syringe.
2. One 2-mL syringe.
3. Three 5-mL syringe.
4. One 20-mL syringe.
5. One 18-gage needle.
6. Three 21-gage needle.
7. One 27-gage needle.
8. One 19-gage winged butterfly needle.
9. Endotracheal tape (50 cm).
10. Sterile gloves.
11. Ten 10-cm gauze swabs (Millpledge, Retford, UK).
12. Masking tape.

13. Five disposable drapes, 90 × 75cm (3 M, Loughborough, UK).
14. One disposable gown (3 M, Loughborough, UK).
15. One 4/0 Sofsilk tie (Auto Suture, Dagford, UK).
16. Four 7/0 Surgipro sutures (9-mm needle) (Auto Suture, Dagford, UK).
17. Three 2/0 Polysorb sutures (Auto Suture, Dagford, UK).
18. 30-mL plastic Gallipot.

2.2.5. Solutions

1. Hibitane 5% (Zeneca Ltd, Macclesfield, UK).
2. 2 mL Heparin multiparin (CP Pharmaceuticals Ltd. Wrexham, UK).
3. 1 mL glyceryl trinitrate (Nitrocine; Schwarz Pharma Ltd, Chesham, UK).
4. 20 mL 0-9% Sodium chloride (Ivex Pharmaceuticals, Lame, UK).
5. 1 mL Buprenorphine (Temgesic; Reckitt and Coleman, Hull, UK).
6. 2 mL Ampicillin (Amfipen) (Intervet UK Ltd.Cambridge, UK).
7. Pentobarbitone solution 20% (J.M. Loveridge plc, Southampton, UK).

3. Methods
3.1. Induction of Anesthesia

1. Sedate pigs in the transport carrier with 0.1 mL/kg (100 mg/mL) intramuscular ketamine hydrochloride. This is best achieved using a butterfly needle and injecting in the muscles at the back of the neck. This causes the least distress and does not require any constraint of the animal.
2. Once sedated, achieve anesthesia by mask inhalation of 5–8% halothane until stage three (surgical level) is achieved. Respiration should be spontaneous with 10–12 breaths/min and no response to pain.
3. Transfer the animal to the surgical table prone position. This will allow the upper and lower jaws to be held open with tape by an assistant while the operator inserts the endotracheal tube (size 7.0 adult) with the aid of a long flat-blade laryngoscope.
4. Once in position, secure the animal, turned supine, with the limbs secured and the head held in place with tape.
5. Maintain anesthesia using a closed circuit with halothane 1%, oxygen, and nitrous oxide in equal parts at flow rates of 2 L/per. We do not routinely require venous cannulation, and monitoring of vital signs is used as a guide to depth of anesthesia. Monitoring of blood oxygen saturation with pulse oximetry on the tail and core body temperature with a nasopharyngeal probe is a useful adjunct.

3.2. Removal of Saphenous Vein and Infection with Recombinant Adenoviruses

1. Disinfect the skin of the leg and neck with an iodine-based solution and drape the animal to provide a sterile operating field. Use unipolar diathermy for vessel cautery.

2. Harvest the saphenous vein from each hindlimb (provides approximately 10 cm length of vein). Make the incision posterior to the lateral malleolus and extend proximally toward the posterior aspect of the knee (**Fig. 2A**). The vein is located deep to the subcutaneous layer and fascia.
3. Once the length of the vein is exposed, identify the side branches (usually 4–10 in number) and ligate with 4.0 silk ties (**Fig. 2B**).
4. Remove the vein, making careful note of the proximal and distal ends (*see* **Note 2**). The vein may go into spasm during the harvesting process, but this is avoided with careful "no-touch" technique dissection.
5. Bevel the vein at either end and make a small incision longitudinally to lengthen the anastomotic area.
6. Place the vein into sterile bathing media (*see* **Note 3**; **Fig. 2C**).
7. Remove the sheath from two 18 gage × 32-mm catheter needles and trim to 2 cm in length with scissors.
8. Insert one catheter sheath into the lumen of the vein to be infected.
9. Wash through with 1 mL bathing medium to ensure unobstructed flow.
10. When unobstructed flow of wash medium is observed, insert the other catheter sheath into the lumen of the other end of the vein.
11. Clamp both catheters at each end using crocodile clips.
12. While still in their sterile wrapping, twist the tap of two 3-way stopcocks to close the stopcocks.
13. Remove both stopcocks from the wrapping and place into the Petri dish containing the vein and wash medium.
14. Attach one stopcock to the vessel cannula.
15. Take up 200 μL recombinant adenovirus solution at 2.5×10^{10} pfu/mL into another 1-mL sterile syringe.
16. Insert the syringe containing the adenovirus into the catheter sheath and inject the contents into the lumen of the vein without distending the vein. Allow some flow-through of lumen contents into the distal 3-way tap (*see* **Note 4**).
17. Carefully remove the 1-mL syringe from the catheter sheath and, using forceps, attach the other stopcock to the catheter sheath.
18. Close both taps and leave for 30 min immersed in the sterile bathing solution.
19. After 30 min, gently flush-through with 2–3 mL bathing media (*see* **Notes 5** and **6**). Ensure the flow-through is decontaminated, as this will contain unused adenoviruses. Also ensure that the flow-through does not come into contact with the outside of the vein.

The vein is now ready for grafting.

3.3. Preparation of the Carotid Artery and Grafting

1. Expose the common carotid arteries on either side of the neck. Make an incision from the lower angle of the mandible to the upper level of the shoulder (± 15 cm).
2. Divide the platysma muscle to expose the submandibular glands.
3. Expose a plane between the submandibular gland and the strap muscles of the neck, which leads directly down to the carotid sheath.

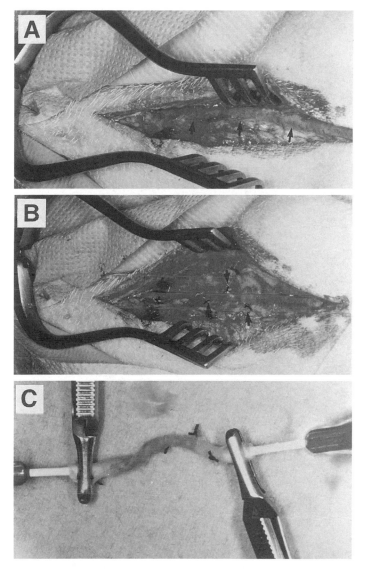

Fig. 2. Removal of saphenous vein and infection with recombinant adenoviruses. (**A**) After exposure of the saphenous vein in the leg. (**B**) The side branches (indicated with arrows) are ligated. (**C**) After removal of the saphenous vein into sterile media, the vein is cannulated and clamped at either end and infused with adenovirus at the luminal surface only.

4. Hold the gland laterally and the muscles medially using tissue retractors while opening the carotid sheath.
5. Clear the carotid artery of superficial adventitial tissue (**Fig. 3A**).

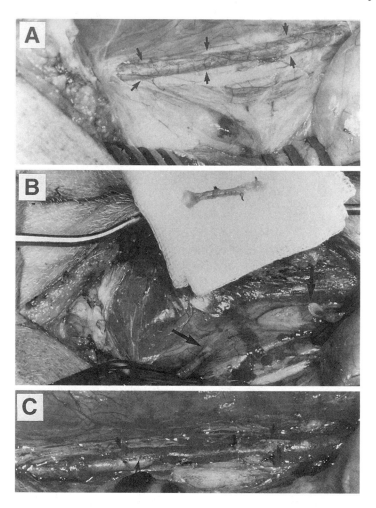

Fig. 3. Interposition vein grafting. **(A)** The carotid artery in the neck is exposed (indicated by arrows) and subsequently bisected **(B)**. The adenovirus-treated vein is then anastomosed into the carotid artery as an end-to-end graft **(C)**. The anastomotic sites are indicated with arrows.

6. Heparinize the animal with 100 IU/kg heparin via the internal jugular vein using a fine-gage needle.
7. Clamp the carotid artery proximally and distally with two artery clamps isolating 10–15 cm **(Fig. 3B)**.
8. A 3–5-cm beveled segment of artery is removed and the exposed ends of artery cleared of adventitia in preparation for anastomosis.
9. Anastomose the vein both proximally and distally to the exposed carotid artery ends in a similar fashion. Use double-ended 7.0 polypropylene sutures for each anastomosis **(Fig. 3C)**.

10. Tie the heel of the vein to the toe of the artery.
11. Using a continuous suture, complete the anastomosis to the toe on either side and fasten the suture (**Fig. 3C**).
12. Release the clamps once both proximal and distal anastomoses are complete and the vein graft has been assessed for hemostasis. Additional interrupted sutures may be required.
13. Once left and right grafts are completed and checked for hemostasis, close the wounds with 2.0 Vicryl suture for the subcuticular layers and skin in the neck and leg. We do not use subcuticular drains. Prophylactic antibiotics (2 mL [200 mg] intramuscular ampicillin) and analgesia (1 mL [0.3 mg] intramuscular buprenorphine hydrochloride) are given.
14. After extubation, return the animal to the pen and allow to recover spontaneously.

3.4. Vein Graft Harvesting

After a predetermined period remove the grafts for analysis.

1. Sedate the animal and anesthetize as above.
2. Expose the graft by careful dissection through the old wound and locate by palpation of the pulsation.
3. Explant the graft with native carotid artery at either end.
4. After retrieval of all grafts, euthanize the animal with 20 mL (4 g) pentobarbitone sodium intravenously.

Fig. 4 illustrates the efficiency of gene transfer using the β-galactosidase reporter gene.

4. Notes

1. The titer of adenovirus required to deliver effective gene transfer to vein grafts or other vascular tissue should be empirically determined in each laboratory. Because of the differences in the methods for titration of recombinant adenoviruses and infection protocols used between laboratories it is important for each research group to test their infection protocols using standard reporter gene expressing adenoviruses. In our hands we have found that infection of the pig saphenous vein with 2.5×10^{10} pfu/mL of adenovirus is sufficient to induce a high level of gene transfer (approximately 40%).
2. It is important to remember proximal and distal ends of the vein for grafting, as valves may hinder infusion of the adenovirus.
3. Bathing medium must be sterile for the infection procedure. We have used infections on the open bench; therefore, the medium becomes nonsterile. However, this has not hindered the graft procedure or promoted bacterial infection in grafts; but, the ideal situation is to perform the entire infection procedure in a tissue culture cabinet, thereby retaining sterility and adenovirus containment.

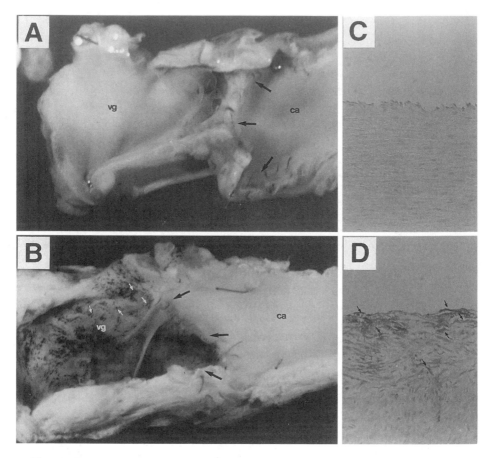

Fig. 4. Gene transfer to vein grafts. Vehicle-treated (**A**) and (**C**) and Ad-lacZ–
infected (**B**) and (**D**) vein grafts explanted and stained for β-galactosidase expression, 7 d postinfection. **A** and **B** show *en face* pictures illustrating the carotid artery
(ca), anastomotic sites (large arrows), and vein graft (vg). **B** and **D** show
hemotoxylin-stained cross-sections of the vein graft region. Dark cells indicate
adenoviral-infected cells (small arrows in **B** and **D** indicate examples) within the
vein graft region only in (**B**) and through the vessel wall in (**D**) but not in vehicle-
treated grafts (**A**) and (**C**).

4. As the saphenous vein is often quite long, it is difficult to know the amount of
   virus required to expose the entire length of vein. We therefore infuse initially
   with the distal tap open and push through until sufficient volume has flowed
   through. Although this results in the use of a larger volume of virus, it ensures
   that the exposure to the virus is consistent throughout the vein.
5. It is important to flush through, following infection, to ensure that all nonbound
   adenovirus is washed from the system. This ensures that the surgeon is not

exposed to unused virus and that following grafting, systemic dissemination of any unused virus is minimized.

6. Be careful to collect the virus solution into a separate container for disposal. This is for safety reasons and also to prevent adventitial exposure of the virus with the vein.

References

1. Baker, A., Zaltsman, A., George, S., and Newby, A. (1998) Divergent effects of tissue inhibitor of metalloproteinase-1, -2 or -3 overexpression on rat vascular smooth muscle cell invasion, proliferation and death in vitro: TIMP-3 promotes apoptosis. *J. Clin. Invest.* **101**, 1478–1487.

2. George, S., Johnson, J., Angelini, G., Newby, A., and Baker, A. (1998) Adenovirus-mediated gene transfer of the human TIMP-1 gene inhibits SMC migration and neointima formation in human saphenous vein. *Hum. Gene Ther.* **9**, 867–877.

3. George, S. J., Baker, A. H., Angelini, G. D., and Newby, A. C. (1998) Gene transfer of tissue inhibitor of metalloproteinase-2 inhibits metalloproteinase activity and neointima formation in human saphenous veins. *Gene Ther.* **5**, 1552–1560.

4. Angelini, G., Bryan, A., Williams, H., Morgan, R., and Newby, A. (1990) Distension promotes platelet and leukocyte adhesion and reduces short-term patency in pig arteriovenous bypass grafts. *J. Thorac. Cardiovasc. Surg.* **99**, 433–439.

5. Campeau, L., Enjalbert, M., Lesperance, J., et al. (1983) Atherosclerosis and late closure of aortocoronary saphenous vein grafts: Sequential angiographic studies at 2 weeks, 1 year, 5 to 7 years and 10 to 12 years after surgery. *Circulation* **68**, II-1s–II-7s.

6. Newby, A. and George, S. (1993) Proposed roles for growth factors in mediating smooth muscle cell proliferation in vascular pathologies. *Cardiovasc. Res.* **27**, 1173–1183.

7. Birkedal-Hansen, H., Moore, W. G. I., Bodden, M. K., Windsor, L. J., Birkedal-Hansen, B. DeCarlo, A. and Engler, J. A. (1993) Matrix metallproteinases: A review. *Crit. Rev. Oral Biol. Med.* **4**, 197–250.

8. Mehta, D., George, S. J., Jeremy, J. Y., Izzat, M. B., Southgate, K. M., Bryan, A. J., Newby, A. C., and Angelini, G. D. (1998) External stenting reduces long-term medial and neointimal thickening and platelet derived growth factor expression in a pig model of arteriovenous bypass grafting. *Nature Med.* **4**, 235–239.

9. Mann, M. J., Gibbons, G. H., Kernoff, R. S., Diet, F. P., Tsao, P. S., Cooke, J. P., Kaneda, Y., and Dzau, V. J. (1995) Genetic-Engineering Of Vein Grafts Resistant to Atherosclerosis. *Proc. Natl. Acad. Sci. USA* **92**, 4502–4506.

Index

From: *Methods in Molecular Medicine*, Vol. 52: *Atherosclerosis: Experimental Methods and Protocols*
Edited by: A. F. Drew © Humana Press Inc., Totowa, NJ